RESEARCH AND CHANGE IN URBAN COMMUNITY HEALTH

Research and Change in Urban Community Health

Edited by
NIGEL BRUCE
Department of Public Health
Liverpool University

JANE SPRINGETT
Centre for Health Studies
Liverpool John Moores University

JULIE HOTCHKISS
Department of Public Health
Wirral Health Authority
Merseyside

ALEX SCOTT-SAMUEL
Department of Public Health
Liverpool University

Avebury

Aldershot • Brookfield USA • Hong Kong • Singapore • Sydney

Published by
Avebury
Ashgate Publishing Limited
Gower House
Croft Road
Aldershot
Hants GU11 3HR
England

Ashgate Publishing Company
Old Post Road
Brookfield
Vermont 05036
USA

British Library Cataloguing in Publication Data

Research and Change in Urban Community
Health
    I. Bruce, Nigel
    362.1042

    ISBN 1 85972 159 1

Library of Congress Catalog Card Number: 95-80520

Printed and bound by Athenaeum Press, Ltd.,
Gateshead, Tyne & Wear.

Contents

v

Figures and tables

List of contributors

Lee Adams, Director of Health Promotion, Sheffield Health Authorities and Healthy Sheffield Board member.

Frances Baum, Director, South Australian Community Health Research Unit and Head, Department of Public Health, Faculty of Health Sciences, Flinders University, Adelaide.

Donald Cameron, Principal Assistant, Housing and Environmental Health Division, Stockport Metropolitan Borough Council.

Cynzia Congiu, Department of Hygiene and Public Health, University of Cagliari, Sardinia, Italy.

Paulo Contu, Department of Hygiene and Public Health, University of Cagliari, Sardinia, Italy.

Valerie Cotter, Assistant Coordinator, Healthy Sheffield Development Unit.

Adrian Davis, Member of Health and Transport Research Group, School of Health and Social Welfare, The Open University, Milton Keynes, UK.

Julie Dawson, Researcher, Liverpool Public Health Observatory, Department of Public Health, Liverpool University.

Kathryn Dean, Independent Consultant in Research and Training, Population Health Studies, Copenhagen, Denmark, and Visiting Professor at Departments of Public Health at Liverpool and Valencia Universities.

Carol Duncan, Director of Communications and Corporate Development, Enfield and Haringey Health Agency, London.

Linda Ewles, Health Promotion Manager, Avon Health, Bristol.

Lynne Friedli, Project Officer, Health Education Authority, London.

Rachel Funnell, Researcher, Wessex Institute of Public Health Medicine, Winchester.

Marleen Goumans, Research Associate, Faculty of Health Sciences, University of Limburg, Maastricht, The Netherlands.

Felicity Green, Deputy Director of Health Promotion, Stockport Health Commission.

Mayer Hillman, Senior Fellow Emeritus, Policy Studies Institute, London.

Alexander Hirschfield, Research Coordinator, The Urban Research and Policy Evaluation Regional Research Laboratory, Department of Civic Design, University of Liverpool.

David Hunter, Professor of Health Policy and Management, and Director, Nuffield Institute for Health, University of Leeds.

Rachel Jewkes, Research Fellow in Women's Health, Medical Research Council, Tygerberg, South Africa.

Margaret Jones, Senior Community Dietitian Co-ordinator, Abercromby Health Centre, Liverpool.

Shirley Judd, Nutrition and Dietetic Service, Abercromby Health Centre, Liverpool.

Ainé Kennedy, Drumchapel Community Health Project, Glasgow.

Rebecca Kilbey, First Bite Theatre Company, Edinburgh.

Maria Koelen, Department of Communication and Innovation Studies, Agricultural University Wageningen, The Netherlands.

Conan Leavey, Centre for Health Studies, Liverpool John Moores University.

Clare Mahoney, Project Manager, Liverpool Child Health Project, Save the Children Fund, Liverpool.

John Middleton, Director of Public Health, Sandwell Health Authority, West Bromwich, West Midlands.

Ursula Miles, Principal Health Promotion Specialist, Bristol Area Specialist Health Promotion Service, Bristol.

Keiko Nakamura, Lecturer in Public Health and Environmental Science, Tokyo Medical and Dental University, Tokyo.

Femi Oduneye, Health Promotion Officer, Department of Health Promotion, Liverpool Community NHS Trust, Liverpool.

Charles Price, Consultant, Healthy Cities Project, World Health Organisation Regional Office for Europe, Copenhagen, Denmark.

Ann Roach, Community Worker, West Everton Community Council, Liverpool.

Peter Smith, Chairman, Environment and Energy Committee of the Royal Institute of British Architects and Director, EC Energy Project Office, School of Architectural Studies, University of Sheffield.

Viv Speller, Director, Health Promotion Division, Wessex Institute of Public Health Medicine, Winchester.

Martlne Standish, Co-ordinator, Heart of our City, Sheffield.

Frances Stillman, Assistant Professor, Medicine, The Johns Hopkins University School of Medicine, Baltimore, Maryland, USA.

Atsuko Tanaka, Department of Public Health and Environmental Science, Tokyo Medical and Dental University, Tokyo.

Takehito Takano, Professor, Department of Public Health and Environmental Science, Tokyo Medical and Dental University, Tokyo.

Sachiko Takeuchi, Department of Public Health and Environmental Science, Tokyo Medical and Dental University, Tokyo.

Joop ten Dam, Research Fellow, Department of Urban Studies, Utrecht University, The Netherlands.

Paul Thomas, Public Health Facilitation Project, Vauxhall Health Centre, Liverpool.

Rascha Thomas, Researcher, Municipal Health Authority, Amsterdam, The Netherlands.

Pat Thornley, Co-ordinator, Croxteth Health Action Area, Croxteth, Liverpool.

Patrick Towe, Department of Public Health, New River Health Authority, London.

Lenneke Vaandrager, Department of Communication and Innovation Studies, Agricultural University Wageningen, The Netherlands.

Gill Velleman, Team Manager, Heart Health, Bristol Area Specialist Health Promotion Service, Bristol.

Peter Whincup, Senior Lecturer, Department of Public Health, Royal Free Hospital School of Medicine.

Mike White, Assistant Director for Arts, Gateshead Libraries and Arts Department, Gateshead.

Lyn Winters, Researcher, Liverpool Public Health Observatory, Department of Public Health, Liverpool University.

Keyvan Zahir, Director of Public Health, Department of Public Health, New River Health Authority, London.

All photographs by Nigel Bruce, except where other source specified.

Foreword

This book is about improving the health of communities, and is based on the view that, important though health services are, substantial improvements cannot be achieved without co-ordinated action to change the many aspects of the social and physical environments which individually and together are the predominant determinants of health. This is the essence of the World Health Organisation's Health for All strategy, and the application of this philosophy through the Healthy Cities initiative.

Two of the most important pre-requisites for improving community health are firstly, good information about what the problems are and secondly, effective strategies for change. Ideally, public health strategy should be based on good information and research, but unfortunately that often is not the case. This is partly because the information available is frequently of limited relevance to those concerned both in communities and in the organisations responsible for change, but also because research has to compete with many other and probably more powerful influences on policy making and implementation. Our purpose is to contribute to breaking down the barriers that have, for too long, prevented a closer relationship between research and public health policy.

A very important focus for this book is the community. It embraces the experience of those living in communities as well as those who work at various levels to support, develop and service those communities. It is through greater understanding of and openness to this experience that we can find ways to build the partnerships necessary to achieve the improvements in health that we seek, especially among those in greatest need.

The value placed on understanding the complex factors that shape people's lives and the choices they make, and on the contribution that participation can make both to research and policy, are among the most important themes that run through this book.

There remain many challenges and obstacles to achieving a closer and more functional relationship between research and policy, but the ideas and experience reported here suggest that a lot of progress in the application of Health for All has already been made, and that a great deal more can be achieved.

A vision of health promotion

So, here I am then, a community health worker on the Bournville Estate, Weston-super-Mare, with a remit to reduce the factors which contribute to morbidity from heart disease over a three year period. I'm interested in heart disease, but my problem is that no-one here gives a toss about it. They're much more interested in other factors in their lives: about how to make ends meet from day to day, how you pay the bills, how they buy food in the afternoon. They don't think about tea-time three weeks in advance, and go down to the local supermarket and fill up the hatch-back with healthy foods. They think about tea-time at half past three, send little Willie over to the chip shop and buy the food then, depending on what's in their purse.

No-one here's interested in heart disease. It's my remit to make them interested - how do I go about that? Do I become the lifestyle thought police following people round the supermarkets, following them home, seeing what they're eating, seeing if they're taking enough exercise, seeing what they're smoking, is that the way?

No. We looked at a completely different approach here. We've not looked at those lifestyle factors at all initially. We've said a healthy community is a community where people feel they're a part of it, they've some control over their daily lives, they feel empowered to make some decisions which affect them.

Traditional health promotion approaches have tended to blame the victim for the diseases they're suffering from. If you're a smoker or drinker, you don't eat the right diet, you're overweight, don't take enough exercise - it's your fault, you've done these things, you contributed to your own ill-health.

What we tried to do on the Bournville is get away from that image of health promotion and instead promote a positive image of people in a community organising for themselves. We feel if they do that, this will be a much more positive approach to improving their health than blaming them for aspects of their lifestyle.

From a community heart health promotion project in Bristol, England, which is described in Chapter 19.

xix

Acknowledgements

The conference on which this book is based was held in Liverpool, UK, in March 1994, with the title "Health in Cities: Research and Change in Urban Community Health". It was planned in collaboration with the World Health Organisation's Healthy Cities Project, which is based at the European Office of WHO in Copenhagen. Particular thanks go to Dr Charles Price, consultant to the project, and to Dr Agis Tsouros, project co-ordinator, for their ideas and support. While WHO collaborated in the preparation of the conference, the views expressed in this book are however the responsibility of the authors and the editors.

Thanks also to Professor John Ashton who originally proposed and scheduled the conference, for his encouragement during the organisation of the meeting, and for his support in the preparation of this book.

A conference such as this depends entirely on the commitment experience of the delegates, and we would like to thank them for bringing a wealth of experience from such a variety of settings to the meeting. Our special thanks go to the contributors who have made the time and effort to prepare their work for publication.

Many thanks to Judie Fairbairn for the long hours and commitment she gave to the preparation of the text.

Finally, we would like to acknowledge the support and encouragement of Pat O'Hare, Andy Bennett and Jenny O'Connor from the Merseyside Drug Training and Information Centre (now HIT), for all their help in organising the conference.

Glossary

Listed here are some of the more technical terms used in the papers, with explanations that relate to the context of community health and the associated research and policy.

Bias - Any systematic error in carrying out research, which may be due to the way a sample is selected, a poorly designed set of questions, or the imposition of preconceived views by the researcher. Whatever the cause, it can lead to incorrect conclusions.

Community - This is a widely used term, and a complex one. The reader is referred to a discussion of the meaning of community in Chapter 8.

Community development - A process of supporting community groups and individuals in identifying issues that they feel affect health, and planning and developing strategies for change. These activities can often lead to greater self reliance and decision making ability.

Empowerment - This is the capacity that people have to make choices. In practical terms, it describes a process in which feelings of being powerless are developed, often through groups, into actions that can achieve changes in the social and physical environment. It is a central idea in community development.

Intersectoral collaboration - This refers to joint working between the different "sectors" at whatever level (national, city, community, etc.), in which sectors are local government, the business community, church, health authorities, higher education, voluntary organisations, community groups such as tenant's associations and health forums, the media, and so on. The important principle is that all these sectors can influence health, and collaboration can lead to more co-ordination, sharing resources and greater health benefit.

Methodology - As distinct from methods (which are the tools of research), methodology is a term that describes (literally) the study of methods.

Paradigm - A view of the world, for instance the view that researchers have about the nature of the reality they wish to study. A paradigm is fundamental because it informs the way scientists view their work, and the methods that they choose.

Positivist - A system of thought which concerns itself only with positive facts and what is observable, and the laws which can be shown to relate them.

Qualitative (research) methods - Methods of inquiry, drawn mainly from the traditions of sociology and anthropology, which rely on observation and in-depth study, to understand experience. Reasoning is achieved through building up an overall picture from the material gained.

Quantitative (research) methods - Research methods, developed mainly in epidemiology, which depend on notions of precise measurement which generally require highly controlled and structured means of collecting information. Reasoning and interpretation is carried out mainly by using statistical techniques to test predetermined hypotheses about how key variables might be related.

Reductionist - An approach which seeks to reduce a situation to its component parts. It relies on the view that the study of the component parts, and how these inter-relate, will allow explanation of the whole situation.

Reliability - A method is reliable if, when repeated in similar circumstances, a similar result is achieved. Assessing reliability may be difficult in community development settings where the situation and people involved are changing.

Validity - Strictly defined, validity in measurement is the accuracy with information is collected and therefore represents the capacity of the method to describe the real situation.

Introduction

In recent years there has been an important shift in the approach being taken to improving the health of populations. While acknowledging the importance of health services, it is now increasingly recognized that major improvements in the public health can only be achieved by changes in social and economic conditions, housing, and the environment. The World Health Organisation's Health for All programme in particular has helped to promote a wide diversity of activities throughout the world which have adopted this new approach (WHO, 1985). This places far greater emphasis on the involvement of communities in needs assessment and strategy development, in moving health services away from the traditional hospital sector, and in bringing together the contributions of the many local government and other agencies whose work on housing, the environment, pollution and transport all have an important bearing on health.

Among the diverse activities stimulated by the Health for All strategy have been the WHO Healthy Cities Project (Ashton, 1992; Tsouros, 1991), and the work of national Health for All and Healthy Cities networks and their constituent cities, mainly in the developed world. The Healthy Cities project started in 1987 with seven European cities, and this has now grown to over 30 with new member cities in the countries of central and eastern Europe. Alongside the WHO project, national and sub-national networks have been set up in hundreds of other cities and towns throughout Europe, and in Canada, USA, Australia and New Zealand, and other large cities including Tokyo and Johannesburg. There is also a wealth of experience from community health projects in developing countries, many of which have a long tradition of working closely with urban communities.

This expansion in recent years of Health for All based activity means that there is now a considerable amount of experience from many diverse communities. During this period it has been recognized that urban health policy needs to be informed by good information and research, but while this

1

was all very well in theory the fact was that in many cases research was missing the point so far as communities were concerned, and all too often policy makers paid scant attention to the findings of the more relevant research. The key issues addressed by this book therefore are as follows:

1.   To examine what type of research is most appropriate for understanding what impairs and promotes health, for assessing community health needs, and for evaluating the processes and outcomes of health promotion.

2.   To understand how research cav be seen as more relevant by communities and the policy making community, and therefore more likely to contribute to and inform a policy development process that is both participative and collaborative.

3.   To examine strategies for implementing effective policies based on these challenging new ways of working which involve real participation by communities, and collaboration between organizations (and sections of those organizations) which have hitherto tended to work independently.

At first, it may seem inappropriate and overambitious to deal with these two sets of questions, that is research and implementation, together. The rationale for doing so is that needs assessment and evaluation, which are among the most important research issues, are integral parts of successful policy planning and implementation. Policy needs good, relevant research based information, and the key to achieving this sheds a good deal of light on many aspects of that research including the methods, attitudes of the research community, and opportunities for funding. Furthermore, the research itself is now recognized as having the capacity to contribute directly to the policy process, so that it is no longer acceptable to examine policy development and implementation without considering the research component. It is unfortunate that up to now research and policy have been rather separate activities. The reasons for this are complex, challenging, and yet at the same time fascinating since they reflect deeply on our political structures and the traditions of scientific enquiry. It is exploration of these issues that underlie the purpose of this book, which seeks to advance the breaking down of the barriers between research and policy in the field of community health development.

Source of material

The papers included and discussed in this book are based on material

2

presented at a conference held in Liverpool, UK, early in 1994, the title of which was Health in Cities: Research and Change in Urban Community Health. This meeting was one of a series over recent years which had dealt, with varying emphases, with the topics of appropriate research and the practical experience of community health development.

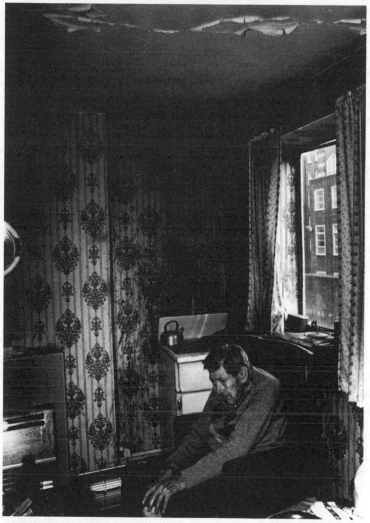

The social, economic and physical environments are the key to improving community health and reducing inequalities

Among the meetings with a particular emphasis on research have been "Research for Healthy Cities", held in Glasgow 1991 (Davies and Kelly,

1993) and the "Formulation and development of a research base for Healthy Cities" held in Tokyo in 1992 (Takano et al. 1992). What was apparent at the 1994 Liverpool conference was that over the last few years there has been a great deal of activity around the practical application of Health for All, including health promotion activity at community level, policy development at community and city levels, and research for needs assessment and evaluation. What we have therefore sought to do is record a selection of that experience in a way that marks what is being achieved, and allows a synthesis of the two main themes of research and strategies for change.

Another focus apparent from the title, and from the close association with Healthy Cities, is that of the urban environment. The city, or any medium to large sized conurbation, is justified as a useful focus because of the concentrations of population, industry, pollution, transport, and in general the extremes of socio-economic deprivation and environmental degradation that follow in the wake of urban development. In addition, the city authorities are more easily identifiable with the area concerned, and there is usually an research community that potentially at least is available as a partner. Although the city may be a helpful focus for this work, the practical experience and theoretical principles that emerge are applicable much more widely. In Canada, for example, healthy cities has also been developed beyond the urban setting as so much of the country is non-urban, and the term "healthy cities and communities" is applied.

Conference organization: a barometer of our readiness to work together

It is of some importance and value to examine the evolutionary course of the "organizational philosophy" of meetings held around these and related topics, since there was quite reasonably a strong sense that they should reflect the participative and intersectoral nature of the underlying strategy (Guidelines for Healthy City conferences; Marie Armitage, personal communication). The experience of trying to apply this philosophy in the situation of the conference is one barometer of the readiness of the delegates, who are more or less representative of the "field", to succeed with the new ways of working.

The 1994 Health in Cities meeting was attempting to work within the Health for All context, and to bring together the research and policy making interests. The issues facing us as conference organisers would inevitably reflect the state of play in the wider community, and the resistance and tensions that were current. The question was how far to "engineer" the circumstances of the meeting beyond the stage at which the wider community ad reached.

The experience of this dilemma at an earlier conference on research for Healthy Cities has been described (Davies and Kelly, 1993):

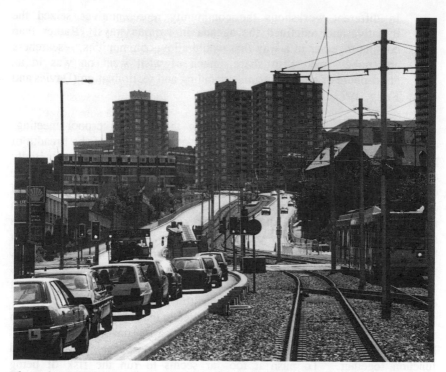

The urban environment provides a useful focus for the application of Health for All principles, but much of the experience is also relevant to non-urban communities

> ... The (1991) Glasgow meeting was convened to bring forward the practicalities of intersectoral working between these groups. The planning committee ... knew what they did not want to happen. They did not want a gathering where "experts", self styled or otherwise, jetted in and delivered papers to a receptive, admiring and passive audience.

What the organizers were seeking was a genuinely participative event, and set about trying to make that happen. They commissioned a number of key papers from people who were familiar with the issues of collaborative working, and these papers were distributed to all the delegates about one week before the meeting was due to start. The idea then was to have discussion about the topics, in groups that were led by someone other than the author of the paper, and that there would be an opportunity the next day to bring the discussion together in a further meeting. In practice however, this plan did not function in the way that had been hoped for:

5

In different workshops the community representatives seized the initiative and redefined the agenda in various ways. Rather than coming together in a way that would allow communities, researchers and policy makers to share, much of what went on was in an atmosphere of mutual misunderstanding and recrimination (Davies and Kelly, 1993).

These problems were largely avoided in the 1994 Liverpool meeting, although it may that this was to some extent at the expense of the breadth of participation. The content and atmosphere of the conference was essentially a reflection of the response to the publicised conference objectives. The delegates were mainly people who were interested in the practical aspects of community health development as well as research, although the interest in the latter for some did not extend beyond a recognition that research in this situation included health needs assessment and was therefore not only relevant but central to the whole process. In contrast to the 1991 Glasgow meeting, the programme was almost entirely constructed from the work submitted: this was the result of a deliberate decision to allow the meeting to reflect current experience of research and community health development.

In retrospect, the level of integration achieved in the conference organisation was probably about right in that it represented a reasonably "comfortable" level of participation and intersectoral working - and hence delegates could function together. To push it too far seems to run the risk of being counterproductive, but of course not to push it at all would be complacent and non-creative. Integration was also achieved by including a strong artistic theme in the main programme, rather than simply as side line entertainment. This included a live theatre performance demonstrating techniques used for school health promotion, and a presentation of art work used in a variety of community health promotion activities. This approach successfully reinforced one of the most important theoretical messages of the conference - that variety in approaches both to research and policy is valuable.

As a result of how the meeting came together, the material presented was, we believe, a fair reflection of the stage reached in terms of participative and collaborative endeavour in research and policy development for urban community health.

Selection of material for the book

Almost 100 presentations were made, and it would have been impractical to report all of these in one book. We have therefore sought to include those which, taken together, would illustrate the breadth and depth of the experience and ideas presented. A deliberate attempt has also been made to achieve

6

variety in style, and for this reason the work of those actively involved in community development work has been included alongside that of those from an academic background. This has been more difficult than might be imagined.

For the professional academic, preparing a paper is part of the job, and is made easier by the existence of preceding work and the accessibility of reference and other support material. For the community health worker it may not be so easy, and we identified two reasons for this. Firstly, some authors tended to lack confidence that their more direct and personal style of writing would be "up to the standard" expected, and some needed reassurance that it was their experience that we were after and no one else would be in a position to write about it. The second reason was pressure of time and the demands of other work which was easily conceived to be of higher priority.

It is most important that those "non-academic" authors who have contributed to this book, or may be thinking of writing for other publications, do not see these comments as in any sense a criticism of them. Their accounts of working with communities are extremely valuable, for it is there that all the fine words are put to the test.

References

Ashton, J. (ed.) (1992), *Healthy Cities*, Open University Press.

Davies, J.K. and Kelly, M.P. (1993), *Healthy Cities: Research and Practice*, Routledge, London, p. 6.

Takano, T., Ishidate, K. and Nagasaki, M. (eds.), *Formulation and development of a Research Base for Healthy Cities*, Kyoiku Syoseki, Tokyo.

Tsouros, A. (ed.) (1991), *World Health Organisation Healthy Cities Project: A Project Becomes a Movement*, Sogess, Milan.

WHO (1985), *Targets for Health for All*, World Health Organisation.

Section 1   Research and change

Research and policy development are two very important elements of the Health for All approach, and while each has its own intrinsic interest and challenges which we shall address in subsequent chapters, there are also some underlying questions about the interrelationship that need to be addressed first. Examining these will inform and colour subsequent exploration of both the research methods and findings, as well as the practical experience of developing and implementing policy.   Among the most important questions are the following:

1.   How can we make research more relevant to the priorities that policy has to address?

2.   How do policy makers view research?   What do they want from research, and are there issues that they rather would not be reminded of by researchers?

3.   Can research and policy become more complementary, or does the reality of political and funding priorities mean that they are destined to remain rather separate activities with each feeding off the other on the occasions that it suits the self interest of the researcher or policy maker?

In the first two papers, Fran Baum and David Hunter provide thoughtful and honest responses to these questions from their own experience.   Fran Baum views the situation primarily from the researcher's angle, while David Hunter draws on his extensive knowledge of the policy making world to offer insights from the other side.   While amply demonstrating the difficulty and complexity of the situation we face, the papers nevertheless offer some direction and guidance for overcoming at least some of these barriers.

Drawing on his experience of the WHO Healthy Cities project, Charles Price describes the vital role that research has to play in policy development for the project cities and sets out an agenda for the years to come. Of particular importance is the growing emphasis being placed on City Health Plans which are a central part of the second phase of the Healthy Cities project. These plans will involve: a variety of types of research from different sectors; community participation and intersectoral collaboration in the interpretation of the research and policy formulation; and, the setting up of appropriate structures to plan and carry out implementation and evaluation.

This provides a clear context for the application of research in the process of change, and in which the challenges and barriers described in the first two papers will be so much a part. The extent and variety of activity in the many hundreds of Healthy Cities projects and network cities will provide the opportunities, energy and commitment to face those challenges and to learn from the experience gained.

1 Research and policy to promote health: What's the relationship?

Frances Baum

Let me start by painting two extreme views on the question I have set for my paper. A hard nosed policy maker sceptical of the value of research may see research as an ivory tower exercise that has little to do with the cut and thrust of the real, dirty, political world from which policies emerge. By contrast a university academic, keen to prove his or her usefulness to the real world, may present research as essential to any policy and believe no policy should see the light of day until all aspects have been thoroughly researched (probably after the provision of many, expensive research consultancies). I would suggest that a more sensible position than either of these extremes is to accept that policy does indeed emerge from, and has to reflect, a heavily politicized context but that research does have an important role in policy development.

Before proceeding any further I should confess my biases. For the past ten years I have worked in community health research in South Australia and for seven of those years I have also held an academic position. So I have a vested interest in supporting the value of research to policy and practice. I have advocated the value of grounded and applied research to bureaucrats who saw the elimination of the South Australian Community Health Research Unit (SACHRU, 1990) as a potential cost saving, to academics who believed the unit's work was not scientific enough and to community health workers who felt research took too long and was too scientific to be of any practical use to them. That the unit has survived and flourished suggests that some people in each of these categories agree with me.

I should also say that my beliefs about the value of research for policy development vary. They vary according to whether the research we are currently engaged on is going well, on whether our previous year's research appears to have made some impact, on whether I've seen research being taken into account in policy formulation and on my more general feelings about the possibilities of change for the better. Most of you can empathize with this

11

optimistic/pessimistic approach to the value of research.

So on my optimistic days I can be very excited about the potential for research to change policy and practice; to make communities healthier places. There seems to be an obvious alliance between policy and research. Both should be concerned with understanding and subsequently improving the current state of affairs. It seems that combining the two will create a powerful partnership to bring about change. So this paper is primarily optimistic. Research has the potential to contribute to all aspects of health promotion in cities: policies for creating supportive environments, encouraging community action, developing individual skills and re-orienting health services. This potential is not always realized, for a range of reasons that I will discuss in this paper.

Policies relating to health establish a framework for public health research. Tesh (1988) has noted the extent to which political philosophies dictate the types of public health questions that are asked. This means researchers have to be aware of policies not only because they hope to change them but also because policies set a framework for research and determine the types of public health questions that obtain formal sanction and those that do not. In the mid 1980s in South Australia, our then Minister of Health, John Cornwall, had a strong commitment to working towards equity in health status, enhancing primary health care including health promotion and establishing a social health office responsible for developing a social health policy. Under this government, a strong policy framework was established for research work which looked at structural determinants of health and which linked health status to household income. This supportive framework contrasts strongly with the UK in the 1980s where government policies appeared to actively discourage analysis of structural factors affecting health and to shift the research focus (together with the blame) to individual causes of illness. The dominant philosophy was individualism and this affected public health as much as any other area of policy.

Tesh (1988) argues that the individualism that dominates disease prevention and health promotion policies in the USA is counter productive. It leads to policies that assume that health education is the best way to prevent disease. Unhealthy behaviour results from individual choice so the way to change such behaviour is to point out to people the error of their ways and exhort them to behave differently. Tesh also points out (1988) that research questions dictated by an individualistic philosophy are different and reflects on the difference between asking "Why do large numbers of people continue to smoke?" and "Why do these particular people continue to smoke?" The first question directs attention to the tobacco culture in which everyone lives: the growing of tobacco, the advertising of cigarettes, the meaning of smoking. The second question directs attention to the psychological and physiological attributes of those people. So policy directions set the parameters for the definition of research questions.

In recent years the focus of the vast majority of public health research has been on what Terris (1980) has termed "the lifestyle approach to health policy". One of the important factors behind the evolution of the Healthy Cities movement appears to me to have been a rejection of such an individualist philosophy. I have argued elsewhere (Baum, 1993a) that the Ottawa Charter provides a strong social democratic framework for the development of health promotion policies - a framework drawing on collectivist roots and one which rejects naive victim blaming. Victim blaming has been pervasive in western democratic society (Ryan, 1972; Allison, 1982). Ryan (1972) describes the absurdity of its focus on individuals in his description of Zero Mostel doing a sketch in the early 1950s in which he impersonated a senator from the deep south of the USA conducting an investigation of the origins of America's involvement in the Second World War. At the climax of the sketch the senator boomed out, in "an excruciating mixture of triumph and suspicion", "What was Pearl Harbour doing in the Pacific?" This is an extreme example of blaming the victim and of how political philosophies can direct lines of inquiry. So even if researchers believe their research is apolitical and value free it is, in fact, almost certainly conducted within a framework dictated by the political and cultural patterns of the society in which it is done.

Definitions of health, selecting research agenda and levels of policy

Health is a crucial part of all our lives. Australian aboriginal people make this very clear with their definition: Health is Life. This means researchers may be concerned with health policy issues at different levels. Before exploring those levels I would like consider the definition of health a little more. Alma Ata, the Ottawa Charter and Healthy Cities have certainly taught us that health is about much more than illness. Most health promoters these days, even those with a behaviourial focus, will acknowledge the importance of structural factors on health. We accept (even if we can not determine the exact nature of the relationship) that transport, housing, urban design, employment or lack of it, income, access to nutritious food and educational opportunities set the parameters for people's health. This social understanding of health with its emphasis on wholeness broadens the health promoter's agenda to a universe of concerns which is quite overwhelming in its extent when compared with the limits imposed by a victim blaming, behaviourial approach. There is no area of life that is not of potential concern for public health. This means that public health researchers have to be increasingly strategic and selective in their choice of what research to do. There are a plethora of research topics that may be of use to policy makers and practitioners but which should be selected and who should select them? This dilemma is present at each level of policy making. In Australia the Commonwealth Department of Human Services and Health appears to be moving more in the direction of commissioning research on specific topics of interest. For example, in September 1993 its Health Advancement Branch advertised three research consultancies concerned with intersectoral action in health, community consultation and information data bases for health promotion. Another of its committees (Research and Development Grants Advisory Committee) has shown a trend towards defining specific research areas rather than simply advertising general grants related to health service and policy research. This shift may be seen as an effort to direct researchers to the areas of most interest to the department and/or as a way of gaining more control over research effort. It is certainly a departure from the more usual notion that useful research topics somehow bubble up from academia in a rather haphazard manner. On the other hand, it could be argued that the bubbling up technique is more likely to lead to independent research and research that is critical of bureaucratic practices and policies. However, despite government attempts to direct research topics public health researchers are left with the problem of how and who selects research agendas. It is a crucial issue to the new public health and one that should be paid more attention by policy makers and researchers. The trick lies in defining research agendas that are of public health importance but maintain and prompt the excitement of researchers in the research topic and process.

The South Australian Community Health Research Unit has a state wide mandate. South Australia is a state of 1.6 million people most of whom are in the capital city, Adelaide, leaving 350,000 in a rural area, about two and a half times the size of the United Kingdom and Ireland. We select our research priorities by consultation with our advisory committee (a majority of whose members are from community health centres) and by holding an annual planning day attended by community health workers, health commission bureaucrats and community members from the South Australian Health and Social Welfare Councils. The priorities are selected with a weather eye to political considerations. These include an assessment of what the current issues of concern to our funders are (the South Australian Health Commission) and whether they will see the priorities as relevant and worth continuing to fund. The process always leaves me with the feeling that what we are able to do is the very tip of the tip of the iceberg. I'm sure this is the case for most research units and institutes. There are always more ideas for research than the resources to carry them out.

When considering the links between research and policy it is important to differentiate local, regional and national public health perspectives. Sometimes the issues and dilemmas will be similar at all levels; other times they may differ markedly. For instance who sets the research agenda is likely to be quite different. Locally, one would hope research is developed in consultation with local communities and service providers; nationally, the players will be determined by those operating at a national level.

The Ottawa Charter is concerned with health at each of these three levels, where different styles of policies are formulated. Locally, policies are likely to be those established by a particular health service or local action group; regionally, State or Provincial health policies and policies determining health funding; and nationally broad policy statements setting frameworks for health promotion. Research has a role in informing policy at the three levels. Relevant research is likely to be either looking back at past initiatives or looking forward and planning for the future. In Healthy Cities projects this has usually involved a strong element of vision. Typical new public health research activities at local, regional and national levels that have been pursued in Healthy Cities projects are shown in Table 1.1.

What factors tend to prevent research from informing policy?

This question will probably receive different answers, or at least answers with different emphases, depending on whether you approach it from the policy or research side of the fence, mirroring the two stereotyped positions I presented at the start of my paper. Policy makers may feel that research too often reflects an ivory tower perspective that is out of touch with "the real world." They may see it as irrelevant.

Depending on their perspective, some policy makers may not use research that does not pay sufficient attention to the communities amongst whom the research has been conducted. In Australia, Departments of Aboriginal Affairs will not give research ethical approval unless it does involve community participation. Research that slips by the ethics committees and does not include significant community participation is extremely unlikely to be given any credibility, or used to form policy or to shape practice. On the other hand, some bureaucrats are not interested in research that they consider presents only a community perspective. Such research may be criticized as "unbalanced" "unrealistic" or "subjective".

Evaluation research raises particular dilemmas. Most policy makers are likely to be at least a little resistant to research that is critical of their department's or service's operation. Evaluation consultants often find this is the case when evaluating services. Departments want to "adapt" the picture or "reframe" it. Policy makers are more likely to be resistant to evaluative research that they have not been involved in. Research that identifies shortcomings in the general fabric of society is usually even more unpopular. A few years ago, one of our reports highlighted the association between low income and health and made front page news in the local paper.

Table 1.1
**New public health research activity and its relation
to policy at local, regional and national levels**

Level	Activity
Local	Local community needs assessment. Researching local people's vision of their community as a healthy one. Presentation of local statistical information. Description of the "feel" of the "invisible" city. Evaluation of local public and community health initiatives. Producing service data that can be used by managers. Barefoot epidemiology. Compiling local knowledge and insight.
Regional/State Provincial	Production of social health atlas to show inequalities in health status between regions. Compilation of service data from across the region. Regional needs assessment to provide information for regional health planning. Environmental and public health surveillance. Epidemiological studies of particular diseases. Studies of collaboration across sectors at the regional level. Evaluation of the effectiveness of illness care services in contributing to disease prevention.
National	Evaluation of national health and illness care system. Evaluation of national public health initiatives. General research (funded by national bodies) that may be conducted in one setting but is applicable nationally. Establishing health promotion to guide research effort.

At each level a framework should be established for determining research priorities and agenda

The fact that the research area included one of the most marginal seats in the State Parliament and that the article appeared shortly before a state election did not help the SACHRU in the popularity stakes!

A further impediment to the use of research is when it is perceived to have been conducted using inappropriate methods. In broad terms most methods derive from two main research approaches: positivism and constructivism. Positivist approaches are based on the methods of the natural sciences and have been viewed by the mainstream scientific community as the gold standard for research since the nineteenth century. They have been particularly dominant in health because medical science made most of its progress by using these methods. Public health, in its quest for medical respectability, has relied heavily on these methods, largely basing itself on the deductive approaches of traditional science. Constructivism, by contrast, puts emphasis on understanding settings and attempts to interpret the complexities of them by using qualitative methods. The approach is based on inductive thinking, deriving theory from periods of observation followed by analysis and leading to slow evolution of theory.

Epidemiology has been the main and most respected tool of public health researchers. Its exclusively use, however, has been increasingly criticized (see for example Brown, 1985; Davies and Kelly, 1993; de Leeuw et al. 1993; Baum, 1993b; Colquhoun and Kellehear, 1993; McKinlay, 1993). The Healthy Cities movement has been important in developing both a critique of epidemiology and complementary research techniques. These critiques do not deny the very real contribution that can be made by epidemiology but rather argue for greater recognition of its limitations, and acceptance of the important contribution that can be made by other methodological approaches. Despite these criticisms, however, positivism's monopoly on research respectability means that only research which is based on its standards will be accepted by some policy makers. Research, especially constructivist, qualitative research, is often dismissed as being unscientific by positivists. In Some cases where the research has not been well conducted the dismissal may be well deserved; in other instances, the research may be dismissed more from political or bureaucratic expediency than for any valid methodological reason. Occasionally, the boot may be on the other foot, when policy makers, reading critiques of epidemiology as meaning no epidemiological study can be of use, disregard useful information. The lesson here is that the acceptability of research findings depends on the eye of the beholder.

People may be cynical about the value of research when they see that it is used inappropriately. It is not unknown, for instance, for research to be used by bureaucracies as a delaying tactic ("a decision will be made once the findings of a review or evaluation are known"). Because research rarely makes a direct and easily discernible impact on policy or practice, people may be cynical about its ability to make any impact at all. Patton (et al. 1977) in an article entitled "In search of an impact ..." make the point that impacts of research on policy are usually subtle. Often good applied research will change practice as it proceeds so that those involved in the change process may be unaware of the ways in which research helped to bring about change.

A vision of the conditions for a world in which research is useful to a new public health policy agenda

I would now like to paint a picture of a world in which the contribution of research to public health policy and practice at a local, regional and national level is maximized. Research is never likely to be any more than one of many voices forming the cacophony from which policy and practice emerge. With the following pre-conditions it could make a more significant contribution than it often does. In this section I put forward five pre-conditions for research to contribute to progressive public health reforms.

Acknowledgement that research is political

The research process and outcome should reflect the principles of the new public health as they are laid out in the Ottawa Charter: health policies should aim at achieving equity in health status, creating supportive environments for achieving health, encouraging individual skills and re-orienting health services towards a focus on prevention. These principles clearly reflect a structuralist perspective on health promotion that sees the importance of environmental and social structures on individual and community health status. Tesh (1988) identifies two main strengths of the structuralist perspective. Firstly it does not mistake political and economic systems for the natural order and so leaves open the possibility of changing them. Secondly, the policies generally imply benefits for the whole community not just for certain individuals. Researchers may find that the implications of doing research that gives foremost consideration to structural factors is that their findings are not always welcome news to existing power holders. Generally, structural research will challenge the status quo more than individually focused research. Therefore, researchers have to decide where their values lie and give up notions that their work can be objective, value free and devoid of political implication. Despite decades of debate on the issues of objectivity in science, and many fine critiques of the notion that science can be removed from social and individual values, public health is still dogged with the idea that the best form of inquiry is the objective. Strong criticism of science and its claim to objectivity has come from the feminist movement. Fee (1981) maintains that the notion of "objective" is often:

18

merely a code word for the political passivity of those scientists who have tacitly agreed to accept a privileged social position and freedom of inquiry within the laboratory in return for their silence in not questioning the social uses of science or the power relations which determine its direction.

For public health the debate regarding the objectivity of research and the social role and responsibility of researchers is crucial. Are researchers primarily technicians who leave the business of policy and practice to others? Or are they activists who have a responsibility to work for change? The Healthy Cities movement appears to see research as a tool for social and political change. Yet public health researchers often present themselves as apolitical and uninterested in the application of their research. Public health draws on both medical and social science. The former is more inclined to present itself as objective and disinterested. An anthropological study of the scientific community in a prestigious Australian institute of medical science noted the dominant view of science in their laboratory:

> Science is characterized by the fact that scientists adopt a completely impersonal attitude. Their own personal (subjective) feelings, emotions, motives, intentions, attitudes and wishes have nothing to do with their scientific activity. In this view the ideal scientist approximates as closely as possible to the status of a pure instrument ... "Pure science" is uncontaminated by the personal and subjective. It may be that in the social sciences - the "soft" sciences - personal and subjective factors play a part in the scientist's mode of theorising, in the selection of an area or research interest and in dictating the style of research; but in the "hard" sciences, so it is claimed, these factors have no place (Charlesworth et al. 1989).

These researchers went on to show that underlying the seeming objectivity of the institute there was a strong political interest in supporting and legitimizing the medical model of health and illness. Thus the scientists were reported as denigrating a view of malaria control by improvement of socio-economic factors and instead promoting the quest for malaria vaccine. This quest brings considerable research dollars to the institute in question. The search for a solution to a particular public health problem is never value free and objective. The authors of this anthropological study refer to Foucault's insight that the establishment of specific discourses also provides access to power and control over the objects of these discourses. Insisting on a particular solution as the "right" one, may bring with it government and public funding, personal and institutional recognition and success, and divert resources from the search for alternative solutions. Their analysis suggests

19

that scientists do play the political game but often behind a screen of objectivity. Science tends to be presented in impersonal ways. Charlesworth (et al. 1989) comment on the impersonality of scientific monographs and suggest that the standard scientific paper gives the impression that the paper has not been written by a human being. Tesh (1988) similarly argues that the language of science tends to strip it of a recognition of its social context. As an example she cites the use of the term "not statistically significant" in medical textbooks. There it is used in cases when the data "fail to provide sufficient evidence to doubt the validity of the null hypothesis" and so implies the null hypothesis is accepted until other evidence is obtained. Tesh (1988) deconstructs the meaning of this:

> This sterile phraseology, besides teaching medical students to use mystifying language avoids acknowledging that "living with the null hypothesis" means "live with" a suspected cause of disease ... It implies that what "one" lives with is merely a hypothesis. Suppose the author had written "When our studies don't show anything yet, they indicate that people have to live with a suspected toxic substance.

She goes on to argue that the sterile language of science (especially the use of the passive voice) makes it less likely that people will ask why an absence of data means they necessarily have to take risks. Medical science has been undeniably effective in dominating the discourse of public health in the twentieth century. This has meant that findings from within this paradigm have found ready acceptance by society in general and by powerful policy makers in particular. The new public health, while stressing consensus, sets an agenda that, if implemented, would challenge many vested interests (Baum, 1993a). The same should hold for new public health research. If the first pre-condition I set for effective new public health research is implemented, then that research will also challenge powerful interests. Inevitably, then, the new public health researcher will be seen as rocking the boat and as being activists for change. This is the result of challenging dominant ideas. Traditional scientists can appear value free, apolitical and objective because they are not generally challenging powerful vested interests with their findings. In public health this challenge to the status quo does not just happen at the social structural level (for example through analysis of patterns of inequity and their relationship to health status) but also at the local level. Feuerstein in her very practical guide to participatory evaluation (1986) reminds us that:

> Evaluation is hard and often painful work. This is because it requires those who are associated with a particular program to be very honest with themselves and with each other. This is not always easy.

The Ottawa Charter stresses the importance of collaboration. This translates as multi-disciplinary research, but in practice this is not straight forward. O'Neill (1993) describes an attempt in Canada to bring together health promotion practitioners and academics from a range of disciplines. He reports that the workshops highlighted the barriers to multi-disciplinary work rather than the breaking down of the barriers. He also comments that the structure of universities tend to preclude co-operation across disciplines. This certainly appears true in Australia where there are few instances of co-operation between the social science and medical disciplines in the interests of public health. AIDS research is, however, one area where there are exemplary instances of collaboration. The need for public health understanding to be broad and to draw on a range of disciplines is contrary to the tendency towards academic specialization, stressing narrow knowledge, extremely detailed about a particular topic but lacking in a wider appreciation of how it fits in the broader scheme of things. A scientist might build an eminent career on the basis of a detailed understanding of the cells in the liver and their pathology yet have little or no awareness of the social, economic and political factors affecting alcohol use and abuse in our community. In public health there needs to be an appreciation of the value of generalists who can pull together and synthesize knowledge from a variety of disciplines and apply it to a particular problem. This may be likened to the revival of general medical practice from the doldrums of the past few decades. The Healthy Cities movement, more than most health promotion initiatives, has emphasized the need to avoid narrow specialization and to think laterally and creatively about public health problems and solutions. Encouraging an appreciation of the value of generalists, who can synthesis and apply knowledge from a range of disciplines is crucial to the future of public health.

Involve the stakeholders in defining the agenda

Research agendas should be determined by those people with a stake in, and responsibility for, achieving healthy cities and communities. These people include members of the public, service providers, policy makers from a range of government departments and politicians. This should help ensure the most relevant research questions are asked. There are few pieces of research that are not in some sense, at least, useful. However, given that resources for research are limited, the usefulness of research should be judged in relative terms. Involvement of a broad range of stakeholders in setting research agendas should help make research relevant. Currently it is researchers and funders of research who have most say over what research is done. Ways of encouraging participation will differ at different levels. Nationally, it can be done through the involvement of consumer and community groups in deciding priorities for national research funding bodies. Regionally, service funders, providers and users and local action groups should work with researchers in deciding what grants should be applied for, what the topics should be for student research projects, and what the priorities should be for public health research in their region. Locally, public health researchers should become accustomed to working with local services and groups to determine research topics. A researcher or research team that is able to work closely with one local community will benefit considerably from building relationships with local people, obtaining a detailed picture of local issues and culture and becoming an accepted and, hopefully, valued part of the local public health effort. One of the advantages of Healthy Cities initiatives is that they enable researchers to tap into a local organization or project that provides a good basis for developing collaborative research.

Most commonly, researchers are based in universities and traditionally have not developed or maintained strong links with those who are devising policy and those who are practising health promotion. There are exceptions, however. The evidence on the impact of environmental lead levels on humans, especially children, has led to public policy change. O'Neill (1993) has described an attempt in Canada to bring academics and practitioners in the health promotion field closer together. The knowledge development project he describes invited academics to play a role different to their usual one of "defining and dominating knowledge development". Rather the project asked them to give away some of this power by working in partnership with practitioners and respecting their knowledge and skills. The project used the term knowledge rather than research to place the focus on the range of knowledge that is developed in service agencies and grass roots organizations. O'Neill (1993) reports that building bridges between the practical and academic world are not easy. He concludes that one of the crucial aspects of a successful recipe is continuity of effort and funding. This ensures that the essential networks and alliances, fuelled by trust and developing knowledge, can evolve. This certainly echoes our experience in South Australia. It has taken years to build up a community health research infrastructure which has real and effective links with community health services and the central office policy makers and funders, and which maintains credibility with the academic (and grant awarding world). The gains tend to be incremental, as the field gains trust in researchers who remain on the scene and become activists on behalf of the community health movement. It is not unlike a community development process.

There are signs that there is a more widespread questioning of the choices made in health research. I came across an example in a women's magazine recently. On the front cover the magazine had the headline "We Want Well Women". I looked inside and instead of finding the usual diet of lifestyle advice read the editorial which indicated that the magazine was adopting a more structural approach to the issue of women's health and had a clear desire to influence research agendas. It asked why, when we make up more than 50 per cent of the population, is much research and testing still being done with men as the models? Why is funding for research into breast cancer, which kills one in eight of us, so much less than funding for research into AIDS? Why, when women go to their doctors with symptoms of, say, high blood pressure, are they treated for stress, when if a man has the same problem he's treated for ... high blood pressure?[1]

One might not agree with all the sentiments expressed by the magazine, but the commitment to influencing national research agendas is striking. The editorial and companion article went to argue the case that women will have to fight to change and influence research priorities. Research agendas have rarely been questioned in the past. They have been accepted as reflecting the objective wisdom of scientists. This needs to change if research effort is to be directed to questions of importance to public health. It is possible that a broader consideration of research agendas will be more likely to led to research that considers the structural as well as the individual factors in health. It is often far easier to identify and conduct research on individual causes of illness. Take, for example, the high incidence of young males killed or seriously injured in motor vehicle accidents. It is much simpler to research questions about driver error than those about the social pressures on young males that encourage them to act recklessly or about the impact of vehicle licensing (the age at which young people are permitted to drive) or the effect of "drinking age" and liquor licensing.

Participatory research

Appropriate research should be conducted in a participatory and/or consultative manner. Since Health for All, there has been an increasing recognition of the potential for community participation in the planning, implementation and evaluation of health programs. The Healthy Cities movement has reinforced this. The emphasis on participation, in part, reflects a disenchantment with reliance on experts for knowledge about particular issues. A further recognition is that professionals can become as concerned about advancing the cause of their profession as they are about the people their profession is designed to serve (Freidson, 1970; Willis, 1983). It also comes from a recognition that local people are often experts on their own needs and those of their communities. It also seems that public health researchers often fail to consult professional workers, let alone communities. However, it is now being recognized that good public health research generally results from involvement of the key groups affected by a particular piece of research. The Healthy Cities network which links researchers around the world has consistently emphasized this aspect of research practice (de Leeuw et al. 1993; Davies and Kelly, 1993; Baum and Brown, 1989).

Much rhetoric has been written and spoken about the benefits of participation. Actual examples of research that is consultative or participatory are rarer. Most research that is sensitive to the need to involve communities in research is consultative rather than participatory. The South Australian Community Health Research Unit generally manages to be consultative. Advisory committees are established for each project undertaken. While it takes time and effort to encourage people to give up their time to be on such a committee, and although using the committee may slow down the progress of a research project, the benefits to the project in terms of grounding it in the concerns of health professionals and community members are real.

In the last decade there has been less tolerance of research practices that are not consultative. Professionals and community members alike express scepticism at vague statements about the likely benefits of research. Participation in research is unlikely these days unless people believe in the value of the research. They are more likely to do this if the research is clearly of benefit to them or their community. This scepticism about research is entirely reasonable. Wadsworth (1984) has dubbed much research a "data raid" in which researchers swoop down from their ivory tower, collect data, whisk back to their tower and never communicate their findings to the people who were the subject of their data raid. Professional workers may also be cynical about research. They know evaluations are often conducted for reasons other than a genuine attempt to review initiatives and that the findings are often distorted by political processes. If, however, they have a sense of control and involvement in a research or evaluation project, they are much more likely to be committed both to the research process and to taking action on the basis of its findings. The commitment of professionals to research is only likely to happen in most busy and usually over stretched service delivery agencies if managers are supportive of the research effort and give it legitimacy and therefore credibility. Researchers should, therefore, seek to establish good working relationships with the managers of services they aim to work with. There are few textbooks on research methods that pay much attention to the involvement in the process of people other than researchers. Other participants tend to be seen as passive. There are some exceptions, most of which relate to developing countries (see for example Feuerstein, 1986; Marsden and Oakley, 1991; Wadsworth, 1991).

Research may be conducted by community groups in a direct attempt to influence policy. In South Australia residents in the north west suburbs of Adelaide conducted their own survey of resident's perceptions of air pollution. Their report "If You Don't Like it Move" proved to be an effective instrument for lobbying government and local industries. While there were attempts to discredit the report's methods, the concerns expressed by residents in the report received some recognition by government and industry. There is now a local environmental forum with local and state government officials, health workers, residents and industry represented. The survey was one of a range of lobbying and activist strategies used by the local action group. Such use of research by local groups on issues of public health importance is an effective way of influencing policy and local public health.

Use of varied research methods

Research to support the new public health should be methodologically eclectic, selecting those methods that are most likely to illuminate issues rather being committed to any particular technique. Data should also be interpreted in the light of relevant theories. In all the types of research listed in Table 1.1, a range of research methods can be utilized to assist understanding and develop knowledge. In particular, the value of qualitative methods has been recognized in recent years. These methods are particularly appropriate for discovering the meaning of social practices and of actions taken by individuals. They help to provide a detailed understanding of public health problems.

Evaluation provides a good example of this. Most evaluations and evaluation textbooks relevant to human services recognize that good evaluation considers both the process of implementing and developing an initiative, and the outputs and outcomes. They also acknowledge that a range of methods are needed to do this. Patton (1990), in what I have found to be one of the most useful texts on evaluation, argues convincingly for an open mind on evaluation techniques so that the full range of qualitative and quantitative techniques available to researchers are used. He warns against an orthodoxy of any particular methodology:

> The establishment of an orthodox evaluation methodology is no different from the establishment of a state religion. Officially telling you what methods to use is only one step removed from officially telling you what results to find. At that point utilization of findings will cease to be an issue - for there will be nothing to use, only orders to follow (Patton, 1990).

What appears to be happening now is that public health practitioners are disestablishing epidemiology as the official methodological religion of public health and recognizing the legitimacy and usefulness of a range of other techniques. Many of these techniques come from the social sciences. They are not new. Most have a long and respectable history. They are, however, often new to public health which has tended to draw on medicine and its scientific premises rather than on the many bodies of knowledge and methodologies within social science. In fact there probably is not a discipline within social science that does not have a significant contribution to make to our knowledge and understanding of the new public health. For example, a political scientist's analysis of power relations within cities could prove to be an invaluable tool for an evaluator of a Healthy Cities project who is trying to make sense of why certain actors within a project dominated the project or why the rhetoric of participation proved so hard to implement. An understanding of decision making theory and organizational culture would be important for an evaluation of an attempt by different sectors to collaborate on a health promotion project. Despite this potential, theories that abound in each social science discipline are rarely used as effectively as they might be by public health researchers. But the need to extend the methodological and theoretical net used by public health researchers is now being recognized (see for example the Leeds Declaration (WHO and Yorkshire Health, 1993). Daly and Willis (1990) present a collection of essays from researchers around the world to argue that the effective evaluation of health care can only be advanced by using a range of qualitative and quantitative techniques. Sage now publishes a journal entitled Qualitative Health Research. Medically trained public health practitioners have recognized the value of methodological eclecticism (Duhl and Hancock, 1988; Scott-Samuel, 1989; Miller and Crabtree, 1992; Holman, 1993; McKinlay, 1993). An increasing number of social scientists have established a career within public health research, becoming strong advocates for the value of their perspectives (Baum, 1988; Wadsworth, 1988; Daly and Willis, 1990; Baum, 1993b; Curtice, 1993; Davies and Kelly, 1993; Hunt, 1993).

Despite some changes, very little research money, compared to that invested in mainstream medical research based on a traditional scientific paradigm, has been dedicated to qualitative research techniques. This is certainly true for Australia and I expect is so for most developed countries. The traditional paradigm has been viewed as an essential pre-requisite for funding public health and medical research in most Western countries. A glance at the application forms for research grants shows that most are designed for hypothesis testing and experimentally based biomedical research. In Australia there are signs that this is changing. The Public Health Research and Development Committee of the National Health and Medical Research Council in recent years has funded a consultancy to look at participatory public health research (Wadsworth, 1988), at least one workshop to consider the methodological debates about appropriate methods, and a number of projects that use qualitative methods. The Australian Health Ethics Committee (a committee of the NH & MRC) is in the process of developing an information paper on the assessment of qualitative research. The Research and Development Grants Advisory Committee (RADGAC) of the Federal Department of Human Services and Health actively encourages applications from researchers working within a range of disciplines using a variety of types of methods. Social scientists outnumber medically trained people on

RADGAC. More research funding to qualitative studies relevant to public health is essential if the application of these methods to public health policy and practice is to improve. Also public health training courses should present their students with a range of methods. Many present only epidemiological methods or, at best, epidemiology with other methods as an afterthought, automatically presenting them as second class. Qualitative research is often seen by traditional science as "soft" research. In fact, good qualitative research is hard to conduct. It requires discipline, a strong analytical mind and acute attention to the detail of a particular setting. All research, within whatever paradigm, has the potential to be inadequate and I suspect this potential may be greater within qualitative research. Devoting more resources to its development and to educating public health practitioners and researchers about how to implement and use its findings will help ensure its quality and applicability.

Reporting research for a wider audience

Research results should be reported in such a way that the opportunities for their application are maximized. Researchers have a responsibility to strive for the application of their results. The image of research reports gathering dust on a shelf and receiving next to no attention from people who could act on their basis is legendary. While the picture is an exaggeration it is uncomfortably near the truth for much research. But all is not lost; researchers can change this. I have already considered the importance of involving key players in selecting research agendas and in the conduct of research. Obviously if people see research as relevant to them, and feel some ownership over it and its product then they are likely to have some commitment to ensuring the results are noticed. The other area in which researchers can help ensure the application of their results is in the reporting. Most textbooks on research give this little attention; they tend to focus on writing for academic journals. The new public health demands that researchers broadcast their results to a wider audience. This means researchers have to acquire the skills of producing reports that are accessible to relevant people. Often these people are service providers and community members. Guidelines for reports suggest that they should be simply written and as free of jargon as possible; be illustrated with pictures, cartoons or other diagrams; present numerical data graphically so that they are comprehensible to people without highly developed statistical skills; and be attractive visually and eye catching. The Healthy Cities movement seems to have implemented these guidelines. Around the world, cities have produced needs assessments and reports on social indicators that conform to the above criteria. My sense is that they stand a better chance of being used in local and regional health planning than would more turgid documents.

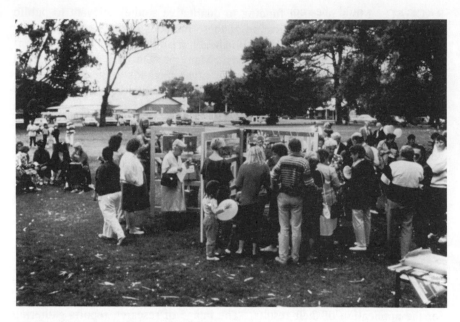

The launch of the Dream Machine

Research can also be reported in creative ways through the use of such techniques as video, strip cartoons and community art. The Dream Machine, developed as part of the Noarlunga Healthy Cities pilot project through a Community arts project, proved to be an effective means of portraying the results from a community consultation on a vision of a healthy Noarlunga. The message is that researchers should seek creative ways of reporting their findings so they are noticed. Having an official launch of a report is another way of doing this. A relevant dignitary can be invited to launch the report and the media used to publicize the report and its findings. None of these techniques can ensure research is utilized but they can increase the possibility that it might be. Reporting is only one aspect of maximizing the chances of research being used. If the message is not well received, however well it is presented it will not make an impact. Although the actions of 19th century public health reformers, such as Virchow and Snow, demonstrated that public health research leads to political action, not all researchers have accepted this. They may still use science as a shield against the political implications of their findings and maintain that the politics is for bureaucrats and politicians. This may mean that they do not follow through on the implications of their research for the public's health. Social scientists are less likely to maintain this notion of objectivity partly because, as noted above, their findings are more likely to challenge accepted notions. In an ideal world public health

28

researchers would be committed to ensuring that their findings and recommendations find practical expression in the policies and practices of the communities and organizations where they work. They would also accept and be reflective about the values and politics underlying their choice of research topics and the ways in which they conduct the research.

Conclusions

The prominence of research in public health has undoubtably increased in the past decade. The Healthy Cities movement in particular has stressed the importance of research to its endeavour. Research has already shown that it can make an impact in many of our cities and communities around the world. Its potential can, however, be increased if the five points outlined in the vision above are taken seriously by researchers. There is little point conducting research if it does not in some way leave the world a slightly different and hopefully better place. As researchers we can only gain if we reject the ivory tower approach to our trade and develop and foster relationships with the communities and organizations which are the focus of our research. By doing this, the output of our endeavours has more chance of being a louder instrument in the orchestra of influences affecting public health policy and practice. So researchers will do well to put more effort into being heard and policy makers into listening.

Acknowledgments

My thanks are owed to the following people for reading and commenting on an earlier draft of this paper: Barry Craig, Libby Kalucy, Ross Kalucy, Paul Laris and Neil Piller. Their comments have improved the paper.

Note

1.   Editorial in New Woman (Australian Edition) January 1994.

References

Allison, K. (1982), "Health Education: Self Responsibility vs Blaming the Victim", *Health Education*, Spring, pp. 11-13.
Baum, F. (1988), "Community-Based Research for Promoting the New Public Health", *Health Promotion*, vol. 3, no. 3, pp. 259-67.

29

Baum, F. and Brown, V. (1989), "Healthy Cities (Australia) Project: Issues of Evaluation for the New Public Health", *Community Health Studies*, vol. 13, no. 2, pp. 140-9.

Baum, F. (1993a), "Healthy Cities and Change: Social Movement or Bureaucratic Tool?", *Health Promotion International*, vol. 8, no. 1, pp. 31-40

Baum, F. (1993b), "Noarlunga Healthy Cities Pilot Project - The Contribution of Research and Evaluation" in Davies, John K. and Kelly, Michael (eds.) (1993), *Healthy Cities Research and Practice*, Routledge, London.

Brown, V. (1985), "Towards an Epidemiology of Health: A Basis for Planning Community Health Programs", *Health Policy*, vol. 4, pp. 331-40.

Charlesworth, M., Farrall, L., Stokes, T. and Turnball, D. (1989), *Life Among the Scientists - An Anthropological Study of an Australian Scientific Community*, Oxford University Press, Melbourne, p. 99.

Colquhoun, D. and Kellehear, A. (eds.) (1993), *Health Research in Practice: Political, Ethical and Methodological Issues*, Chapman and Hall, London.

Curtice, L. (1993), Chapter in Davies, John K. and Kelly, Michael (eds.) (1993), *Healthy Cities Research and Practice*, Routledge, London.

Daly, J. and Willis E. (eds.) (1990), *Social Sciences and Health Research*, Public Health Association of Australia, Canberra.

Davies, J.K. and Kelly, M. (eds.) (1993), *Healthy Cities Research and Practice*, Routledge, London.

de Leeuw, E., O'Neill, M., Goumans, M. and F. de Bruijn (eds.) (1993), *Healthy Cities Research Agenda. Proceedings of an Expert Panel*, Maastricht, The Netherlands: Research for Health Cities Clearing House, University of Limburg.

Dulh, L. and Hancock, T. (1988), *A Guide to Assessing Healthy Cities, WHO Healthy Cities Papers no. 3*, FADL Publishers, Copenhagen.

Fee, E. (1981), "Is Feminism a Threat to Scientific Objectivity?", *International Journal of Women's Studies*, vol. 4, p. 385.

Feuerstein, M.T. (1986), *Partners in Evaluation*, Macmillan, London, p. 168.

Freidson, E. (1970), *Professional Dominance: The Social Structure of Medical Care*, Aldine, Chicago.

Holman H.R. (1993), "Qualitative Inquiry in Medical Research", *Journal of Clinical Epidemiology*, vol. 46, pp. 29-36.

Hunt, (1993), Chapter in Davies, John K. and Kelly, Michael (eds.) (1993), *Healthy Cities Research and Practice*, Routledge, London.

McKinlay, J.B. (1993), "The Promotion of Health Through Planned Socio-Political Change: Challenges for Research and Policy", *Soc. Sci. Med.*, vol. 36, no. 2, pp. 109-17.

Marsden, D. and Oakley, P. (1991), "Future Issues and Perspectives in the Evaluation of Social Development", *Community Development Journal*, vol. 26, no. 4, pp. 315-28.

Miller, W.L. and Crabtree, B.F. (1992), "Primary Care Research: A Multi-Method Typology and Qualitative Road Map" Chapter 1 in Crabtree, Benjamin F and Miller, William, L. *Doing Qualitative Research*, Sage, Newbury Park, California.

O'Neill, M. (1993), "Building Bridges Between Knowledge and Action: The Canadian Process of Healthy Communities Indicators" chapter 10 in Davies, John K. and Kelly, Michael (eds.) (1993), *Healthy Cities Research and Practice*, Routledge, London.

Patton, M.Q., Grimes, P.S., Gutherie, K.M., Brennan, N.J., French, B.D. and Blyth, D.A. (1977), "In Search of Impact: An Analysis of the Utilisation of Federal Health Evaluation Research" in C.H. Weiss *Using Social Research in Public Policy Making*, Lexington Books, New York.

Patton, M.Q. (1990), *Qualitative Evaluation and Research Methods*, Sage, Newbury Park, California, p. 494.

Ryan, W. (1972), *Blaming the Victim*, Random House, Vintage, New York, p. 3.

Scott-Samuel, A. (1989), "Building the New Public Health: A Public Health Alliance and a New Social Epidemiology" in Martin, Claudia and McQueen, David V. *Readings for a New Public Health*, Edinburgh University Press, Edinburgh, pp. 29-41.

Terris, M. (1980), "Epidemiology as a Guide to Health Policy", *Annual Review of Public Health*, vol. 1, pp. 323-44.

Tesh, S.N. (1988), *Hidden Arguments - Political Ideology and Disease Prevention Policy*, Rutgers University Press, New Brunswick, pp. 80, 163, 170.

South Australian Community Health Research Unit (1990), *Planning Healthy Communities*, SACHRU, Adelaide, South Australia.

Wadsworth, Y. (1984), *Do-It-Yourself Social Research* Victorian Council of Social Services, Melbourne, Victoria.

Wadsworth, Y. (1988), *Participatory Research and Development in Primary Health Care by Community Groups, Report to the NH & MRC, Public Health Research and Development Committee*, Consumers Health Forum, Canberra.

Wadsworth, Y. (1991), *Everyday Evaluation On the Run*, Action Research Issues Association (Inc.), Melbourne.

Willis, E. (1983), *Medical Dominance*, George Allen and Unwin, Sydney.

World Health Organisation and Yorkshire Health (1993), *The Leeds Declaration - Principles for Action*, Nuffield Institute for Health, University of Leeds, Leeds.

2 The pragmatic approach in British public policy – can research make a difference?

David J. Hunter

My perspective in this short paper is the view point of the policy maker - what does he/she expect, or want, from research? Although I am not myself a policy maker, the nature of the work in which I am engaged, and that of the institute of which I am director, brings me into direct and frequent contact with the activities and concerns of policy makers and managers. Although the arguments and examples which follow are drawn from the British experience of research, I anticipate that what I have to say will apply to many other countries and therefore have a more universal appeal. Indeed, I know this to be the case from my involvement in the activities of many European countries and several developing countries. Nevertheless, I think it is fair to say that the British NHS research and development strategy, introduced in 1991, does offer an exemplar to other countries (Department of Health, 1991). It may prove to be one of the more successful outcomes of the NHS changes also introduced in 1991 (Secretaries of State for Health, 1989).

In addressing the question posed in the title - can research make a difference? - I want to make a distinction between biomedical research on the one hand and health systems research (HSR) on the other (Hunter and Long, 1993). Without getting caught up in complicated definitions over the precise meaning of these terms I think it is possible to contrast the impact of biomedical research on the direction of health policy and health care services with the rather disappointing impact of health services research which is concerned with the effective application of biomedical developments and with the organization, management and delivery of health and health care services.

There is, therefore, in most health care systems (and related areas) no concerted attempt to encourage the systematic use of research results, and little understanding of how to characterize health services or health problems as research questions. Policy makers and managers have persistent difficulty with such matters. Why? In general, they are not recruited for such skills or come from a background where they form part of their training or development. But the reasons also go deeper. In my view, the most plausible explanation is actually quite simple and goes to the heart of why policy makers and managers, and some practitioners, are dismissive, implicitly if not explicitly, of much HSR. The reason has its basis in stakeholder interests and the politics and power of the research endeavour. Whereas most biomedical research follows and supports the existing medical order and hierarchy of stakeholder interests, HSR is no respecter of such matters and is invariably more challenging and potentially threatening to the status quo and the vested interests which derive benefit and succour from it. Much HSR involves the revelation of conflict (covert as well as overt) and competing perspectives and the interplay of power between different stakeholder groups. It also cuts across compartmentalized policy and organizational arrangements which can affect health. HSR is diffuse and knows few boundaries. It can therefore be regarded as threatening for precisely this reason (Hunter, 1988; Pollitt et al. 1990).

The key issues affecting HSR are set out in Figure 2.1. There is no doubt in my mind that the pragmatic tradition in Britain has been a powerful antidote to the efforts of researchers, in particular social science researchers, to challenge policy assumptions and the impact of much policy on the health of communities. What we get instead from conviction politicians, and their appointed agents in the form of managers and members of health authorities and trust boards, is unwarranted confidence and synthetic enthusiasm for what they believe is right. But their unbounded enthusiasm is not grounded in empirical evidence nor, in some cases, would they wish it to be.

- Pragmatic tradition of public policy in UK

- Politicization of public policy

- The challenge posed by research to policy-makers

- The illusive search for clear prescriptions

Figure 2.1   NHS R and D strategy: key issues affecting health systems research

I suspect these trends are present in all countries to some degree but they are evident in Britain to a degree that may be considered quite unhealthy. There is virtually no connection between the products of researchers and the intentions or needs of policy makers. The politicization of public policy inhibits such a dialogue and I would argue that such politicization has gone much further in Britain than in many other countries around the world which are similarly engaged in reorganizing their health care systems. The paradox is that such overt politicization has occurred at the same time as the arrival of the NHS Research and Development (R and D) strategy and its commitment, signed up to by ministers, to knowledge based decision making.

It is possible to give various examples of the politicization process at work. For example, there is the case of the suppression of certain kinds of AIDS research through the personal intervention of a former Prime Minister; the government has steadfastly averted its gaze from the growing volume of studies reaffirming the link between poverty and deprivation and ill health - it remains to be seen how serious ministers are about the issue of health inequalities following the setting up of a working party to study the latest evidence; research on family structures and child rearing has been ignored and government policy is, for what its worth, basically, if unintentionally, anti-family. Inconvenient or potentially threatening research may tempt politicians to manipulate statistics, refuse (or restrict) publication, blacklist researchers or attack their motives or personal beliefs. All these devices and tactics have been deployed at one time or another.

When policy makers do turn to research they want instant, clear prescriptions. They do not want to be told how difficult and complex it all is or to have the questions redefined and the problems reinterpreted. The apparent, though often quite unfounded, certainty of biomedical research constitutes its chief appeal. HSR does not carry such certainty unless it is very tightly focused on specific questions of a largely technical nature. Since most HSR is concerned with understanding decision making and organizational processes and practices, and since it is directly concerned with offering interpretations of, and explanations for, why things happen or do not happen it is bound to be the case that HSR will not come up with hard and fast conclusions that can be readily implemented. More often than not, therefore, the outputs of such research can be uncomfortable for policy makers and managers.

As mentioned earlier, in the British NHS since 1991 there has been an R and D strategy (Department of Health, 1993). As the first such strategy, its very existence is testimony to the irrelevance of most research on policy and on practice over the last 45 or so years of the NHS. The absence of good evaluative research throwing a critical spotlight on health policy and health care services has been largely absent (Robinson, 1994). The (then) director of the R and D initiative has conceded as much. Most decision making in the NHS and related areas proceeds according to hunch or guesswork. Rarely has it been knowledge based. This is the major challenge to the R and D strategy. For it to be effective it must demonstrate not only that research can provide possible solutions to problems but also that it can be implemented in terms of changing the way people behave or operate (Haines and Jones, 1994; Harrison, 1994). Moreover, the R and D strategy needs to be seen in a wider context than simply health care services so that it addresses the Health of the Nation agenda and the whole notion of health gain.

The main objectives of the R and D strategy are set out in Figure 2.2. But even this strategy risks being hijacked by an unhealthy politicization of public policy. Moreover, the managerial agenda in public policy could result in the R and D effort being sidetracked into narrow, technical issues. If this happens, it will avoid some of the major, political strategic issues in health policy and health care systems, notably, health gain, the move to primary care, the links with community care, and intersectoral strategies to develop healthy alliances.

Main objectives

- To base decisions - clinical, managerial and policy - on research based information

- To provide the NHS with the capacity to identify problems that may be appropriate for research

- To improve relations between the health service and the science base

Key challenge

- Getting R into D

Figure 2.2 NHS research and development strategy

The other risk comes from the pace of change. Policy risks being ahead of the capacity of the research community to deliver on the complex questions which are, in the end, not technical but political and subjective. Time is not on the side of researchers as politicians, hungry for rapid results, and impatient with lengthy research timetables put pressure on the research community to deliver the impossible within impossible timescales. If they fail, which is a real possibility, these very same politicians can then blame researchers for being incompetent or unable to deliver what is required of them.

What needs to change if policy makers are to turn to research for genuine reasons and take it seriously? I put forward four propositions for consideration:

1. Depoliticize policy (not in all ways because the health care system in Britain and politics can not be readily separated but at least there could be less dogma and less ideology driving the changes in the system).

2. Develop a research culture among policy makers in which research is truly valued and connected into the management process at all levels.

3. Provide opportunities to raise awareness of research and its potential (and limitations) among managers.

4. Ensure that the research agenda links into the development agenda to enable the effective management of change; it is not enough for knowledge to exist - it has to be applied (see Figure 2.3).

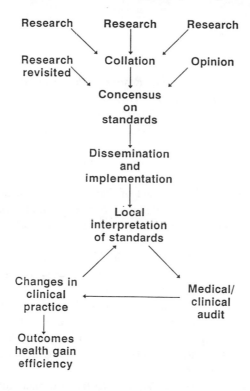

Figure 2.3 Pathways for translating knowledge into practice

I remain to be convinced that policy makers and managers do actually want research. Experience, I suspect, will still be taken as the trustiest guide - to solve a policy problem simply tap the advice of those who have extensive practical experience of the issue in question. Given the scale and complex nature of the problems confronting all of those who work in and around health care services such resort to existing expertize may not be appropriate.

More worrying, perhaps, is the notion that managerialism places the emphasis on data driven prescriptions and devalues interpretative approaches, even if (or perhaps because) it is the latter which form the basis of much managerial action. I would argue that it is interpretive approaches that we need to value in respect of much HSR (Hunter, 1994). Regrettably, it is unfashionable in these days of quick fixes and instant solutions. There is a need to separate the rhetoric from the reality about research and its contribution to policy. Much symbolic posturing is evident in this area as in so many others. We need to move beyond that and actually make the connections between the research process and the decision making process that will then lead to developments in health care services that will result in improved outcomes.

References

Department of Health (1991), *Research for Health - a Research and Development Strategy for the NHS*, Department of Health, London.

Department of Health (1993), *Research for Health,* HMSO, London.

Haines, A. and Jones, R. (1994), "Implementing Findings of Research", *British Medical Journal*, vol. 308, pp. 1488-92.

Harrison, S. (1994), "Knowledge into Practice: What's the Problem?", *Journal of Management in Medicine*, vol. 8, pp. 9-16.

Hunter, D.J. (1988), "The Impact of Research on Restructuring the British NHS'" *Journal of Health Administration Education*, vol. 6, pp. 537-53.

Hunter, D.J. (1994), "Are We Being Effective?", *Health Service Journal*, 16 June, p. 23.

Hunter, D.J. and Long, A. (1993), "Health Research" in Sykes, W., Bulmer, M. and Schwerzel, M. (eds.), *Directory of Social Research Organisations in the United Kingdom*, Mansell, London.

Pollitt, C., Harrison, S., Hunter, D.J. and Marnoch, G. (1990), "No Hiding Place: On the Discomforts of Researching the Contemporary Policy Process", *Journal of Social Policy*, vol. 19, pp. 169-90.

Robinson, R. and Le Grand, J., (1994) *Evaluating the NHS Reforms*, King's Fund Institute, London.

Secretaries of State for Health, Wales, Northern Ireland and Scotland (1989), *Working for Patients*, Cm 555, HMSO, London.

3 Research for healthy cities: Where are we now?

Charles Price

It is ten years since the conference "Beyond Health Care" took place in Toronto, and the idea of the Healthy Cities project was conceived. During that time research for Healthy Cities has received much attention. The agenda has stretched from supranational policy making to family dynamics, and the methods from geographical mapping to participant observation. There have been vigorous discussions on the ethics of research, the application of health promotion principles to research work and several research frameworks have been proposed. But despite this interest we are still at the beginning of the research effort which needs to be made to inform policy and provide knowledge about how to reverse health inequalities and improve the social and physical environments of our cities with the resources we have available. There are of course examples of progress, some of which I will refer to, but we need to ask ourselves whether the current research effort really matches the importance of the questions and whether research policies and research agendas need to be altered to reflect health priorities.

Growing inequalities

Today many cities are experiencing declining health of their populations. Life expectancy is falling in many central and eastern European countries after steady increases for a generation. Health inequalities are increasing in the United Kingdom and inequalities are also increasing in other parts of the world - not only in the rapidly expanding cities of developing countries but also amongst disadvantaged groups in the industrialized world. In fact the term the "fourth world" is being used to characterize the huge disparities which exist between some of the chronically disadvantaged groups and others in the major urban areas of Europe and North America. In some instances these disparities are as great within a single city such as New York as between countries such as the UK and Bangladesh (McCord and Freeman, 1990).

The existence of such health inequalities is widely acknowledged. So too is a central tenet of the Health for All strategy that health is created in people's everyday lives. But where is our real understanding of how our physical and social environments affect our health or what should be the best ways of going about improving the situation? Where is our understanding of how to generate health and well being in our societies? Where is the advice to give to policy makers eager to build a new dawn for the 21st century? In short just what contribution can research make to the reduction of health inequalities? This is the first challenge for the research agenda.

In addition to the fundamental questions of tackling health inequalities, this conference rightly focuses on relationships between three key areas - research, policy and community. To create the best health outcomes we need strategies which link these three together. We need not only research which can inform policy, but policies which stimulate and support relevant research and we need research and policy making prepared to work with and for communities.

What research is needed?

Researchers and public health professionals need to be able to advise policy makers on the answers to three questions - where is health created?; which investment strategies produce the largest health gains?; which investment strategies help to reduce health inequalities? To answer these questions we need information on the processes and outcomes of health promotion interventions and detailed evaluations of the health impact of actions in areas ranging from housing and transport policy to community development, from job creation schemes to screening programmes. Altogether there have been perhaps half a dozen meetings to discuss research for Healthy Cities and there have been a number of proposals for research agendas and frameworks (Davies and Kelly, 1993). There is a research network and even a research newsletter co-ordinated by the University of Limburg in Maastricht. But how far have we come in the six years since the Healthy Cities project was formerly established? Well perhaps on the basis of McKnight's (1987) observation that communities learn by stories, institutions learn by studies, we have a mixture of both stories and studies. There are many descriptions of city based action both published and presented in Healthy Cities symposia. Evaluations are far fewer. Carefully constructed studies are rare indeed. During the first phase of the project WHO carried out systematic assessment visits and interviews and Curtice and McQueen collected structured information from cities (WHO, 1994). Knowledge gained from these exercises was converted into the mid term review (Curtice and McQueen,

1990) and the booklet "20 steps for developing a Healthy Cities project" (Tsouros, 1992) which has now been translated into 17 languages. Semi structured interviews and analyzes of materials from cities were conducted as part of the five year review exercise. This gave information on the uptake of the ideas and of the application and was important in securing continuation of the project into the second phase.

Comparative indicators for cities were an issue from the outset. But choosing the indicators and collecting the data from cities proved a long process. Finally the opportunity of the start of the second phase of the project was used to put together the work done so far into a questionnaire. We were able for the first time to collect data on a wide range of issues from cities in 25 European countries. In spite of problems of definition and comparability which are still being tackled there are some interesting early comparisons to be made. The percentage of low birth weight babies for instance can be looked at geographically with cities in North and West Europe on the low end of the scale and high percentages being reported from cities in Poland, Czech Republic and Hungary. The percentage of households without sole access to a bathroom can also be examined: some of the least well provided cities are in Western Europe. Copenhagen, Liege and Vienna all have more than 20 per cent of households without their own bathroom. Liverpool, is towards the lower end of the range just ahead of Glasgow, but behind Maribor in Slovenia. Evidently the relationship between health and physical environments is complex and such comparative data is already exciting interest from researchers from around Europe as well as support from the European Commission.

Research and city planning

The current phase of the Healthy Cities project from 1993-1997 concentrates on policy - in particular on developing comprehensive city health plans based on health for all and on accountability for health - particularly in developing ways of assessing the impact on health of policies outside of the health service and moving towards health audits in a similar vein to environmental audits. Some cities have already produced proposals for city health plans. Aspects of Healthy Cities policies and research can clearly be seen in some of these plans. For example the conceptual framework for the Healthy City Plan of Copenhagen has its main roots in the Health for All policy, the principles of intersectoral co-operation and community participation. But the main approach is based on strengthening social networks particularly in the settings of schools, work places, local communities. These settings will act on "traditional" problem areas including alcohol, accidents, physical exercise, abortion and urban ecology (WHO, 1992).

41

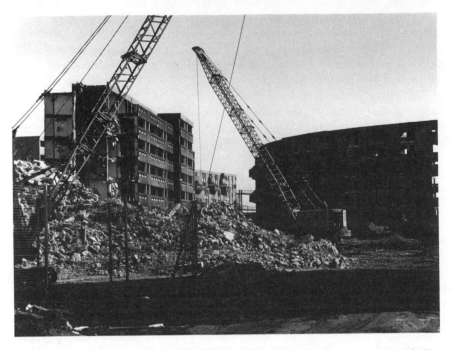

Research is needed on the health impacts of actions in many areas, including housing such as this inner city redevelopment in Manchester

It is interesting to note here that the analysis used in support of the plan has drawn on work of participants at this conference - including the work of Kay Dean from the University of Copenhagen on social networks. The level of research activity in relation to individual Healthy Cities projects has varied enormously. A few projects could almost be said to be research driven while others are at the other end of the spectrum. Case studies and small scale evaluations have been mentioned but there have also been some city wide initiatives. Rotterdam for example has developed an ambitious geographical information system to integrate health, environment and service information to allow relationships to be examined in small areas (Copenhagen Health Services, 1994). A similar exercise is being undertaken in Tokyo as part of its long term planning exercises which include the development of an active health promotion movement as one of its ten priorities. Nakamura and Takano have reported how a variety of disciplines including epidemiology, architecture and economics have worked together to build up data on the city and to integrate this with many specialized studies to allow the relationship between health, environment and service provision to be investigated (Van Oers, 1993).

Community involvement is an important goal of Healthy Cities but how often is it measured? The city of Horsens tried a simple way to measure it by incorporating two questions into a poll done by the city to assess a wide range of services. Based on a survey of 1,500 adults they estimated that over 90 per cent of adults in the city had heard of the project and 13 per cent had taken part in activities connected to the project. There was little variation by age with similar numbers of 18-19 year olds taking part in activities as people over the age of 70 (Nakamura and Takano, 1992).

Healthy Cities is entering a new phase. New research is needed. Although there are examples of progress we are only scratching the surface of what is needed and what is available to be discovered. We need research to take place at the local level and we need research to take place internationally. Although research is driven by curiosity it is clear that the major driving force is national research policy and the funding which goes with it.

Target 32 of the updated Health For All targets makes some recommendations on research policy which few countries have yet implemented (Moller and Hansen, 1992). We need research policies which put the focus firstly on health as well as on the sectors which contribute to health. Maybe there is a case for "health research councils" - to compliment medical research councils. The research agenda needs contributions from a range of disciplines - social science, economics, medicine, public health to name but a few - and should include the views of community representatives and policy makers as well as researchers.

Priorities for research funding need to be determined with consideration for the potential impact of the findings on health. Funding needs to be adequate to the task and communication needs to be improved between the researchers, policy makers and the communities which they serve.

The research arena of the Healthy Cities project has generated many sparks. Let us hope that this meeting will help some of these to ignite into a flame which can lead the way for development of the research initiatives we need for the 21st century.

References

Curtice, L. and McQueen, D.V. (1990), *The WHO Healthy Cities Project: An Analysis of Progress Working Paper No. 40, Research Unit in Health & Behaviourial Change*, University of Edinburgh, Edinburgh.

Davies, J.K. and Kelly, M. (1993), *Healthy Cities Project Research and Practice*, Routledge, London.

Healthy City Project (1994), Copenhagen Health Services, *City of Copenhagen Healthy City Plan* (english edition), Copenhagen.

McCord, C. and Freeman, H.P. (1990), "Excess Mortality in Harlem", *New*

England Journal of Medicine, vol. 322, no. 3, pp. 173-7.

McKnight, J.L. (1987), "Regenerating Community", *Social Policy*, winter edition.

Møller, F.R. and Hansen, E.B. (1992), *Borgernes Vurdering af Horsens Kommune*, AKF Folaget, Copenhagen.

Nakamura, K. and Takano, T. (1992), "Image Diagnosis of Health in Cities: Tokyo Healthy City" in Takano, T., Ishidate, K. and Nagasaki M. (ed.), *Formulation and Development of a Base for Healthy cities*, Kyokiku, Syoseki, Tokyo.

Tsouros, A. (1992), *World Health Organisation Healthy Cities Project: A Project Becomes a Movement*, (ed.), FADL, Copenhagen.

Van Oers, J.A.M. (1993), *A Geographical Information System for Local Public Health Policy*, Den Haag.

World Health Organisation Regional Office for Europe (1992), *Twenty Steps for Developing a Healthy Cities Project*, World Health Organisation Regional Office for Europe, Copenhagen.

World Health Organisation Regional Office for Europe, (1994), *Action for Health in Cities*, World Health Organisation Regional Office for Europe, Copenhagen.

Section 2   Philosophy and methods of research for health promotion

In section one, it was argued that there are a number of reasons why research for better health is frequently not translated into policy, and some of the reasons are very political and not easily or directly influenced by the researcher. There are however another set of issues that do fall very much more within the influence of the research community, and which concern the appropriateness of the methods and the ways in which the research is carried out. In particular, there is a need to make research more relevant to the experiences of individuals, communities and policy makers, and this will involve a shift in the approach used.

There appear to be two main aspects to this: first, the question of what are the most appropriate techniques for studying what damages or promotes health; and second, how research to promote health should be planned and carried out so that the people and communities concerned can gain the most benefit in terms of relevance to their lives and involvement in the implementation process that should follow.

These threads in both scientific thinking and practice of health promotion have been brought together in the "Leeds Declaration", described by Alex Scott-Samuel. This initiative seeks to define the important principles that are required for research in public health, with particular emphasis on the understanding of the social structures and process that influence health, and an acceptance of a "plurality" of research methods. The paper emphasizes the urgency with which this refocussing of attitudes to public health research is required.

In the second paper, Jane Springett and Conan Leavey examine the evolution and contemporary relevance of participatory action research. This emphasizes the value that derives from participants being involved in carrying out the research which is actually an integral part of the process of change in their community. There are a number of ways in which this brings benefit, some of which are explored in the following sections, but one particularly valuable outcome is the way in which this can break down the barriers between research and policy. While that potential benefit does exist, there are also dilemmas which those practising research in this setting experience and need to cope with. They tend to be caught between the "scornful approach of scientists toward any claim of validity ...", while those involved in community action may be "equally scornful about the relevance of research and its ability to challenge the status quo." Those experiencing this dilemma will recognize it only too well, while others who are exploring this field will see the tension and uncertainty that is very apparent in the accounts that follow. Research of this type poses threats to existing professional roles and structures, including those of researchers, and this is also explored through an example of collaborative research with a professional group.

We have seen that it cannot be helpful to use research methods which deny participation of those whose circumstances are the subject of research, or to use measurement techniques which are unresponsive to the realities of people's lives. In the third paper, Maria Koelen examines why research for health promotion must pay more attention to the so called "qualitative" methods, techniques which employ indepth interviews and discussion, observation, and other ways of expressing experiences. The benefits of doing so follow on from the very fact of describing people's circumstances as they really are - for it is only then that the people concerned will feel the value of sticking with the process, of working with the statutory agencies to develop and implement new policies. As noted above, one problem of these qualitative techniques is their perceived lack of scientific objectivity: that is, the view that the results are too easily influenced by the prejudices of the investigators and the needs of the subjects. Traditional epidemiology has made us very aware of the many sources of bias in research, be it from sampling technique, non-response, inconsistent techniques for conducting interviews and measurements (see for example: Bruce et al. 1988), or inaccurate equipment. This awareness should be carried forward into these new areas of research, and Maria offers a number of techniques for assessing the validity of the work. It is of interest that at the time of going to press, a series on qualitative research appeared in the medical press, marking the growing awareness of the value of these techniques (Mays and Pope, 1995a; Mays and Pope, 1995b).

One other important area for population research is the investigation of the complex interaction of factors which lead to illness or the adoption of certain health related behaviours in some people while others remain healthy or avoid these behaviours. In the final paper, Kay Dean argues that traditional epidemiological methods, while useful for identifying factors which "on average" promote or harm health (for instance, cigarette smoking), are inadequate for studying the effects on health of the much greater complexity of circumstances that individual lives are subject to. Being able to describe the health consequences of more realistic life circumstances should lead to policy that is more relevant, believable and therefore more likely to be acted on. These ideas are then illustrated with an analysis of factors which influence the will and ability to give up smoking, drawing on data collected in a lifestyle survey. It is interesting that this analysis emphasizes the different values placed on smoking by people in differing social circumstances, findings which are highly relevant to health promotion policy and which also accord with some of the experience from community development work such as that in Bristol (see Chapter 18).

The ideas described in these three papers represent an extension to, rather than a denial of, traditional epidemiological concepts and research methods. These have provided much of value and can continue to do so, but what is nevertheless urgently required for public health research is a refining of this epidemiology, the inclusion of sociological and other approaches, and an openness to active involvement by participants - especially the community. This broader picture of methods and attitudes, although challenging to the existing somewhat polarized research traditions, has the potential to offer much greater understanding of community health and relevance to policy making.

References

Bruce, N.G., Shaper, A.G. and Wannamethee, G. (1988), "Observer Bias in Blood Pressure Studies", *J Hypertension*, vol. 6, pp. 375-80.

Mays, N. and Pope, C. (1995a), "Rigour and Qualitative Research", *British Medical Journal*, vol. 311, pp. 109-12.

Mays, N. and Pope, C. (1995b), "Observational Methods in Health Care Settings", *British Medical Journal*, vol. 311, pp. 182-4.

4 A new synthesis: Population health research for the 21st century

Alex Scott-Samuel

Advocates for the idea that a "new public health" has emerged in developed countries during the past fifteen years share a common understanding that people's health is primarily determined by a complex ecology of social, economic, and political influences. The familiar medical model of agent, host, and environment, which served the cause of infectious disease epidemiology so well in the past, is no longer tenable. But the development of a new public health worthy of that name has been retarded by the continuing absence of new models of epidemiology capable of explaining the multi-causal and multi-dimensional complexity of the new ecology of health.

Two key tasks need to be undertaken if such new models are to be developed. The first of these is the transformation of orthodox disease epidemiology, with its roots in nineteenth century positivism. The ways in which health research has begun to tackle this question include the application of approaches giving greater primacy to subjective and biographical knowledge. Medical sociology and anthropology have much to offer here. Of equal importance are the social relations of ill health and of the research process. The World Health Organisation has begun to promote participatory research, which involves those being studied in all stages of the research process, from the formulation of hypotheses and the design of instruments through to the implementation of findings.

The second, and perhaps greater, challenge of exponents of the new public health entails the elaboration of an epidemiology of health itself. This body of knowledge will need to take in both the dynamic processes of achieving and maintaining health (what Antonovsky and others have termed salutogenesis) and also the determinants of the health outcomes analogous to the disease outcomes studied by clinical epidemiology (Scott-Samuel, 1992).

The above paragraphs constituted one of the "problem statements" requested from participants prior to a three day workshop which took place in Leeds in July 1993. The workshop was jointly sponsored by the Nuffield Institute for Health at the University of Leeds, the World Health Organisation's Regional Office for Europe and the former Yorkshire Regional Health Authority. The 30 participants represented three continents and a range of disciplines which included epidemiology, sociology, anthropology, education, management, social policy and public health medicine. What brought them together was a common concern that, after more than a decade of discussion of the ecological concepts of the new public health, "Research on the health of populations is still dominated by experimental designs based on simplistic notions of causality that try to remove the variation and complexity of real life health and disease processes" (Lancet, 1994).

The problem statements and the opening session of the workshop identified a range of problems with contemporary epidemiology relating to its underlying paradigm, methods and purpose (Long, 1993). It was also pointed out that similar problems could be identified in other health related fields such as sociology or social policy. The key issues of the workshop related not to any one discipline, but to the current scientific basis, policy and practice of public health. Thus the major question to be answered was "What is the appropriate knowledge base for public health action?" The wide ranging discussions raised many issues and left many points unanswered, but there was broad consensus around a set of action principles and around the idea that a declaration embodying these would be helpful in taking the discussion into a wider arena. The Leeds Declaration (see Appendix 4.1), which sets out these principles, has been widely disseminated and readers are encouraged to use it as the basis for continuing debate around the appropriate knowledge base for public health action as we move into the 21st century.

In contrast to the continuing focus of public health on a clinical model of intervention at the level of the individual, the first principle reflects Zola's notion of "refocussing upstream" (McKinlay, 1974). This refers to the metaphor of the villagers who are forever devising more elaborate equipment to fish drowning people from the river rather than looking upstream in order to discover who is pushing them in. The reductionist focus on disease rather than on health, which is another element in the refocussing metaphor, is referred to in the second principle. There is a need for health itself to become a major focus within the public health knowledge base (Brown, 1985) and for the development of research which attempts to understand health inequalities rather than disease inequalities (Lundberg and Nystrom Peck, 1994).

The elaboration of an appropriate knowledge base for public health implies also the definition of appropriate methods. The fourth to seventh principles refer to the substantial reliance of present day public health research on quasi-experimental and other quantitative methods. While study designs such as randomized controlled trials can be highly effective in isolating single causal variables, they are often wholly inappropriate and inadequate for studying the complex and multi-dimensional structures and processes which cause health and disease. In areas such as these, qualitative approaches (such as ethnographic interviewing, participant observation, case studies, and focus groups) are often the methods of choice, frequently in combination with quantitative approaches. Both sets of approaches require equal care, thought and rigour.

The third principle refers to the importance of lay knowledge and perspectives in public health research. In addition to people's health knowledge and practices being crucial determinants of health outcomes, there is also a need for the subjects of public health research to become its practitioners. In participatory research, (Starrin and Svensson, 1991) lay people take part in hypothesis generation, study design, research implementation and policy development. The World Health Organisation (1988) has recommended that "research should provide ample opportunities for the people affected by the studies to take part in defining their aims, conducting the investigations and using the results."

Reference to the knowledge base for public health is a reminder that the time has long since passed when epidemiology was the only public health science. Management science, economics, sociology, psychology, anthropology, geography, political science and statistics are only the most obvious additions to the long list of public health disciplines. The eighth principle refers not only to the pluralist approach which this implies, but also to the importance of interdisciplinary research which integrates theory and methods and which incorporates new analytical models (Dean, 1994).

The effective implementation of appropriate research for public health action depends on the final two principles: the redirection of research and development funds to reflect the emerging consensus which I have described, and a commitment to ensuring that the findings of the new public health research are properly applied to influence policy and practice. This emphasizes that the successful implementation of the Leeds Declaration must involve managers, politicians and other health related policy makers well beyond the research disciplines. Success in implementing the Declaration will be no easy task, but it is an essential one if research on the health of populations is to provide the basis for effective health policy in the 21st century.

References

Anon, (1994), "Population Health Looking Uupstream", (Editorial) *Lancet*, vol. 343, pp. 429-30.

Brown, V.A. (1985), "Towards an Epidemiology of Health: A Basis for Planning Community Health Programmes", *Health Policy*, vol. 4, pp. 331-40.

Dean, K. (1994), "Integrating Theory and Methods in Population Health Research" in Dean, K., (ed.), *Population Health Research: Linking Theory and Methods*, Sage, London.

Long, A.F. (1993), *Understanding Health and Disease: Towards a Knowledge Base for Public Health Action. Report of a Workshop Held at the Nuffield Institute for Health University of Leeds, 30 June-2 July 1993*, Nuffield Institute for Health, University of Leeds, Leeds.

Lundberg, O. and Nystrom Peck, M. (1994), "Sense of Coherence, Social Structure and Health", *European Journal of Public Health*, vol. 4, pp. 252-7.

McKinlay, J.B. (1974), *A Case for Refocussing Upstream: the Political Economy of Illness, Proceedings of American Heart Association Conference on Applying Behavioural Science to Cardiovascular Risk*, American Heart Association, Seattle.

Scott-Samuel, A. (1992), "Complex Interactions", *British Medical Journal*, vol. 305, p. 593.

Starrin, B. and Svensson, P.G. (1991), "Participatory Research: A Complementary Research Approach in Public Health", *European Journal of Public Health*, vol. 1, pp. 29-35.

World Health Organisation (1988), *Regional Office for Europe, Priority Research for Health for All*, WHO, Copenhagen.

Further selected reading

Black, N. (1994), "Why We Need Qualitative Research", *Journal of Epidemiology and Community Health*, vol. 48, pp. 425-6.

Paterson, K. (1981), "Theoretical Perspectives in Epidemiology - a Critical Appraisal", *Radical Community Medicine*, no. 8, pp. 21-9.

Scott-Samuel, A. (1989), "Building the New Public Health: A Public Health Alliance and a New Social Epidemiology" in Martin, C.J. and MacQueen, D.V. (eds), *Readings for a New Public Health*, Edinburgh University Press, Edinburgh, pp. 29-44.

Stallones, R.A. (1980), "To Advance Epidemiology", *Annual Review of Public Health*, vol. 1, pp. 69-82.

Watterson, A. (1994), "Whither Lay Epidemiology in UK Public Health

Policy and Practice? Some Reflections on Occupational and Environmental Health Opportunities", *Journal of Public Health Medicine*, vol. 16, pp. 270-4.

Wing, S. (1994), "Limits of Epidemiology", *Medicine and Global Survival*, vol. 1, pp. 74-86.

DIRECTIONS FOR HEALTH
NEW APPROACHES TO POPULATION
HEALTH RESEARCH AND PRACTICE

THE LEEDS DECLARATION

New approaches to understanding and managing public health problems are urgently required. Traditional epidemiological methods provide instruments that are too blunt to dissect the complexities of today's health problems. Many other methods are available from different disciplines which can and should play a complementary role. At present these remain seriously underutilised or are not recognised as having a contribution to make.

At a recent international workshop in Leeds, it was agreed that reconstruction of the principles of public health is urgently required.

The academic and service public health practitioners who have worked to produce the **LEEDS DECLARATION** have done so in the expectation that it will be used as a focus for discussion and debate in the widest arena. Only by doing so will we begin seriously to address the real issues confronting contemporary public health. Consequently, we will make a positive contribution to improve the public health as we move towards the twenty first century.

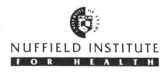

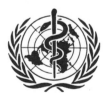

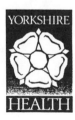

For further information, contact:

• Professor David Hunter or Mr Andrew Long at the Nuffield Institute for Health on 0532 459034

• Dr Frada Eskin at Yorkshire Health on 0423 500066

• Dr Alex Scott-Samuel at Liverpool Health Authority on 051 236 4747

THE LEEDS DECLARATION
PRINCIPLES FOR ACTION

- There is an urgent need to re-focus upstream, to move away from focusing predominantly upon individual risks towards the social structures and processes within which ill-health originates.

- Research is needed to explore the factors which keep some people healthy despite their living in the most adverse circumstances.

- Lay people are experts and experts are lay people - lay knowledge about health needs, health service priorities and health outcomes should be central to public health research.

- The experimental model is an inadequate gold standard for guiding research into public health problems.

- A plurality of methods is required to address the multiple dimensions of public health problems.

- Not all health data can be represented in numbers - qualitative data have an important role to play in public health research.

- There is nothing inherently 'soft' about qualitative methods or 'hard' about quantitative methods - both require rigorous application in appropriate contexts and hard thinking about difficult problems.

- An openness to the value of different methods means an openness to the contribution of a variety of disciplines.

- Public health problems will only be solved through a commitment to the application of research findings to policy and practice.

- Research funding should address the new directions that follow from these principles.

5 Participatory action research: The development of a paradigm, dilemmas and prospects

Jane Springett and Conan Leavey

The aim of this paper is three fold. Firstly, to argue that participatory action research provides a solution to the practical problem of crossing the boundaries between the two conflicting cultures of research and policy making. Secondly that it is an approach to research that can be a real catalyst for change. Thirdly, to demonstrate with reference to a research project on health promotion in primary health care, the dilemmas and problems generated by such an approach. It can turn out in practice to be a messy process but an instructive learning experience. It will be argued that this is inherent in action research which is essentially dialectical and by its very nature contains within it certain contradictions that create very real tensions in its pursuit.

What is action research?

The notion of action research can be traced back to work done by Lewin in 1945 (Lewin, 1946). Since then it has been pursued with greater or lesser success in three main areas, development research, management science and education, generating tremendous variety in form as it has been applied to increasingly complex problems (Elden and Chisholm, 1993). Many of the papers in this book and workshops at the conference on which it is based could be classified as some form of action research.

In development research it has been extensively used as a vehicle for rural development and is closely associated with Frierian approaches to popular education (Kroeger and Franken, 1981). This southern focus, as Brown and Tandon (1993) calls it, emphasizes mobilization, conscientizing and empowering the oppressed to achieve community transformations and social justice i.e. understanding and changing communities and grass roots. It has much to offer, therefore, urban community health projects. In the 1960s and

1970s in western Europe action research was seen as an important feature of community development approaches. However it differed from the southern tradition in that it was seen more as the involvement of the local community in research which had been initiated by the researchers rather than real collaborative inquiry where the identification of the problem and the production of knowledge is community led.

In management science, classical action research has come to be seen as a form of action learning which encourages the systematic collection of data and information, combining rigour and relevance in moving towards high levels of performance in organizations as well as leading to innovation (Margerison, 1987). As such therefore it is geared to solving major job/organization issues or problems on a group basis and its focus is decision makers. A key feature of recent research in this area is the emphasis on participation, use of action research to generate networks to support economic development and on bringing about change in multi-level systems rather than single units or organizations (Ledford and Mohrman, 1993).

The emphasis on practitioners becoming researchers in order to become more reflexive and improve practice is a feature of educational action research (McTargart, 1991). Here the focus is on the systematic collection of evidence as well as collaborative and collective enquiry, motivated by the quest to improve and understand the world by changing it and learning how to improve it from the effect of the changes made, particularly in the class room. This also has tended to be the main focus in nursing action research where the emphasis is on day to day practice on the ward (Meyer, 1993).

From these different traditions one can identify three types of action research relevant to creating change for community health depending on who is involved in the creation of knowledge as the result of the process:

1.   Participatory action research which is knowledge created by the community and the researcher.

2.   Action research which is knowledge created by the practitioner and the researcher.

3.   Collaborative inquiry which is knowledge created by the researcher, practitioners and the community as equal co-researchers.

In each of these categories practitioner could mean policy makers or the key managers involved in the implementation of policy within organizations that impact on community health.

What unites these different definitions of action research is that they all focus on knowledge creation in the context of practice and the development of what is called local theory (Greenwood et al. 1993). It is an approach that is in direct conflict with orthodox methods in social science and challenges dominant knowledge based systems. It is based on a completely different conception of the relationship between science, knowledge, learning and action. It assumes that people can generate knowledge as partners in a systematic inquiry process based on their own categories and frameworks. This, it can be argued, enhances scientific validity producing richer and more accurate data, creates active support for the results of the process of inquiry and therefore greater commitment to change as well as the greater likelihood that ideas will be diffused (Reason and Rowan, 1981).

Learning, is the raison d'etre of action research and it draws heavily on the notions about the way adults learn which form the basis of Kolb Learning Cycle (Kolb, 1984) which suggests that in order for learning to take place all elements of the cycle have to be present. In traditional research the emphasis is on theory creation and testing while in traditional practice the emphasis is on action. In action research the entire cycle is addressed with the production of knowledge resulting from collaboration between insider practitioner and outsider researcher.

It is the emphasis on change which is another distinguishing feature of action research. Those engaged in traditional social research rarely become involved in linking their research to action and whilst their findings may have practical significance it is primarily the responsibility of others to make use of what social researchers discover. Social researchers should be alert, of course, to the danger of imposing their own values and meanings on the interpretation of the data. However, action research does not accept the positivist assumption that "involvement" in the research setting is incompatible with good social "science" (Susman and Evered, 1978).

The aim of action research is to make change and learning a self generating and self maintaining process which continues after the researcher has left. It seeks to bring about change that has a positive social value e.g. a healthy community. Moreover, process is seen as a product which is just as important as any solution to a practical or scientific problem. The essence of action research is that it is an emergent process controlled by local conditions. It involves the collective production of knowledge and seeks to empower those involved in the research in such a way that encourages change from within. As such it would appear to be a excellent vehicle for breaking down the boundaries between research and policy. No longer would the production of knowledge be retained in the hands of experts and lodged on the shelves of offices and libraries as interesting but not relevant to day to day practical problems of the here and now. Rather by being involved in the research process, policy makers would own both the ideas of the research and its results so that they would be ready to implement the appropriate action because it is already an innate part of their consciousness and the process of doing the research has already begun to change the way they act and what

59

they believe. The key to the process is dialogue (Hazen, 1994). By creating situations whereby thoughts are communicated and exchanged a new social reality starts to be shaped as argued by Habermas (1984/87). The role of the researcher is to create those situations through various techniques such as workshops and allow the joint product, a more integrated and higher form of consciousness to emerge from the interplay between the actors (Reason, 1988). A new set of social relations is created and the new knowledge is the result of that process.

This approach represents a fundamental challenge to the conventional scientific view about the way knowledge is constructed. Conventional science is predicated upon a principle of objectivity, inherited from the positivist natural sciences, that does not translate favourably into the social sciences. Whilst we must, indeed, be careful not to let the values of the researcher dominate the data it is an illusion to assume that we can conduct objective, value free research which will yield immutable "facts" about the way things really are in the social world. To paraphrase Schutz (1954), from a memorable passage, what distinguishes us from electrons and sub-atomic particles is that the process of being researched means something to us. The social sciences have a reflective subject matter; other thinking, feeling human beings who will construct meanings, hold values and have a dynamic relationship with those studying them. And if this is the case then surely the relationship between the researcher and the researched must be central to the research process itself rather than excluded from it.

The tenets of action research, therefore, appear strangely counter intuitive to researchers schooled in conventional research methods, so deeply ingrained is our general commitment to maintaining barriers between the researcher and the researched. Action research tells us that the researcher/researched dichotomy should be broken down, that we are all co-researchers and co-subjects producing the data which constitutes the object of research. Furthermore, analysis of this data is no longer the sole domain of the researcher but should be a collaborative venture between all the participants. Such an approach is yet to have an impact on the mainstream in the production of health policy. The potential, however is there.

Dilemmas inherent in action research

Action research, therefore, is profoundly challenging. At an epistemological level it reaffirms that social meanings are not fixed. They emerge from active interaction between participants in any given context, and research can never be exempt from this because it is in itself a context that will influence the meanings constructed by researcher and participants alike. There is no underlying positivist reality waiting to be revealed. We will never devise a set of research tools, having controlled for every possible source of bias and distortion, that will enable us to hold up a mirror to social reality and say with any degree of confidence "this is how things really are."

The resultant knowledge and outcomes in terms of change cannot be predicted at the start of the process since they are a product of the social relationships involved in the process. Who is included in the process, history, the existing power relations, the nature and type of communication that takes place and the arena in which it takes place, all influence the process. The journey will be a choppy one and rarely follow an ideal model. Tensions will be created which stem from the inherent contradictions involved in bringing theory creation and practice directly together. Action research explicitly challenges the scientific method of inquiry based on the authority of the outside "observer" and the "independent" experimenter and it claims to reconstruct both practical expertise and theoretical insight on the different basis of its own inquiry procedures (Winter, 1990). Thus, criticisms of the approach can come from both ends of the spectrum. Scientists are scornful of claims of validity and deplore the lack of theoretical base while practitioners are either scornful of its claims of relevance and question its authority or suggest its ability to challenge the status quo is illusory. Both and neither are right because while action research is an explicit challenge to positivism's version of the relation between theory and practice, it rests on the belief that through the process of critical reflection new theory can be generated. However this is an illusion. That process is informed already by theory since each social actor is embedded in an particular institutionalized authoritative structure and ideology (Rahman, 1993). Moreover, how can the existing status quo be challenged or the theory created be analytically different if the participants are embedded in existing institutional structures that negate "democratic dialogue" without the action researcher intervening in the process in a way it wishes to avoid.

At a political level, action research challenges orthodox power structures. Subjects no longer passively produce data for researchers to interpret and hand over to decision making elites. Participants define their own problems, collaborate in the inquiry and have an equal say in the implementation of the findings. This undermines the professional expert model that preserves the autocracy of the researcher and attempts to democratize the whole research process.

It is in the nature of action research that it generates a high level of uncertainty and lack of control over the research process. The investigators do not know in advance the exact pattern of the inquiry that will develop. Although action research is distinguished by its adherence to a collaborative ethic, that process is not a clear cut one. Much depends on the parties involved, who initiated the agenda, who has sponsored the work, what the relationship between the parties is and how the research problem is defined.

In some cases the roles need to be negotiated and as the research process unfolds, and will change. Quite often the roles are overlapping and there can be confusion as to which interest group is being served. All parties are changed in the process. The researchers will also suffer the transformations of the process they initiate.

Embedded in the notion of action research is dialogue, feedback and change as a spiralling process rather than a series of static episodes. Research is clearly situated as a precursor for action not merely information for its own sake; the whole context is seen as being relevant and the traditional distance between the researcher and researched is abandoned with the intention of developing methods for promoting intersubjectivity rather than subject/object relations. This gives rise to a series of conflicts at every stage in the process and far from producing a clear framework, that framework is a permeable one changing as the research cycle unfolds. Gone therefore is the false dichotomy defining the separation of subject and object, researcher and researched, detachment and involvement, rationality and intuition, logic and emotion: instead one is faced with the real production of knowledge on its own battle ground (Rahman, op cit.). The following case study illustrates some of these points.

Health promotion in primary health care

As has been noted, action research has been predominately employed in hierarchical settings where traditional research has served to perpetuate inequalities by silencing others even when trying to speak out on their behalf. It is only recently that action research has been employed among the powerful, literate, professional cultures who ordinarily exercise power in society, implement change and establish social norms.

This research represents a collaboration with four Liverpool general practices interested in improving attendance rates at health promotion clinics. In conjunction with the Liverpool Primary Health Care Facilitation Project, the Department of Health and Liverpool John Moores University, a project was established to investigate the situation, particularly in inner city areas where attendance was perceived as being something of a problem. It was our intention to work with the practices rather than do research on or into them. We wanted to use the research findings as a platform on which to create change in the organizational culture of general practices.

Although we make no claims that our methods represent a completely participatory programme, we feel that genuine measures were implemented to democratize the research process. Initial meetings were held at the onset of the two year project to allow practice staff to decide the focus of the research and volunteers enlisted to share the collection of the data. Cycles of feedback (workshops, news circulars and revitalization meetings) allowed information to cascade, enabling practice teams to produce and review action plans that addressed issues arising from the research. Towards the end of the project a one day conference brought the four practice teams together to share their experiences, discuss what they had learned and exchange ideas about how to improve clinic attendance.

Implementing these participatory measures was an extremely instructive process. We encountered directly the dilemmas that action research engenders among professional elites, allowing us to make a realistic assessment of the ways in which participation can be sustained in a project of this duration and intensity.

Action research as a "choppy" experience

As has been stated previously, action research is not predicated upon an ideal model. It revolves around coming up with workable solutions to self defined problems. Over time it is likely that these problems may shift with the political climate, disappear altogether or be superseded by more pressing concerns. During our project, government recommendations for health promotion clinics changed significantly, necessitating some serious re-evaluation of the relevance of the research to the daily life of the practices. After lengthy discussions practice staff decided that whilst the context of health promotion in primary health care had changed, practices would still experience problems of non-attendance whatever structure replaced the current clinic system. This dilemma exemplifies the point that action research must be flexible if it is to address issues germane to all those taking part. Constant reassessment of what these issues actually are is vital if the research is to remain relevant to its participants.

Action research challenges the traditional method of scientific inquiry

Action research rejects the autocracy of the researcher and blurs traditional distinctions between researcher and researched, theory and practice. It is overly optimistic to assume that this approach will be embraced unconditionally by its participants, particularly among professional elites accustomed to traditional research methods. Using general practices as a point in case, the researcher is attempting to initiate an action research programme in a setting that largely anticipates traditional research. General practices may be comfortable with the professional/expert model and expect results to be submitted in an acceptable format i.e. in a way which will be acceptable to policy makers and planners. In such a context action research may represent to participants a set of extra tasks which should be the researcher's job to perform. It should never be underestimated that participation takes time and effort and professionals are forced to prioritize responsibilities given finite resources of time and energy. Essentially there is a clash of expectations about what constitutes legitimate research and valid knowledge. The researcher is attempting to implement ideas that are openly challenging in a setting that is highly accustomed to and conversant with traditional methods of producing scientific knowledge. This potentially fractious situation can be eased by compromise. In this project, findings were fed back continuously in a variety of different formats, mixing formal reports with participatory workshops, quantitative with qualitative data, so as to optimize the usefulness of the data to all the stakeholders. However, getting stakeholders to attend important steering group meetings was a struggle.

In conclusion, this example of implementing action research in general practice showed the need for time and patience because it involved effecting a change in the way powerful elites think about research. These distinctions are perpetuated by the structures in which organizations operate so we can only expect attitudes towards research to change gradually. Whilst acknowledging that action research directly challenges positivist assumptions concerning the production of scientific knowledge this challenge should include qualities of compromise and negotiation, producing a gentle fusion of ideas and processes.

Prospects for change in health: the role of action research

Full participation in action research is rare. Indeed the convergence of professional researchers who are advocates of participatory action research, an organization willing and able to commit to a demanding research process and the environmental conditions that permit a sustained process of participatory discussion is also rare. A key feature is its emergent character. The project design is not fixed but evolves over time and will be dependant on circumstances and the methods are used to enable through "democratic dialogue" the social construction of reality. It can range from researcher dominated to client managed. But wherever it is along that continuum, it has great potential. Firstly, because its main intention is to bring about change and secondly, because it attempts to integrate two strengths, the outside researcher with social science knowledge and insider in depth understanding of the community or organization and how to get things done, and finally, because it utilizes eclectic and multi-disciplinary models rather than seeing multi-causality, history and diversity as an obstacle to be overcome (Greenwood et al. op cit.).

Action research is the production of new social knowledge, and can be defined as objective in that by its very nature it has passed the process of social verification i.e. it is verified within its own paradigm just as conventional science is. The difference is that it is argumentative and dependent on consensus rather than pre-established rules applied systematically. It distinguishes itself from orthodox science by being open about its social value bias i.e. that it aims to create a new social construction of reality through democratic dialogue (Gustavsen, 1992). Since orthodox science has increasingly demonstrated its inability to solve practical problems in a rapidly changing world, the prospect for acceptance by funders of action research as a valid way of doing research becomes more tenable (see for example Charles et al. 1994). However, it will have to be accompanied by training and education. What action research can contribute to is bridging the huge gap between theory and practice, a gap which has severed the links between social research and the surrounding world over the years. Finally, by involving public sector policy makers in the research process, it can also play a key role in bridging the other large divide in urban community health which exists between innovative small scale community led projects and the organizations which are responsible for service delivery and public policy.

References

Brown, L.D. and Tandon R. (1983), "Ideology and Political Economy in Inquiry: Action Research and Participatory Action Research", *Journal of Applied Behavioural Science*, vol. 3, pp. 277-94.

Charles, C., Schalm C. and Seradek, J. (1994), "Involving Stakeholders in Health Services Research: Developing Alberta's Resident Classification System for Long Term Care Facilities", *International Journal of Health Services*, vol. 24, no. 40, pp. 749-61.

Elden, M. and Chisholm, R.F. (1993), "Emerging Varieties of Action Research: An Introduction to the Special Issue", *Human Relations*, vol. 46, no. 2, pp. 121-41.

Greenwood, D., Whyte, W.F. and Harkavy I. (1993), "Participatory Action Research as a Process and as a Goal", *Human Relations*, vol. 46, no. 2, pp. 171-91.

Gustavsen, B. (1992), *Dialogue and Development*, Van Gorcum, Assen.

Habermas, J. (1984/1987), *The Theory of Communicative Action*, vol. 1-2, Polity Press, London.

Hazen, M.A. (1994), "A Radical Humanist Perspective of Interorganisational Relationships" *Human Relations*, vol. 47, no. 4, pp. 393-415.

Kolb, D.A. (1984), *Experiential Learning Experience as a Source of Learning and Development,* Prentice Hall.

Kroeger, A. and Franken, H.P. (1981), "The Educational Value of

Participatory Evaluation of Primary Health Care Programmes: An Experience With Four Indigenous Populations in Ecuador", *Social Science and Medicine*, vol. 15B, pp. 535-9.

Ledford, G.E. and Mohrman, S.A. (1993), "Looking Backwards and Forwards at Action Research", *Human Relations*, vol. 46, no. 11, pp. 1349-59.

Lewin, K. (1946), "Action Research and Minority Problems", *Journal of Social Issues*, vol. 2, no. 4, pp. 34-46.

Magerison, C.J. (1987), "Integrating Action Research and Action Learning in Organisational Development" in Winter (ed.), *Organisational Development*, pp. 88-91.

McTaggart, R. (1991), "Principles of Participatory Action Research", *Adult Education Quarterly*, vol. 41, no. 3, pp. 168-87.

Meyer, J.E. (1993), "New Paradigm Research in Practice - the Trials and Tribulations of Action Research", *Journal of Advanced Nursing*, vol. 18, pp. 1066-72.

Rahman, M.A. (1993), *People's Self Development. Perspectives on Participatory Action Research*, Zed Books.

Reason, P. and Rowan, J. (1981), *Human Inquiry*, Wiley.

Reason, P. (1988), *Human Inquiry in Action*, Wiley.

Schutz, A. (1954), "Concept and Theory Formation in the Social Sciences", *Journal of Philosophy*, vol. 51, pp. 257-73.

Susman, G.I. and Evered, R.D. (1978), "An Assessment of the Scientific Merits of Action Research", *Administrative Science Quarterly*, vol. 23, pp. 582-602.

Winter, R. (1990), *Action Research and the Nature of Social Inquiry*, Avebury.

6 Health promotion requires innovative research techniques

Maria A. Koelen and Lenneke Vaandrager

Over the last few decades there have been rapid and fundamental changes in our conception of health and health promotion. However, the development of research techniques have lagged behind. In this paper we describe the development of health education and health promotion as a professional and scientific field and the role of research, and then pursue the question of why conventional research techniques are no longer sufficient and argue that participatory research techniques, although not meeting the criteria for conventional research, can result in data of high quality, both for practice and for science.

A brief history

The development of health education and health promotion as professional and scientific field is fascinating. Health education started from making people aware of the consequences of their behaviour for health. The approach was based on medical practice at the time, that is, prescriptive and uni-directional. Individuals were expected to process information in a logical manner and subsequently act accordingly. Changes in individual's opinions, attitudes and behaviour were seen to result from information and knowledge. However, information and knowledge are important but not sufficient factors in behaviour change. Individual motivation, skills and the influence from the social environment appeared to be very important conditions as well (see for example Ajzen and Fishbein, 1980; Green et al. 1980; Kok, 1986). We now realize that individuals cannot be isolated from their material and social environment and that a single behaviour can not be isolated from its context, and consider the (social) function of behaviour in the wider context of lifestyles (Koelen, 1988).

Related to these developments in the practice of health promotion, the research questions have also changed. First the questions could be categorized with the label "How to change people's knowledge?" to be operationalized as for example "How to convey a particular message?" Next we wondered about the fact that, even though a message was very clear, it did not lead to significant changes in opinions and behaviour. This led to research on determinants of behaviour (including factors such as knowledge, attitudes, social influence and opportunities), the modifiability of such behaviours, and characteristics of the target population. However, health is affected by a multitude of factors, including (the organization of) health care services and the availability of means and facilities (Lalonde, 1974; Blum, 1982). Over the years, it became evident that health education can only develop its full potential if it is supported by structural measures, such as legal, environmental and regulatory ones (Kickbush, 1986). Health education nowadays is covered by the umbrella of health promotion. Central to the principles underlying health promotion is the notion that it demands coordinated action by governments, health and other sectors, non-governmental and voluntary organizations, local authorities, as well as by industry and the media. In addition, active participation of the public is relevant (WHO, 1986; Ottawa Charter, 1986). But although the approach shifted from a prescriptive and uni-directional to a more interactive and participative one, the research methodologies did not develop at same rate and certainly not in the same direction.

What is the problem for research?

At present the dominant research strategy still appears to be to document the frequencies of involvement in different health behaviours (Anderson, 1988), and then to seek to understand the patterns of behaviour by exploring its determinants.

There are a number of problems related to this strategy. Firstly, although the selection of health behaviours (for study) may be determined by contemporary understanding of the role of behaviour in the aetiology or prevention of illness (Anderson, 1988), the appropriate level of different behaviours for good health are quite often subject to debate (Koelen, 1988). Technical knowledge is either lacking or disputed (Dean, 1990), for example the controversy over health effects of low cholesterol, or the role of alcohol in preventing heart disease. A second problem stems from the desire to count, to make number and frequency observations and recommendations. This tendency may have led to more research in "countable" areas, whereas much less attention has been paid to the less concrete areas. It is much easier to study concrete behaviours (e.g.

number of cigarettes smoked per day) than to study behaviours such as information seeking or social participation.

More important however is the fact that the search for explanation is the dominant strategy. Quantitative research is a process of reductionism, which involves breaking down components of a complex world into discrete parts, analyzing them, and then making predictions about the world, based on interpretations of these parts (Pretty, 1994; Chandler, 1992). Investigation with a high degree of control has become equated with good science, and quantitative research leading to explanations summarized in "universal" generalizations (i.e. theories) is most valued. But there are economic motives as well, since health promotion programmes cost money. In order to find funding, one organization or another has to be convinced of the necessity of the project and of the health-benefits to be gained. A pre-condition then is that interventions are accompanied by sound scientific research which can show that the programme increased knowledge, and positively changed attitudes and behaviour: the indicators against which performance is measured.

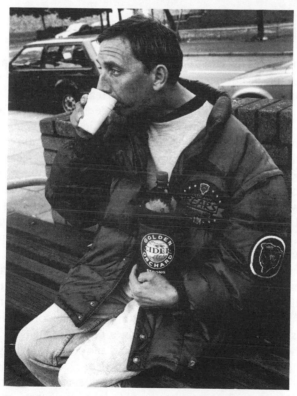

Behaviours that affect health cannot be isolated from their social contexts

A researcher then is more or less obliged to choose the quantitative approach, to collect large amounts of data using at least a quasi-experimental design, and trying to contol as much as possible for interfering variables in order to be able to declare certainty. Researchers have to be sure that nothing else will happen other than what has been planned, other one cannot make any proposition about what has actually caused eventual observed changes. This approach however, is at odds with the principles of health promotion, for which the key issues are:

1. There should be active involvement of communities, including volunteers and professionals from different institutions and organizations in the health, social and economic area.

2. It is based in the setting of everyday life.

3. That positive effects depend particularly on public participation in the research and interventions.

Experience from nutrition health promotion

We have experienced this conflict between prevailing research methods and the principles of health promotion with the SUPER-project, a study of nutrition promotion, in which six European Healthy Cities are cooperating (Vaandrager et al. 1993). It took some considerable effort to find financial resources to carry out the project, the most difficult part being to convince potential funders that the study would yield both health benefits and research results of high quality, without satisfying the demands of the positivist research paradigm. We found the solution in saying that we were not in search for explanations but trying to solve practical problems. However, we did opt for a quasi-experimental design, selecting an experimental and a control area. The central place for action was to be the supermarket, and guided by the principles of health promotion, we involved several professionals and volunteers from different institutions working in the selected neighbourhoods, as well as local citizens. In planning the activities they came up with many good ideas, much better then we could have ever thought of from our academic position, including activities which could take place in settings like schools, neighbourhood centres and street fairs. At first we felt in a difficult situation, caught in a struggle between the demands of science and our knowledge of what constituted good health promotion practice. From the research methodology point of view it seemed to be a disaster as we grappled with how to determine which action would lead to what consequences.

70

However, from health promotion point of view it was the best that could happen: participation, enthusiasm, collaboration, every day life situations. After careful consideration we opted for the principles of health promotion.

Where are we up to?

What is good for science and the individual scientist may not be good for those on whom the research is based. What needs consideration is not what makes research good within the tenets of dominant theories (including research methods) but what makes research good for health promotion. The breaking down of a complex world into components and reducing the components to their most specific parts presupposes that:

1.   The research components could be determined in advance.

2.   The sum of the parts would equal the whole.

3.   Explaining the essential elements objectifies the research and thus makes it more valid (Chandler, 1992).

This however opposes the holistic nature of health as we wish to see it in health promotion. As Ashton (1988) states: "Above all health promotion is about synthesis; about holism rather than reductionism ...". We are not saying that person centred variables and individual behaviours are less valid or aetiologically less important than situational variables in accounting for health problems. Neither are we blindly enamoured of an approach that stresses environmental factors to the exclusion of person centred factors and individual behaviour. That would be an error in the opposite direction. However, health promotion research has special reason to consider a more balanced approach in the selection of variables and of research techniques.

Health promotion deals not only with the theoretical explanation of certain phenomena, but also has to solve practical problems of achieving change. There is a need for participatory action research, which follows the route of problem - diagnosis - plan - intervention - evaluation. Health promotion is an ongoing process of decision making that requires a flow of regular inputs rather than a one intervention - evaluation situation. Therefore, a combination of research techniques is required. As far as the measurement of knowledge and attitudes are concerned, there is nothing wrong with scientifically validated instruments. However, since health related behaviour is rather complex, influenced not only by individual factors, but also to a great extent by social, cultural and economic factors, those measurements are far from complete. Other measurements are necessary. Rapid appraisal of knowledge networks (WHO, 1991; Engel, 1994) and a combination of other techniques are necessary to measure process planning, development and outcome. Action in the quest for positive health does not demand full certainty before intervening, although it should make uncertainties explicit.

Health promotion embraces the principles of participation and collaboration. These principles are not only essential for health promotion activities, but also for health promotion research. The community is the focus of research, and there should be a dialogue, on an equitable basis between researcher and community (McQueen, 1991). Participative research gives us the opportunity not only to create scientifically validated knowledge but also to benefit from the knowledge by experience. Research techniques need to be developed that combine understanding complex and dynamic situations with taking action to improve them, in such a way that the actors and beneficiaries of the research are intimately involved as participants in the whole process (Sriskandarajah et al. 1991; quoted in Pretty, 1994).

Criteria for evaluation of health promotion research

The research methods in participatory research are more qualitative than quantitative in nature. Although the practical value of the results may be clear, the question remains whether the findings of such inquiry are of good quality. How certain can we be that the interpretations of results reflect the real situation, and are not biased by the researcher? How do we know that they are scientifically relevant - that is - do they have any predictive value, and can we generalize the results to other situations?

It is commonly asserted that participatory methods constitute inquiry that is undisciplined and sloppy, quick and dirty, of poor quality and no more than second rate work. Conventional research uses four criteria in judging confidence and applicability of the findings: internal validity, external validity, reliability and objectivity; criteria based on the underlying assumptions of the traditional research paradigm (Cook and Campbell, 1979). From our point of view these criteria are difficult to measure and difficult to meet, but there are nevertheless a number of ways in which the research can be judged. We will mention six criteria which are based on the work of Caplan and Nelson (1973), Guba (1990), Chandler (1992), Engel and Salomon (1994), Pretty (1994), and, maybe more important, on the underlying principles of health promotion. The criteria pursue the route of planning, implementation, adjustment and reconsideration of health promotion activities and follow the line from practice to theory.

Continuing collaboration and debate

In health promotion projects we aim at the involvement of a wide range of actors. Health promotion demands co-ordinated action from national and local governments, the health, social and economic sectors, research centres, and volunteer organizations. Each of them has its own specific domain of knowledge and information, but also its own philosophy, objectives, standards, need for protection of its domain and its own finite horizons (Koelen and Brouwers, 1990). In collaboration between all those actors the focus is on cumulative learning by all participants. Exchange of ideas and debate about differences leads to sophisticated information and definitions of the situation at hand and gives insight in situations requiring improvement. The result can be a research agenda agreed upon by all participants, in which they recognize their own position and in which they feel involved.

Triangulation

With triangulation we refer to a cross check of information, using multiple sources, multiple methods and multiple investigators.

Multiple sources refers either to the use of multiple accounts of one source (for example interviews with members of one social group), or to the use of different sources about one topic (for example interviews with local people, professionals working in a community, volunteers and supermarket managers about food habits and healthy eating).

Multiple methods refers to the comparison of results derived from a range of methods. For example comparing the results of observation in a supermarket with the results of interviews or group discussions with clients. Once a proposition has been confirmed by more than one or two methods, the uncertainty of interpretation is greatly reduced.

The idea of multiple investigators is especially strong in participatory research, with those involved in activities are involved in the inquiry as well. We have to deal with a variety of professions, backgrounds and standards, which increases the range of perspectives and biases. When the participants agree on interpretations of results, the threat of biased interpretations is much less.

Participant checking

Among the multiple investigators are the participants. Participant checking involves checking the data, interpretations and conclusions with people with whom the original information was constructed. If the reconstructions by the inquirers are recognized by the group of participants as adequate

73

representations of their own realities, the credibility of the findings is established. Participant checks can occur both during the course of inquiry, and formally by presentation in meetings towards the end of the research. Participants then have the opportunity to hear a summary of what investigators have learned and constructed, investigate discrepancies and challenge findings, and to volunteer additional information.

Differing views about the interpretation of results

In participatory research a wide range of actors are involved, not only in gathering information but also in the analysis and interpretation. Discussions of the findings and their meaning from different perspectives results in some common interpretations but also to disagreement. Interpretations with a high level of agreement can be considered reliable, while disagreement should lead to further enquiry.

All of these steps so far are essentially parts of the working process of health promotion, and the benefit for research is that the trustworthiness of results is increased. These steps serve two goals: first, they provide the criteria against which the information can be judged, much like statistical analyses provide grounds for judgement in conventional methods, and therefore provide a sounder basis for developing work programmes and agendas. Second, they motivate those involved to take action, and to implement the desired changes. This action includes local institution building or strengthening, so increasing the ability of people to participate and to initiate action on their own.

The forum

So far, we stayed more or less "indoors" in the community under study. More certainty about the value and validity can be achieved by external presentation, which gives the opportunity for external checks. In the SUPER-project, annual business meetings are organized where all participating cities present their recent research, with critical exploration of aspects of the inquiry that might still be implicit in the minds of the individual researchers and subject to bias.

Multiple cases

With multiple cases we mean parallel investigations in different settings, and are essential as they can demonstrate replication. Experience is affirmed if other research teams proceed with parallel investigations using similar techniques and come up with similar results. The SUPER-project is an example of a multiple case study, with six European Healthy Cities following the same working plan and line of research.

For parallel investigations to succeed however, there must be regular communication between the research groups. Multiple case studies can also provide a basis for generalizing the results to other situations, and that is a very important aspect of validity so far as the usefulness of this research is concerned.

Final remarks

In this paper we have pointed out that it is difficult to meet the norms of conventional empirical scientific research in health promotion projects. This is due to the nature of health promotion, involving multi-sectoral collaboration and public participation in problem definition, planning and implementation of activities. Participatory research therefore, is more or less a pre-condition. We have argued that, despite the prevailing conflict between scientific method and the needs of health promotion, this approach to research can make relevant contributions to both practice and to science.

References

Ajzn, I., and Fishbein, M. (1980), *Understanding Attitudes and Predicting Social Behavior*, Prentice Hall, Englewood Cliffs.

Anderson, R. (1988), "The Development of the Concept of Health Behaviour" in Anderson, R., Davies, J.K., Kickbush, I. and Turner, J. (eds.), *Health Behaviour Research and Health Promotion,* Oxford Medical Publications, Oxford.

Ashton, J. (1988), "Health Promotion and the Concept of Community" in Anderson, R., Davies, J.K., Kickbush, I. and Turner, J. (eds.), *Health Behaviour Research and Health Promotion*, Oxford Medical Publications, Oxford, p. 192.

Blum, H.L. (1982), "Social Perspective on Risk Reduction" in Faber, M.M. and Reinhardt, (eds.), *Promoting Health Through Risk Reduction,* Macmillan Publishing Co. Inc., New York.

Caplan, N. and Nelson, S.D. (1973), "On Being Useful: The Nature and Consequences of Psychological Research on Social Problems, *American Psychologist*, vol. 28, pp. 199-211.

Chandler, S. (1992), "Displaying our Lives: An Argument Against Displaying our Theories, *Theory in Practice*, vol. 31, pp. 126-131.

Cook T.D. and Campbell, D.T. (1979), *Quasi-Experimentation: Design and Analysis Issues for Field Settings*, Rand McNally College Publishing Company, Chicago.

Dean, K. (1990), "Nutrition Education Research in Health Promotion", *Journal of the Canadian Dietetic Association*, vol. 51, pp. 481-4.

Engel, P. and Salomon, M. (1994), *RAAKS: A Participatory Action-Research Approach to Facilitating Social Learning for Sustainable Development,* Paper presented at the International Symposium on System Oriented Research in Agriculture and Rural Development, Montpellier, France, 21-25 November 1994, Department of Communication and Innovation Studies, Agricultural University Wageningen, The Netherlands.

Green, L.W., Kreuter, M.W., Deeds, S.G. and Partridge, K.B. (1980), *Health Education Planning: A Diagnostic Approach*, Mayfield Publishing Company, Palo Alto.

Guba, E.G. (1990), *The Paradigm Dialog*, Sage Publications, Newbury Park.

Kickbush, I. (1986), "Health Promotion: A Global Perspective, *Canadian Journal of Public Health*, vol. 77, pp. 321-6.

Koelen, M.A. (1988), *Tales of Logic: A Self-Presentational View on Health-Related Behaviour*, Dissertation, Department of Extension Science, Agricultural University, Wageningen.

Koelen, M.A. and Brouwers, T., "Knowledges Systems and Public Health, Knowledge in Society", *The International Journal of Knowledge Transfer*, vol. 3, pp. 50-7.

Kok, G.J. (1986), "Gezondheidsmotivering: GVO als Wetenschapsgebied", *Gezondheid and Samenleving*, vol. 7, pp. 58-68.

Lalonde, M. (1974), *A New Perspective on the Health of Canadians,* Government of Canada, Ottawa.

McQueen, D.V. (1991), "The Contribution of Health Promotion Research to Public Health", *European Journal of Public Health*, vol. 1, pp. 22-8.

Pretty, J.N. (1994), *Alternative Systems of Inquiry for a Sustainable Agriculture*, Paper for ICRA, February 1994.

Vaandrager, H.W., Koelen, M.A., Ashton, J.R and Colomér Revuelta, C. (1993), "A Four-Step Health Promotion Approach for Changing Dietary Patterns in Europe", *European Journal of Public Health,* vol. 3, pp. 193-8.

World Health Organization, (1986), *Health Promotion - Concepts and Principles - In action - A Policy Framework*, Copenhagen.

World Health Organization, (1986), *Ottawa Charter of Health Promotion*, Health and Welfare Canada, Canadian Public Health Association, WHO, Copenhagen.

World Health Organization, (1991), *Improving Urban Health. Guidelines for rapid appraisal to assess community health needs. A focus on health improvements for low income urban areas*, Geneva.

7 Combining relevance with scientific quality in health research: Reconsidering the criteria of rigour

Kathryn Dean and Julie Dawson

Over the past century, rather rigid stereotypes developed about what constitutes scientific soundness in health research. These stereotypes have associated beliefs about types of research design and methods that are more rigorous, and thus provide more certain knowledge about causation. Deep divisions between research disciplines and even between approaches to research within the same discipline have developed around these beliefs. The beliefs originated from traditions in the philosophy of knowledge that culminated in the positivistic science that dominated research in the first half of this century (Suppe, 1977; Dean, 1993).

The emphasis in positivistic science on separating phenomena into elements (reductionism) that can be observed and manipulated for predicting an outcome is no longer the driving force at the forefront of knowledge development. It is now known that prediction does not provide explanation about causation. That indeed predictions about any one influence will usually be overcome by the multiple interacting influences that constitute true causation. At the forefront of scientific endeavour today, researchers work to understand causal processes in dynamic systems, to illuminate complexity, rather than seek simplicity.

In research on human health, experimental research or research attempting to approximate the experimental model, e.g. case control designs or random sampling with statistical control of confounders, for the purpose of predicting the statistical effects of specific factors, continues to dominate the research agenda. Theoretical and empirical traditions remain separate in some places, quantitative and qualitative research are often pitted against each other and it is difficult to obtain recognition and funding for the new types of interdisciplinary research that are needed to study the interacting systems that shape human health over the life course (Dean et al. 1993).

Public health workers are concerned with promoting health in communities. The knowledge needed for their work is an understanding of the forces in communities that protect health or contribute to its deterioration. These forces involve complex causal processes that differ for sub-groups of the population. Public health work thus requires the expertize and skills of various academic and professional disciplines.

The research needed to inform public health practice must deal with levels of causation and the interactions among the multiple influences that affect health among groups of people living their daily lives. There is now a growing recognition that the imbalance in the types of research conducted on population health issues is not providing the range of knowledge needed for public health policy and action (WHO, 1992; Anon, 1994; Dean, 1994). The need for more relevant knowledge does not, of course, negate the need for scientific soundness in research to provide the knowledge needed for action.

Redressing the myths about what is sound research

In the reductionistic experimental model the highest aim is rigour or "parsimony". The goal is to identify the cause which will predict the outcome of interest and, in turn, find the definitive treatment. Extensive bodies of research and clinical experience discredit this model for maintaining or improving the health of populations (WHO, 1992; Alvarez-Dardet and Ruiz, 1993; Hulley et al. 1992). It is difficult to modify long term assumptions and traditions, especially when the status quo favours researching biological causes and treatment of already existing disease.

Experimental design and attempts to push other types of research into experimental frameworks do not provide the best way to conduct research on many subjects. Experimental approaches actually inhibit knowledge development when they are used inappropriately, or are not followed by the range of complimentary types of research. The goal of experimental design, to remove by randomization or statistical control of "confounders" the multiple influences involved in causal processes, precludes the types of knowledge needed for public health work. Rather than rigour and parsimony, understanding the complex workings of many forces needs to be the knowledge goal.

Both the "gold standard" status of the experimental model and the tendency to grant quantitative information superior status in health and social research are dysfunctional. Myths about the value of numbers are so pervasive that "... sometimes we may suspend our critical faculties when faced with quantitative information, whether derived from routine or ad hoc sources" (Black, 1994), a problem with serious consequences for both knowledge and practice. At the same time that numbers have been given magic power, the serious consequences of interpreting numbers superficially or manipulating them inappropriately are generally ignored. Myths about the superiority of specific research designs and analytic approaches interfere with the range of research appropriate for studying public health problems.

Identifying relevant aspects of health issues: a behaviourial example

Over the past decade, many population health policies and programmes have focused on behaviourial practices that are considered dangerous to health. Based on the widely documented health damaging effects of smoking (Bottomley, 1992; Royal College of Physicians, 1991), consensus about the danger of smoking habits and the need to develop policies to reduce the use of tobacco developed. Considerable expenditures of public and private resources are used for health education campaigns to convince people to not take up smoking or to stop if they are already smokers.

Policies directed toward smoking reduction have been successful to a certain degree. However, for a segment of smokers, perhaps those with the heaviest and most dangerous consumption patterns, smoking cessation campaigns are not very successful and recidivism rates are high. In recent years a great deal of attention has shifted to social class differences in smoking based on the idea that these differences may contribute to social class differences in health and longevity (Marmot et al. 1992; Blaxter, 1990). While it is known that behaviourial differences do not explain the (statistical) variance in social inequalities in health (Smith et al. 1994), it is possible that dangerous routine behaviourial habits interact with other causal influences to contribute to the differences.

Many people start or continue smoking even though they are aware of the health damaging consequences of the habit and in spite of their desire to quit (Dawson, 1993). Existing approaches to changing smoking behaviour have little influence on people already convinced of the dangers of smoking. The processes of influence that support and reinforce the habit in daily life must be understood to design programmes that facilitate behaviourial change among people that want to stop smoking. For these reasons, we conducted a secondary analysis of data collected from people motivated to give up smoking in order to study the influence of the social situation on the reasons people gave for being unable to quit.

Data and methods

The study uses data from the investigation of Health and Lifestyles in the Cheshire and Wirral areas of England. The details of the study design and characteristics of the sample are published elsewhere (Dawson, 1993). In summary, the register of the patients of General Practitioners was used to draw a random sample of persons aged 16 and over from the geographic area mentioned. A postal questionnaire was used to collect data from 5,943 respondents, with an overall response rate of 64 per cent. Females and younger persons were over represented among those who returned the questionnaire.

The analysis presented here concerns only smokers motivated to quit smoking (N=1,269). The multivariate analysis could only include the smokers for whom information was available on all the variables included in the analysis, 1,094 respondents. Seven perceived barriers to giving up smoking that had been included in prior regional surveys conducted in Oxford and Trent were studied. Each has two categories: yes, reported as a reason for not stopping/reducing smoking on a closed list of barriers to quitting or reducing smoking, and no, not reported a barrier to changing smoking behaviour. Other variables included in the analysis were: General Health Questionnaire 12 (Goldberg and Williams, 1988) scores, a measure of psychological distress (disorder), with three categories using a GHQ scoring system (0, 0, 1, 1) - no psychological distress (score: 0), low to moderate distress (score: 1-3), and high level of psychological distress (score: 4-12); three categories of social class; gender; and five age categories: 16-24, 25-34, 35-44, 45-54, 55 and older.

The GHQ12 variable is included to examine interactions among an "objective" measure of distress and the perceived barriers. Social class, gender and age are included to study social situational influences on the relationships among the perceived barriers and psychological distress.

Graphical interaction regression models, a sub-class of log linear statistical models were used for the multivariate analysis of the data. Building on the statistical notion of conditional independence, the graphical methods analyze the relationships between all pairs of variables given all other variables in the multivariate statistical problem without making any assumptions about the parametric structure of the data (Whittaker, 1990; Whittaker, 1993). They are particularly suited to the goals of this project because of their ability to elaborate direct and indirect relationships among the variables.

Barriers to changing smoking habits

The reasons given by 20 per cent or more of the respondents for not giving up smoking are shown in Table 7.1. The table is based on 1,269 smokers, including also the 175 persons for whom not enough information was available to classify on the social class variable. Seventy five per cent of the smokers reported that a major barrier was not enough will power. Enjoyment, the second most frequently given reason, was reported by 53 per cent, followed closely by the 47 per cent who gave stress reduction as a barrier. Smoking among friends or family were given as reasons by 34 per cent and 32 per cent respectively. Fear of weight gain was a reason given by 27 per cent, while 25 per cent believed that an attempt to stop would not succeed.

Table 7.1
Reasons cigarette smokers who would like to stop or
reduce smoking gave for finding it difficult to succeed

	Number	Percentage
Not enough will power	955	75%
Enjoyment	676	53%
Too much stress, smoking calms my nerves	602	47%
Friends smoking	437	34%
Members of family smoking	404	32%
Fear of gaining weight	339	27%
Belief that attempt would fail	315	25%

The seven perceived barriers differ in character ranging from perceived strength or control over the habit through pleasure, fears, stress reduction and exposure to the substance in daily life. Will power, the force considered necessary for action, was reported as insufficient by over three-quarters of the smokers who consider the habit dangerous and want to give it up. Lack of will power may be considered the proximate and global barrier to change. It would seem that lack of will power and belief that an attempt would not succeed are parallel barriers, but given the great discrepancy in the frequency of reporting the two (75 per cent and 25 per cent), this is clearly not the case. It is relevant to study the influence of the other types of barriers on will power and determine if their influence changes in the context of different life situations.

Using methods to increase relevance

The graphical interaction models are well suited for examining the relationships among the perceived barriers and studying the statistical influence of the social situation variables on the barriers to changing behaviour. The models can be used to simplify the complexity of multi-dimensional contingency tables by identifying the log linear generators or graphical "cliques" that compose the statistically related variables found in the analysis (Whittaker, 1993; Kreiner, 1992). It is possible to analyze the data in directed graphs specifying a theoretical framework for levels of influence among the variables to guide the analysis (Wermuth, 1993). The methods used for this study include procedures that examine the conditions under which the relationships among the variables change in subcategories of the other variables included in the multi-way interactions identified in the independence graph (Kreiner, 1992).

The structure defined for this study places age and gender on the first level. These fixed variables exert influence on all those on subsequent levels. Social class as a fundamental influence is assigned to the second level. The perceived barriers having to do with exposure to smoking in daily life, personal feelings, beliefs and functioning, along with the GHQ scores make up the third level, and will power as the outcome variable is placed on the last level. This structure assigns directionality and a theoretical logic to the analysis to avoid, or at least reduce, the problems of data drudging that can occur in the statistical analysis of complex multi-dimensional data. No interpretations are made about directionality of relationships among variables within the structural levels, and these associations are therefore represented in Figure 7.1 as lines without arrow heads.

The network of statistical relationships among the variables produced by the graphical analysis is presented in Figure 7.1. The "independence graph" provides an overview of the statistical relationships found in the multivariate contingency table. It can be seen that only three variables, belief in one's ability to succeed (gamma=0.50, p=0.000), fear of gaining weight (gamma=0.23, p=0.005) and smoking by members of the family (gamma=0.15, p=0.038), are directly related to will power. The belief variable exerts the dominant influence of the three variables with a statistical correlation over twice that found for family smoking and more than three times greater than that for fear of gaining weight.

Social class differences in barriers to smoking reduction

The independent relationships between social class and perceived barriers to changing smoking behaviour are also seen in Figure 7.1.

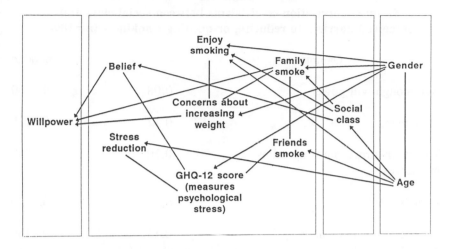

Figure 7.1   Life situation influences on barriers to changing smoking behaviour: the independence graph following graphical modelling

There is no statistically independent relationship between will power and social class. Belief in the success of an attempt to reduce or stop smoking, enjoyment of smoking and the smoking of family members are independently related to social class. The relationships between social class and each of the perceived barriers are shown in Table 7.2. Persons in the lower categories of the social status variable more often felt they would not succeed in an attempt to reduce or quit smoking and were bothered by members of the family smoking, while higher social status was positively related to reporting enjoyment as a barrier to smoking reduction. The statistically significant relationship between friends smoking and will power is a marginal rather than an independent relationship. That is, it is a "spurious" relationship arising from the strong statistical connection between the variables measuring the smoking of family and friends (gamma=0.71, p= <0.0001).

An advantage of the graphical models is the ability, not only to determine "independent" and spurious statistical connections among variables, but also to readily find meaningful indirect relationships and identify important partial relationships. Self confidence to succeed in an attempt to quit smoking emerged as an important barrier to changing smoking behaviour for disadvantaged persons. While reported by only 25 per cent of the smokers who want to quit, lack of belief in the success of attempting the behaviourial change was both more common in the lower social class groups and by far the most important variable related to perceived will power.

Table 7.2

Gamma correlation co-efficients between social class and perceived barriers to reducing or quitting smoking - (n=1094)

Gamma		p-value
Not enough will power	0.08	0.1100
Enjoyment	0.12	0.0138
Too much stress, smoking calms my nerves	-0.10	0.0650
Friends smoking	0.12	0.0350
Members of family smoking	-0.13	0.0150
Fear of gaining weight	0.03	0.2625
Belief that attempt would fail	-0.19	<0.0001

Another finding casts important light on these relationships. The GHQ12 scores are also related to confidence in self. Indeed, the results of the analysis show that these three variables form a graphical clique, meaning that the relationship between belief and social class can (and should) be examined in relation to GHQ scores without having to consider the other variables in the total multi-dimensional statistical problem for valid results.

Examining this three way interaction, it is found that the gamma correlation of -0.19 (p < 0.0001) between belief that an attempt would fail and social class increases to -0.27 (p = <0.0001), in category two, mild psychological distress, of the GHQ variable, while reducing in strength to -0.16 with a marginal p value of 0.0450 among those with no psychological distress, and becoming non-significant among those with moderate to severe psychological distress. These findings seem to indicate that disadvantaged circumstances contribute to distress and reduce self confidence. For those persons in the highest GHQ score group, more likely to be actually mentally disturbed, social class is not related to the belief variable. These findings suggest that there may be some kind of distinction between mental distress and actual psychological disturbance that is not recognized.

The interaction of social class with environmental smoking as a barrier to changing behaviour is also complex and must be examined for meaningful interpretation. While social class is not directly related to friends smoking, among those smokers who do not consider family smoking a barrier, the smoking of friends is perceived as a barrier, but the relationship is in the opposite direction. That is, while family smoking is more often a barrier for members of the lower social class categories, the smoking of friends is more often perceived as a barrier by members of the higher social class category.

The relationship between enjoyment and social class is even more complex, being embedded in a five variable graphical "clique" with fear of gaining weight, gender and age. The greater tendency of upper social class persons to report enjoyment as a barrier to quitting smoking is significant only among women, especially those who do not name fear of weight gain as a barrier. At the same time, proportionately more males than females report enjoyment as a barrier and the relationship between enjoyment and gender, 0.15, (p=0.0275), increases to 0.38, (p<0.0001), in the lowest social class group. Also, the gender difference in enjoyment is significant in the 25-34 age group and among those who do not consider fear of weight gain a barrier. Overall the findings in this five way interaction suggest that gender is more important than social class in finding enjoyment a barrier to changing smoking behaviour, and that males in the lower social class groups find enjoyment an especially important factor, while for females enjoyment is a more important factor in the higher category of social class and fear of weight gain is an important factor for females.

Discussion

The health and lifestyles survey documented, like many others, the larger proportions of smokers found in lower social class groups (Dawson, 1993). The data available from that survey provided the opportunity to study perceived barriers to quitting or reducing smoking in relation to the social situation. The findings point to the need to study subgroup differences in variables influencing smoking in order develop relevant interventions for effecting behavioural change.

While the barriers studied were identified in prior research and selected by at least 20 per cent of the respondents motivated to reduce smoking in this investigation, the variables do represent only a limited range of influences that may affect smoking and there was no opportunity for the respondents to elaborate on the meaning of the closed ended items. This research would be fruitfully supplemented by qualitative interviews building on the findings in order to explore their meaning and identify other possible avenues of influence creating barriers to changing smoking behaviour.

Nevertheless, the social class and gender differences in the perceived barriers suggest different approaches for supporting changes in behaviour, making these findings relevant to consider in programmes designed to facilitate smoking reduction. Twenty five per cent of the smokers reported that lack of belief in the success of an attempt to quit smoking was a barrier. The extremely high correlation between the belief variable and will power suggests a strong influence that appears to be a type of self confidence or self efficacy affecting a core of smokers who want to quit. That members of lower categories of social class are over represented in this group with no direct statistical relationship between social class and will power, along with the finding that the negative relationship between belief in self and social class increases considerably among moderately distressed persons, suggests that for this group of smokers some form of empowerment strategy is appropriate for designing interventions.

The findings with regard to gender are also relevant to consider in programme development. Women more often reported fear of weight gain as a barrier to reducing or quitting smoking. Body image and social role stereotyping affecting women can be very powerful forces affecting the behaviour of women. It may be necessary to build weight control components into effective smoking reduction interventions for women.

The greater proportion of males who report enjoyment as a barrier to smoking reduction, especially among 25-34 year olds and in the lower category of social class suggests a culture of young male behaviour that may be important to consider when working with this group of smokers.

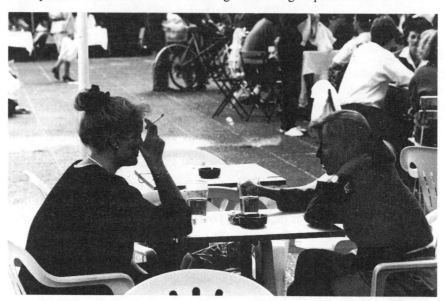

Exploring the complexity of social interactions in research helps us to understand those aspects of peoples lives that determine behaviour and what it means to them

The findings with regard to the GHQ12 variable are interesting and suggest that research to study possible multi-dimensionality and item bias (that is, some items may be biased with regard to certain population groups) in this measure would be useful. Women were over represented among persons who scored higher on the GHQ12 scores. Also, the negative relationship between belief in the success of attempted smoking reduction and social class was much stronger among persons in the moderate distress category on this measure. At the same time, reporting stress reduction as a barrier to smoking reduction was strongly correlated with the GHQ scores. This correlation, the biggest found in this investigation, of 0.68 ($p < 0.0001$), increased with age, reaching gamma values of 0.81 and 0.78 respectively in the two oldest groups, while smoking for stress reduction was not related to the other perceived barriers or to social class and gender. It appears that this measure may tap some dimensions of both the real distress found in the life situations of disadvantaged people and the distress of mental illness that need to be separated and understood.

In conclusion, the results of this analysis suggest that the stereotypical views about the superiority of specific research designs and analytic approaches are inappropriate. The perspective of removing or "controlling" for intervening and moderating variables in experimental or quasi-experimental research can actually take away the opportunity to explore the causal processes that shape health and health related behaviour in the real world. Qualitative research that provides new insights into causal processes and barriers to change, and quantitative approaches that elaborate direct, indirect and moderating influences in population studies, are both needed if we are to advance public health knowledge. Traditionally rigid attitudes towards the different types of research also tend to interfere with the funding and training needed for the appropriate range of research required to obtain both relevant and scientifically sound knowledge for health programmes.

References

Alvarez-Dardet, C. and Ruiz, M. (1993), "Thomas McKeown and Archibald Cochrane: A Journey Through the Diffusion of Ideas", *British Medical Journal*, vol. 306, p. 1252.

Anon. (1994), Population Health Looking Upstream (editorial), Lancet, vol. 343, p. 429.

Black, N. (1994), "Why We Need Qualitative Research", *Journal of Epidemiology Community Health*, vol. 48, p. 425.

Blaxter, M. (1990), *Health and Lifestyles*, Routledge, London.

Bottomley, V. (1992), *The Health of the Nation*, Department of Health, HMSO, London.

Dawson, J. (1993), *Health and Lifestyles in Cheshire and Wirral*, Observatory Report Series, no. 16, Liverpool.

Dean, K. (1993), "Integrating Theory and Methods in Population Health Research" in Dean, K. (ed.), *Population Health Research: Linking Theory and Methods*, Sage Publications, London, p. 9.

Dean, K., Kreiner, S. and McQueen, D. (1993), "Researching Population Health: New Directions" in Dean, K. (ed.), *Population Health Research: Linking Theory and Methods*, Sage Publications, London, p. 227.

Dean, K. (1994), "Creating a New Knowledge Base for the New Public Health", (editorial), *Journal of Epidemiology and Public Health*, vol. 48, p. 217.

Goldberg, D. and Williams, P. (1988), *A Users Guide to the General Health Questionnaire*, NFER, Nelson.

Hulley, S., Walsh, J. and Newman, T. (1992), "Health Policy on Blood Cholesterol: Time to Change Directions", *Circulation*, vol. 86, p. 1026.

Kreiner, S. (1992), *Notes on Diagram Version 2.10*, Danish Institute of Educational Research, Copenhagen.

Marmot, M., Kogevinas, M. and Elston, M. (1992), "Socioeconomic Status and Disease" in Badura, B. and Kickbusch, I. (eds.), *Health Promotion Research: Towards a New Social Epidemiology*, WHO Regional Pub. Series, no. 37, Copenhagen.

Smith, G., Blane, D. and Bartley, M. (1994), "Explanations for Socio-Economic Differentials in Mortality, *European Journal of Public Health*, vol. 4, p. 131.

Suppe, F. (1977), *The Structure of Scientific Theories*, University of Illinois Press, Chicago

The Royal College of Physicians, (1991), *Preventative Medicine*, London.

Wermuth, N. (1993), "Association Structures with Few Variables" in Dean, K. (ed.), *Population Health Research: Linking Theory and Methods*, Sage, London, pp. 181-203.

Whittaker, J. (1990), *Graphical Models in Applied Multivariate Statistics*, Wiley, Chichester.

Whittaker, J. (1993), "Graphical Interaction Models: A New Approach for Statistical Modelling" in Dean, K. (ed.), *Population Health Research: Linking Theory and Methods*, Sage, London, pp. 160-80.

World Health Organization, (1992), "The Crisis in Public Health: Reflections for the Debate", *Scientific Pub.* no. 540, WHO Pan American Health Organization, Washington D.C.

Section 3   Community needs assessment

The assessment of community health needs is absolutely key to the Health for All Strategy, and other (mainly derivative) health policy initiatives of recent years.   The methods being used are varied and evolving, and a range of techniques being explored is reported in this section with a number of examples from different settings and countries.   This is however not intended to be a comprehensive review of the methods and theoretical background to community needs assessment, and the emphasis is primarily on approaches which involve local people in the process.

Understanding and representing the community

If involving the community in the process is so important, then it is important at the outset to ask how "the community" can be represented in whatever group is established to manage the process of needs assessment.   Rachel Jewkes has examined the issue of what is meant by community, and the implications that this has for attempting to represent what is in effect a very complex and heterogeneous entity with different meanings for those living in the area concerned and those whose job it is to provide support for or a service to local people.

Representing the community in the process of assessing need may be achieved in a variety of ways.   Pat Thornley explains how a period of community development work in a poor suburban estate in north Liverpool laid the foundations for a new model of primary health care, in which needs assessment played a central part.   The techniques used for the needs assessment included focus groups and a household interview survey, with the project managed by a multi-sectoral team that included community representatives.   This project was the main subject of an evaluation reported by Nigel Bruce and Lyn Winters, with particular emphasis on the experience of participation and intersectoral working in this complex project. The role of the community development workers was very important in maintaining participation and trust, and it was also clear that participation has to be achieved through a variety of methods, and through a variety of channels that are built up over time.

Assessing the needs of minority groups

The provision of appropriate services that are directed towards the needs of minority groups also demand good information. The discussion about identifying and representing the "community" is of particular relevance with minority groups since within any city there may be a large number of culturally distinct communities. Femi Oduneye describes some of the difficulties faced in carrying out a needs survey for AIDS/HIV service development among the ethnic minorities in Liverpool. Among the issues identified were the difficulties in sampling, and the importance of careful selection and training of interviewers, a point noted by others (Hughes et al. 1995). Needs assessment studies in these circumstances are not cheap, quick or easy, but have the potential to be valuable if the research process itself contributes to building relationships with the communities and the capacity of local people.

Another important issue that arises when planning to initiate needs assessment work, particularly with a relatively disempowered community, is a dilemma that arises for the researchers and the service providers. They must achieve a balance between waiting for the community to begin the process, which may be slow, and moving in to start things off which runs the risk of imposing their own perceptions and priorities. Joop ten Dam describes a programme in a poor immigrant community in central Amsterdam, which used a participative Delphi technique with individual health profiling for needs assessment and policy development. This approach has helped to achieve a successful balance between the community and the health services, and has led on to implementation of policy ideas. Another project in a poor area of Amsterdam in which research has formed the basis for change, is described in Chapter 32 (section 5).

A comparison of methods

Among the themes running through this section are representation and participation. Representation may be viewed by the scientist as a technical requirement of valid research, and by the health promotion worker more as a desire to ensure that those most in need are not excluded by those who choose to respond or are better able to speak up. These are in essence two ways of viewing the same goal, or at least should become so, but achieving representation in poor, ethnically diverse urban areas is not straightforward. So what method seems to represent the community best? And which provides the best opportunity for participation of local people that can lead on to policy development and implementation? Drawing on their experience of needs assessment on the Broadwater Farm estate in north London, Carol Duncan and colleagues describe the use of a random sample survey using interview questionnaires, compared to a focus group approach.

Integrating other sources of information

Needs assessment for any given community must draw on information from a wide variety of sources, in addition to the views and experiences of the local residents. These other sources of information include demography, socio-economic information, indicators of environmental quality, health services, transport, leisure, and many other aspects of daily life. One powerful and emerging means of integrating and analyzing this information are geographical information systems (GIS). Alex Hirschfield describes some of the ways in which GIS can handle and present information that is relevant to the communities concerned and to those involved in policy development. If routinely available data can be criticized for lacking the depth and insight of qualitative information, then GIS may be seen as contributing to bridge building through the capacity to integrate data representing a wide range of influences on health.

In the final paper in this section, Keiko Nakamura and colleagues report on how the Tokyo Healthy Cities initiative has brought the research community together with the city authorities and citizens to develop a very broad range of information to promote participation and policy development. Geographical analysis played a part in this, as did the development of more efficient indicators of health and the determinants of health, and the modelling of health effects of various policy options. What is most important though, is that underlying all of the information and analytical work, are the commitment and structures for collaboration. This is manifest through, for example, collaboration with local residents in collecting information about their community amenities, as well the city level Citizen's Council for Health Promotion.

91

Reference

Hughes, A.O., Fenton, S. and Hine, C. (1995), "Strategies for Sampling Black and Ethnic Minority Populations", *J Public Health Medicine*, vol. 17, pp. 187-92.

8 Representing the community?

Rachel Jewkes

Introduction and research methods

The idea of "community" is one of the most important and frequently occurring in the arena of Health for All by the year 2000. People who work in this area continuously operationalize it in the process of activities to generate "community development", "community participation", "community involvement" and so forth. Sometimes there are prolonged and occasionally agonizing discussions of what is meant by "community", but very often it is seen as self evident, after all "community" is part of popular vocabulary and many organizations and workers have definitions incorporated into their aims and objectives or job descriptions. Yet the ease with which people engaged in community participation derive working definitions of "community" should not be interpreted as concordance, nor would anyone familiar with the debate around the definition of "community" in the disciplines of sociology, anthropology and philosophy expect it to be so. For the meaning of community has been one of the most contested debates in the social sciences, stretching over at least two centuries (Frankenberg, 1960; Bell and Newby, 1971; Cohen, 1985; Plant, 1974). One of the most important products of this debate was the realization in the 1950s and 1960s that an agreed and substantiated definition of community would not be found (Bell and Newby 1971). This was exemplified by a review published by George Hillery in 1955 which examined 94 definitions of community found in community studies and concluded that they only thing they all had in common was that they all dealt with people.

This lack of consensus on definition presents considerable difficulties for researchers seeking to develop a generalizable framework for evaluating community participation in health promotion. Those authors, such as Rifkin (et al. 1988), who have tried to devise mechanisms for doing so have focused on the notion of "participation". Yet without an agreed definition of

93

community, one of "community participation" cannot be constructed. The classical framework for evaluation which measures success in achieving objectives, cannot therefore be employed as the objectives cannot be clarified.

Nonetheless "community" is given meanings continuously by those who work in health promotion, ones which are translated into actions, which in turn have implications, particularly in so far as one of the intentions behind community participation in health is that of extending democracy (Adams, 1989; Kickbusch, 1986). Understanding the meanings given to community and the consequences of these meanings is an important object of study for those involved in Healthy Cities research, but it is necessary to look to ethnography to provide the methodological framework for such research so that conscious and unconscious meanings can be revealed and their implications considered in the context of use. This paper is based on such a study which sought to explore meanings of community and some of their consequences (Jewkes, 1994). In it, the notion of community is explored and implications for representation on Health for All steering groups discussed.

Data was collected via in depth interviews with 50 informants from the health, local authority and voluntary sectors who were involved in activities around community participation in health promotion. The settings were four boroughs in south east England, three of which had Health for All steering groups, whilst the fourth was reported to have close intersectoral working relationships. In each location the informants were identified with the help of a key informant who was either the co-ordinator of the project or the Director of Public Health. The interviews were tape recorded, transcribed and the transcripts analyzed as "text". The researcher was a public health physician who had herself been at one stage an active member of a Health for All steering group.

Meanings of "community"

Cohen, in his seminal work "The symbolic construction of community", presents an interpretive representation of meaning of community for its "members". He identifies two central ideas within the notion of community, one relational and the other aggregational (Cohen, 1985). "Community" implies that people have something in common which distinguishes them in a significant way from members of other groups. What is shared depends on the particular circumstances at the time, it may be location, ethnicity, a work place and so forth. The relational idea encompasses the opposition of one community to others. His central thesis is that "people become aware of their culture when they stand at its boundaries: when they encounter other cultures, or when they become aware of other ways of doing things, or merely of contradictions to their own culture."

An understanding of boundary is a necessary precondition for valuing culture and community.

It follows from this interpretation that perceptions of "community membership" are context specific and temporal. The boundaries of communities are mental constructs and as such people on opposite sides or even the same side, may perceive them differently. For groups of people, "community" and "community membership" are thus ideas rather than uncontestable, concrete forms.

In this study none of the informants regarded themselves as members of the community with which they work. Metaphors of distance ("go to", "meet with", "get access to", "tap into" the community) are employed when talking of the community, which indicate that it is a notional "community" of which they are not members. This is important as the meanings of community understood by non-members may differ from those of members. It is also surprising, not least because many "non-members" have attributes which are often colloquially identified as objective manifestations of community, some live in the locality of their work, some are local activists, others are from ethnic minorities, gay or lesbian.

Examination of the use of "community" by people who are involved with community participation reveals continuous switching between meanings, sometimes with several being juggled simultaneously. In a formal sense most Health for All projects, as most local government, health authority and voluntary sector employees, have formal definitions of community to which they work. These usually encompass the population ("everybody") who lives within a defined geographical boundary (usually a borough) and sometimes also include those who work and use services within it.

"Community" is also used to refer to clusters of people who share certain characteristics with others. Sometimes they are identified in a tautological manner, as groups or people identified through the use of the word "community". In this way "the people who community workers work with" or "the people who use or could use a community centre" are referred to as a "community". So for an employee of a Somali Women's group "Somali Women" are the community; for a north London office of the mental health charity MIND it is "people who receive services or even social services"; for a community centre serving an electoral ward it may be the population of that ward. Health Promotion Officers and others often regard themselves a point of reference, in which case their target group becomes the "community". As one observed "I suppose its whoever you are aiming to work with at the time". These diverse groupings are all constructed around a point of reference which is the community worker, association or Health Promotion Officer.

Sometimes communities are defined through what they are not. In the National Health Service "community" may mean "not hospital" e.g in "community nurses" or "non-statutory", and usually encompasses a notion of an implicit geographical boundary. In certain circumstances it may mean "not the voluntary sector" or can be a particular place: for example, one informant said "I live in the community". Community is also used to refer to people at an elementary and unorganized level, again within an unstated but implicit geographical boundary, as in "the public at large", "the general population", "people" or "the grassroots".

Although these communities are constructed in different ways they share in common a central relational idea, the opposition of one group "the community" to others. Often their construction is based on assumptions which are fundamentally aggregational (for example the sharing of residence, ethnicity, mental health service use or being "non-NHS") however their construction does not take into account how the putative "members" perceive their community boundaries. Indeed this is clearly not a constraint on the ability of non-members to construct communities in the course of their work. People working in community participation have almost complete freedom to construct and deconstruct communities as they desire. This was indicated by 28 different types of definition which can be identified in the transcripts. One Health Promotion Officer working with minority ethnic groups explained how she constructed "communities" for the purpose of her work by aggregating ethnic groups, nations, regions and even continents. No matter how disparate the final grouping, at no stage does it cease to be a "community". If the "members" were to perceive themselves to be a "community" it would surely be coincidental.

Nonetheless discourses of sharing form an important part of discussions of community within parts of the sociological literature and body of literature related to Health for All. To cite a few examples, Willmott (1984) in his discussion paper Community in Social Policy reviews published material and activities with "community" labels and whilst highlighting a huge diversity in the word's use, argues that the essence of each was "sharing". The Alma Ata Declaration (Mahler, 1981) itself, whilst not defining community, suggests that it is a locality bound aggregation of people who share economic, socio-cultural and political characteristics, as well as problems and needs. Rifkin (et al. 1988) discuss three definitions of community. It could be used geographically to refer to "people living in the same area and sharing the same basic values and organization" or people who share the same basic interests. They observe that for health personal, it was an "at risk group" or target group. When they define community participation they imply a fourth definition, "specific groups with shared needs living in a defined geographical area".

The extent to which people who construct "communities" in the course of Health for All work believe the envisaged "members" perceive themselves to share important characteristics is unclear. However analysis of imagery that is used when discussing communities reveals that the idea of sharing, expressed as "spirit" or "sense" of community, is an important one and sometimes so much so that it is used to distinguish "community" from "non-community". An example of this was provided by one Environmental Health Officer who said of local drug users "I'm not sure they form a community at all ... there isn't a community spirit". The notion of sharing is further reinforced by the metaphors of personification which are repeatedly used when referring to "community". Indeed the community is represented as having the qualities and competencies of a living person when reference is made to "speaking to" the community, "meeting with" the community, or when people speak of its "expertize", its "views", its "wants", "needs" and its "voice".

An apparent, but important, contradiction is seen to emerge. In delineating the boundaries of the communities which they construct in their work, a relational idea is employed in order to distinguish one section of the population which they would call the "community" from another. However the notion of sharing amongst members of these "communities" is shown through the imagery used and in the literature still to be an important one. Yet the views of the putative "members" themselves on their own sense of sharing are not taken into account in the construction of these communities.

Representatives on steering groups

With the above discussion in mind we will now look at the Health for All steering group. The notion of "community" representation on steering groups is that the group of representatives together should be able in some way to represent the "community". A varying number of "community representatives" (between two and five) were identified to serve on the groups. One of the mechanisms employed to avoid tensions and contradictions which might arise from the simultaneous use of different definitions of community, is a folk model of "lots of communities within the community" or alternatively a notion of a "whole" community made up of "bits" or "parts" or "fragments", which at times can also be "communities" in their own right. The different representatives on steering groups are often selected because they are regarded as being able to represent different "communities" within the community or "parts" of the community, where "the" community is the population of the Borough. The precise numbers chosen reflect institutional desires for "balance" between the numerical representation of different sectors on the steering group, rather than an attempt to enumerate the "communities" or "parts" which should be represented.

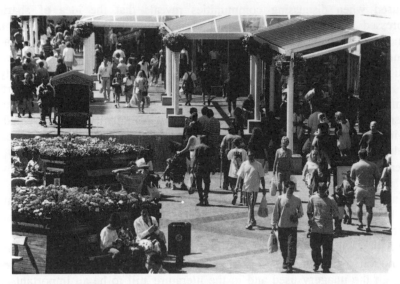

What is a "community"? Is it in reality too complex for a few people to represent in situations such as Healthy Cities steering groups?

When asked whether the community representatives did represent the community, informants from all sectors on every group expressed dissatisfaction with their performance. There were not enough of them ("I don't know that we have enough people yet"), they were not selected properly ("we would like to see nominated people from the voluntary organizations"), or they were the wrong types of representative ("I'd like to see users on the steering group"). The comments imply that with some fine tuning, they would be representative of the community. The "problem" of the representatives not being deemed to be representative is perceived as serious and often a source of endless discussion in the groups, but is not apparently seen as sufficiently grave to undermine the institution. It is something which will be improved on in the future, something still to be "addressed".

Some informants identify the Community Health Councils, community workers and community groups as examples of institutions which do not represent "the community". These remarks appear as specific criticisms, but since these were the only sources of community representatives informants had worked with on the groups, it might be hypothesized that what is being reflected was not criticism of these three sources per se but an inherent dissatisfaction with their experience of the construct of the "community representative".

Set in the context of the foregoing discussion of meanings of community, what is surprising is not that "community representatives" are invariably considered not to be representative, but that anyone could consider that a small group of people could represent these relationally constructed "communities" in any sort of scientific or political meaning of the word. Perhaps one way of understanding this would be if informants imagine that the communities which they construct do incorporate a sense of sharing, in which case we would be bound to suggest that this is "misconceived", not least because it contradicts their own daily experiences of working with the "community" which they characterize as being dominated by expressions of heterogeneity. Viewed in this way the "problem" of the representativeness of the community members of steering groups can be seen not as one of the specific people involved, nor the sources from which they are drawn, but rather the very notion that to "represent" the community is truly attainable.

Acknowledgements

This chapter arose out of research undertaken for an MD, awarded by the university of London. It would not have been possible without the support of my supervisor Prof Anne Murcott, North East Thames Regional Health Authority and my informants. The work was undertaken whilst an Honorary Lecturer in the Health Promotion Sciences Unit at the London School of Hygiene and Tropical Medicine. The author is currently at Women's Health, CERSA, Medical Research Council, PO Box 19070, Tygerberg, Cape Town 7505, South Africa.

References

Adams, L. (1989), "Healthy Cities, Healthy Participation", *Health Education Journal*, vol. 48, pp. 178-82.
Alma Ata Declaration (1978) in Mahler, H. (ed.) (1981) *The Meaning of "Health for All by the Year 2000"*, World Health Forum, vol. 2, pp. 5-22.
Hillery, G.A. (1955), "Definitions of Community: Areas of Agreement", *Rural Sociology*, vol. 20, pp. 111-24.
Jewkes, R. (1994), "Meanings of "Community" in Community Participation in Health Promotion", Unpublished MD Thesis, University of London.
Kickbusch, I. (1986), "Introduction to the Journal", *Health Promotion*, vol. 1, pp. 3-4.
Plant, R. (1974), *Community and Ideology: An Essay in Applied Social Philosophy*, Routledge and Kegen Paul, London.
Rifkin, S. and Muller, F. and Bichmann, W. (1988), "Primary Health Care: on Measuring Participation", *Social Science and Medicine*, vol. 26, pp. 931-40.

Willmott, P. and Thomas, D. (1984), *Community in Social Policy*, Discussion Paper no. 9, Policy Studies Institute, London.

9 Community health needs assessment for the development of a new model of participative and intersectoral primary health care in north Liverpool

Pat Thornley

The Croxteth Health Action Area Project (CHAAP) was a Liverpool Healthy Cities initiative set up in 1989. Following the initial phase of compiling health, demographic and socio-economic data for the area, the project became fully operational in January 1990 with the employment of three community development workers. The project boundaries encompassed the outer city council estates of Croxeth and Gillmoss and a small section of the Norris Green estate of traditional houses, built in the 1920s. Further information about the evolution of CHAAP can be found in the brochure "Croxteth Health Action Area" (Green and Thornley, 1992), which traces the background of the project and describes the varied health promoting initiatives developed during the community development phase.

The very fruitful community development phase provided the foundations for the implementation of a primary care strategy, which had been planned for the third stage of the project. This was to involve a community wide effort which aimed at including everyone living and working in the community; all the people who contributed to the promotion and maintenance of health in the widest sense. The health status of a community may be said to reflect both the personal lifestyles of its residents, as well as the social, economic and environmental conditions of their every day lives. However, communities may have little if any control over their poor housing, low income, and the provision of services and facilities etc., all of which can impact on individual or collective health status. Nevertheless, people in the community can bring about change by influencing the way in which local services and facilities are provided and delivered, albeit within the constraints of central government policy.

A community development approach to health is about working with local people to enable them to gain control of their day to day lives, and the way in which they live these. It takes as its starting point the problems, issues and solutions which are identified by local people. This process of empowerment provides the impetus and framework for change in the community.

Community development as a foundation

Community development alone cannot bring about the changes which are necessary to have a real impact on people's health status. What it can do is to help to create the conditions which will enable this, in terms of strengthening the social, economic and environmental structures of support in the community. The next step is working in effective and constructive partnerships with the statutory and private sectors.

These partnerships are crucial to achieving long term change and maintaining the impetus of community development approaches. However, in order for this process to be effective, organizations also need to develop and change, not only in terms of how they work with each other, but also how they will respond both individually and collectively to the community. This is particularly so in terms of what the community sees as its needs and solutions, and how these needs and expectations can be balanced with the needs and goals of the organizations concerned.

Primary care, as conceived in the Health for All strategy, presents us with a prime opportunity to creatively harness the skills, talents and energies within the community, and to effectively deploy available statutory sector resources where they are most needed. Therefore, the model which was to be developed in Croxteth, Gillmoss and Norris Green took as its starting point, the contribution that everyone makes to promoting and maintaining the health of the community. Central to this, were the residents themselves who, it may be argued are the major providers of care for their families, friend and neighbours, a role which is all too often undervalued and unacknowledged.

First steps

During the summer of 1991, a small working group met to explore how this theoretical concept of primary health care could be put into practice. The first stage was to organize a series of workshops, with the goal of bringing together informal and formal providers. The idea was to initiate a process of debate about how primary health care (PHC) could be enhanced and developed in the future to include not only the environmental and social agencies outside the traditional health service, but also the community itself as major providers of health and social services.

This was achieved with the attendance of 64 participants, including representatives from the following: community and voluntary organizations including tenants associations; Church; Police; Family Health Services

Authority; General Practitioners, Pharmacist; Community Dentists; Community Services Managers, Health Visitors, Midwives, School Nurses, District Nurses; Local Authority Councillors, Environmental Health Managers, Social Services, Probation Services, Youth and Community Service, Education Department, Health Education Advisers, teachers and pupils from local schools; Liverpool University and Polytechnic. These participants attended a series of sessions which explored their contributions to primary health care, the similarities and overlaps in their activities, how they could work together to improve what they were able to contribute, and how could they overcome any obstacles. The workshops required a great deal of planning. The facilititators were given detailed guidance notes to enable members to make the connections between their role and contribution to primary health care, in the widest sense. The result was a general agreement and commitment to taking forward the development and implementation of a new concept of primary care (Green, 1993).

Management and organization

Under the aegis of the CHAA project team, a body known as the Neighbourhood Health Action Management Team was drawn together.

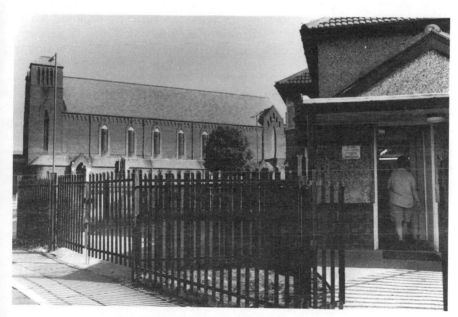

The new primary care strategy was set up to go beyond the health centre to include all whose work and activities contribute to health in the community

103

This was comprised of representatives from: the Healthy Cities project; community and voluntary sector; health sector which included community health services; a local General Practitioner; Family Health Services Authority; District Health Authority; City Council Directorates of Social Services, Education, Housing, Environmental Health Services together with Merseyside Police and Merseyside Probation Service.

Following this, a statement of intent was drawn up. This included the team's agreed overall and specific aims together with its operational objectives. In order for the team to make progress, it was thought that there was a crucial requirement to establish an understanding of the views and wishes of local people. This would ensure that the strategy developed was grounded upon the needs of the community.

In order to fill in some of the gaps in information about the area, it was decided to commission two major studies, one of which would examine community needs (Hotchkiss, 1993), and the other existing PHC provision (Stafford, 1993). The main aims of these two pieces of research were:

1.   Needs assessment - to establish a data base on the community's perception of health need and the services already provided by the statutory and voluntary sectors, together with the gathering of information about the contribution of informal carers.

2.   PHC provision - to identify the resources currently deployed within the area, in terms of the statutory, voluntary and informal services. This work would complement the community needs assessment and would contribute to the formulation of the recommendations which followed.

This paper is primarily concerned with the needs assessment study, which was undertaken by Merseyside Information Services (a local government information resource) in conjunction with the Liverpool Public Health Observatory. It was funded jointly by the CHAA Project, North Mersey Community (NHS) Trust and Liverpool District Health Authority.

Participation in designing the survey

The needs survey was planned to be carried out by interview, using a questionnaire administered to a random sample of around 1,000 residents within the three estates. For the purpose of the survey and to meet the future information needs of Norris Green residents, the Health Action Area boundaries were extended to include the whole of the Norris Green estate (Figure 9.1).

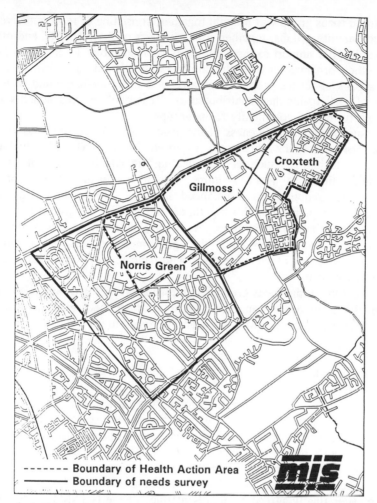

- - - - - - Boundary of Health Action Area
——— Boundary of needs survey

mis

Figure 9.1 **Map of north east Liverpool, showing the boundaries of the Health Action Area, and that of the needs survey which was extended to cover the whole of the Norris Green area**

It was crucial to ensure that the process of designing the survey was participatory, so that it also reflected the community's rather than the professionals perceptions and priorities. So often in the past, professionals have imposed an agenda by asking only those questions which have reflected their priorities. In order to avoid this problem, the questionnaire development was preceded by a series of focus groups, made up of local people, which were designed to identify the issues people wanted to study.

105

An initial focus group was brought together, consisting of representatives of local community groups, together with members of the NHAMT and others who would give support to the community representatves when it was taken back to their organizations. Following this initial group, an information and training pack about the proposed research was made available and with this the initial participants then contributed to a "cascade" process which was to involve a further 15 community focus groups.

The issue of representativeness of the groups was of concern, and various options for addressing this were explored by the NHAMT including recruitment techniques such as "snowballing" in which initial contacts use community links to identify more participants using quotas of the charactersitics required for a balanced sample. However, the practical difficulties of implementing this together with financial constraints proved an insurmountable barrier at the time. As it was, the main issue was to ensure that the focus groups represented the age composition of the community, particularly in terms of young people, who have few opportunities to make their needs known.

Following the initial focus group, the information pack was amended in the light of the participants' comments. A total of 15 focus groups were held including one with people who had learning disabilities.

Achieving a balance

The information gathered from the groups was turned with some difficulty into a questionnaire. This difficulty arose partly because of the practicalities of translating the information, which had been gathered primarily through "brainstorming", into key themes. Another important aspect of this was the need to achieve a balance between the issues arising from the focus groups and the specific issues that the NHAMT wanted to include. The questionnaire was however finally agreed by representatives of the NHAMT. It included the various issues raised by the focus groups, additional questions relating to the carers and their perceived health status, and some questions taken from other surveys concerning disability and illness.

A team of four trained interviewers employed by Merseyside Information Services administered the questionnaire. In all a total of 1,173 households were approached and 704 agreed to interview, giving a response rate of 60 per cent (68 per cent if properties thought to be uninhabited are excluded). A detailed report on the results of the survey is available (Hotchkiss, 1993).

The results of the survey were explored by the NHAMT in another series of groups involving many of the people who had been originally involved, with the purpose of developing policy recommendations. It was agreed by the NHAMT that it was important to try to ensure that the recommendations put forward were, in the main, achievable, if not immediately, then in the forseable future.

This policy development phase involved a lengthy and difficult process with each agency representing the various sectors being given responsibility for drafting their particular section. The community representatives probably had the biggest task, since they needed to identify where and how they could respond to all the sections of the report, and then draft the appropriate recommendations. These were finally all drawn together and agreed by the NHAMT, and reported to the city authorities. In addition, the report was presented and discussed at a well-attended launch in the area, to which community leaders and representatives of the service providers were invited.

Outcomes of the project

A crucial question has to be whether the structures and processes that evolved through the NHAMT were actually able to deliver the concepts of primary health care that informed its development. In some ways the original primary care project has been overtaken by events in policy development. The original NHAMT no longer exists, but some of its recommendations are being acted on (for instance in the training and support of carers), but more generally it has been a powerful learning experience that is continuing to contribute at local and city level. In concrete policy terms there are two ways in which this is the case at the present time:

Neighbourhood health planning

Over the last few years, the Health Authority has established neighbourhood planning for the whole city. Recognising the importance of a foundation of community development, already five neighbourhood health development workers have been appointed (three local authority funded, and two health authority funded), and in due course it is proposed to appoint one health authority and one local authority funded worker to each neighbourhood in due course.

Objective 1

Following the recent designation of Merseyside for Objective 1 status by the European Commission, a wide variety of proposals are being prepared by communities throughout the city of Liverpool. The key to these proposals is partnerships, of community, statutory agencies and business. The experience of the NHAMT has been of assistance in this work, partly through identifying needs, but particularly through what has been learned about negotiating the balance between the goals of the statutory sector officers and the community representatives.

Some strengths and weaknesses of the process

Amongst the strengths of this project has been the way it has enabled the community to determine its own needs, priorities and solutions. It has provided the foundations for developing neighbourhood planning, and provided a framework for negotiating competing needs and priorities, together with the setting of realistic and achievable targets. We found that it also enabled the statutory agencies to build a constructive partnership with the community and to recognize and acknowledge their major contribution. One tangible benefit arising from partnership was the joint funding of the health needs survey, which gave all three partners a stake in the exercise and access to the findings. Not only has this been a relatively efficient use of resources, it has in the process brought the goals of the three partners that much closer together. In other ways, the report still functions as a working document, so that elements have been built into the locality business plan, and where possible opportunities are taken to develop the services recommended in the report.

This initiative has not been without its difficulties however, among which lack of time and resources were important. Time constraints placed limitation directly on the process, for instance it was not possible to select and train local residents to carry out the interviews. Lack of time also constrained the contribution of some of the statutory sector officers for whom this initiative was seen as an "add on" to their existing responsibilities, while for other it was built into their objectives. Limited funding placed very tight restrictions on the survey work, and in general it is important to emphasize that these activities cost money. There is a tendency to press ahead with policy on local needs assessment and local development of primary care without thorough or realistic costing of the financial implications of what is being initiated.

Conclusion

Looking back from the position of the work that is now going on in Croxteth, Gillmoss and Norris Green, makes us more aware of what projects such as the NHAMT have given us. It is a sense of a "history" that is proving to be of value now. Of course, it is very difficult to separate out the extent of the NHAMT contribution from other activities in the area, and wider initiatives in the city, but it has played a part. This is particularly so because it was primarily about partnerships, and it is partnerships that are central to the development of primary care and for special programmes such as Objective 1, and which seem to offer the best way of sharing finite resources in a more efficient way.

Acknowledgement

We would like to acknowledge the commitment and time given to this project by all those involved in the Neighbourhood Health Action Management Team, and in the focus groups.

References

Green, G. (1993), "Auditing Community Health Needs & Resources", *Healthy City Project*, Liverpool.

Green, G. and Thornley, P. (1992), "Croxteth Health Action Area", *Healthy City Project*, Liverpool.

Hotchkiss, J. (1993), *Croxteth Health Action Area Community Needs Survey and Response, Croxteth, Gillmoss and Norris Green, Public Health Observatory Report Series No 15*, Liverpool University, Liverpool.

Stafford, B. (1993), *An Audit of a Community's Health Resources in the Croxteth, Gillmoss and Norris Green Areas of Liverpool*. Department of Economic and Related Studies, University of York, York.

10 Building community action: Experience from the Croxteth Health Action, Liverpool

Nigel Bruce and Lyn Winters

Community participation and intersectoral collaboration are fundamental to the WHO Health for All programme (WHO, 1985), and received further impetus in England with the publication of the national strategy, "Health of the Nation" (HMSO, 1992). The subsequent policy document, "Local Voices" (NHSME, 1992) - regarded "making health services more responsive to the needs and preferences of local people as being a central objective of District Health Authorities and Family Health Services Authorities' new roles as purchasers of health." It is in this process that the experience of the Croxteth Health Action Area (CHAA) in north Liverpool, described more fully below, has so much to offer.

The Croxteth Health Action Area was established in 1988 partly in response to the findings of a working party set up to consider the needs of this disadvantaged post war estate near the north eastern edge of the city (Croxteth Area Working Party, 1983). The action area also covers part of the neighbouring community of Norris Green, which had been built some 20 to 30 years earlier. The World Health Organisation's Healthy Cities (HC) project, seen as a practical method of implementing the Health for All 2000 (HFA) programme (WHO, 1985; Ashton, 1992), had been recently established and the Health Action Area was to be an important focus for local action. The CHAA has attempted to bring about change by facilitating community participation in activities that respond to locally expressed need, and by encouraging the co-ordination of action between the city's statutory agencies. Four phases of the programme were envisaged, as follows:

1. Research on health status, housing and the environment, and setting up a small area data base.

2. Community development, in which a Neighbourhood Health Team would have a central role.

3.   Changes in the organization of primary care to bring together the community and statutory sectors in the assessment of need and development of policy.

4.   Implementation of new policy initiatives.

The CHAA is based in an office in Croxteth Family Health Clinic, and employs a full time manager, two full time support staff and has been joined by a research worker. The Neighbourhood Health Team (NHT) has used a variety of techniques for community involvement, including public meetings, work with voluntary groups, focus groups, forums, a wide range of community initiatives, and surveys for needs assessment (Habib, 1993; Hotchkiss, 1993). Almost 30 identifiable projects or activities have been organized or facilitated by the NHT, and examples of these are listed below (Table 10.1):

Table 10.1
Examples of the activities in the CHAA

-     Community chest
-     Credit Union
-     Carer's group
-     Environmental improvements
-     Women's health groups
-     Domestic violence forum
-     Counselling group
-     Action newspaper
-     Independent living for people with learning difficulties
-     Neighbourhood Health Action Management Team (needs assessment and strategy development for re-oriented primary care)
-     Multi-purpose centre (Norris Green Community Health Forum)

While the experience of all of these activities is of interest and relevance, it is the work of the Neighbourhood Action Management Team (NHAMT) that is perhaps of the most direct and pressing relevance to contemporary health policy in this country and more widely. Planning of the NHAMT began between May and June 1991, and the project began actively in January 1992 with the following aims and objectives (Table 10.2).

Table 10.2
Aims and objectives of the neighbourhood health
action management team

Overall aim

To implement an integrated model of Primary Health Care which promotes, enables and supports everyone's contribution to the promotion and maintenance of health within the community.

Specific aims

To explore and develop ways in which all participants in Primary Health Care can integrate their services, at a neighbourhood level.

To promote and encourage the active involvement of all partners in the planning, delivery, development, organization, management, monitoring and accountability of health promotion and care.

Objectives

1. To identify and enhance joint areas of working.

2. To develop improved systems of communications between and within agencies, including community groups.

3. To raise awareness about the services provided.

4. To identify and assess the resources available within the community.

5. To identify and assess individual and community care needs, within the community.

6. To identify and assess the gaps in the services provided.

7. To manage all available resources to meet assessed needs and maximize health gain.

8. To help people in the community take control of and make informed choices about their health.

9. To identify, monitor and evaluate progress towards the above aims and objectives.

The NHAMT met on a regular basis on the site of a former secondary school, a building identified by the community as the base for their plans to create a multi-purpose centre. A series of focus groups were held in order to inform the development of a random sample questionnaire survey among local residents covering health status, service use and perceived need. In addition, a survey of existing provision in the area was also carried out. The results of this work were then fed back for the group to discuss and reach consensus on policies which could address the issues identified. This work is described in more detail by Pat Thornley in chapter nine.

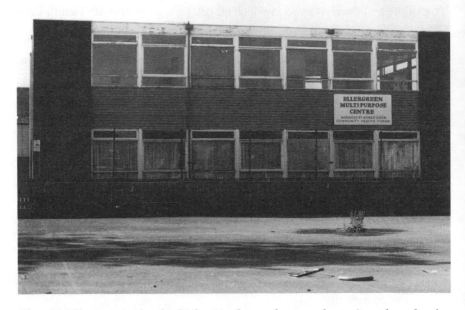

The old Ellergreen school which served as a focus and meeting place for the primary care development project

Purpose of study

The aim of the study is to evaluate the work of the Croxteth Health Action Area and the NHT, with particular emphasis on the strengths and weaknesses of methods used for needs assessment, promotion of community participation, and collaboration between agencies with responsibility for the area, in order to inform the future development of the project and the development of contemporary health strategy for the city. The study had the following specific objectives:

1. To complete a systematic record of the objectives, structure, activities, strengths and weakness, and outcomes of the 26 projects that have been supported and/or initiated by the CHAA.

2. To carry out a more detailed evaluation of one of the projects, the primary care development initiative (Neighbourhood Health Action Management Team) concentrating on the key processes of (i) community involvement and (ii) intersectoral collaboration, in needs assessment and policy development, and the potential for more general application.

3. To consider the implications of the CHAA experience for the future development of the project and other initiatives based on this approach in Liverpool and elsewhere.

Methods

A review of background information on the CHAA and the philosophy of Healthy Cities as applied in the CHAA was carried out, and is reported elsewhere (Bruce and Winters, 1994). The context of the evaluation is of importance in considering the methods and limitations of these. The work was carried out on behalf of the city's Joint Public Health Team, a high level committee overseeing public health policy, and combining health authority, local government, trades unions, the business community and voluntary sector. As evaluation had not been planned in advance as part of the CHAA work programme, time and resources were limited, and this placed constraints on the degree of participation achieved in developing the methods used and the opportunity for interviewing key persons who were on leave during the short period available. For the current purposes, attention will be focused on the study of the primary care development project

Study of the neighbourhood health action management team

The study of the NHAMT was carried out using a semi structured interview with key informants who were selected from all of the interests represented (Appendix 10.1). The interview schedule was developed after consultation with a number of individuals from different sectors who were associated with the NHAMT project in order to identify priority issues, and by reference to literature on the evaluation of community participation (Bjaras et al. 1991;

Cooke, 1992; WHO, 1988), and expertise in intersectoral collaboration (Dr Jane Springett, personal communication).

The interviews were carried out by LW, using the main headings listed in Appendix 10.2, and were conducted in a manner that encouraged exploration of respondents' views. All interviews were tape recorded and transcribed. The key issues have been identified and summarized, with verbatim quotations which have been selected to illustrate the most important points.

Findings

The results of this analysis are presented under key headings which identify the processes underlying the objectives of the programme, as well as those which arose through the experience of implementation.

The neighbourhood health team (NHT)

Role

The role of the NHT in community development was clearly identified, and regarded as indispensable in a situation which involved conflicting interests, the need to build trust, and perhaps more straightforwardly the need for time, persistence and patience.

> Community groups need more direction ... If it is left to the community, it takes them a long time to develop their ideas.

> You need people who can work in the community, that it is their role to make it happen ... people with a professional background do come with established views on what is right, and they will very possibly think in a certain way.

> A problem with a community development approach is that it does take resources, time and people to help it along and statutory agencies have not got that time or those people.

What the NHT has achieved and done well

In summary, the NHT was reported to have built up trust in quite difficult circumstances, and laid the basis for genuine community participation.

They (the statutory sector) tend to be in the market for quick fixes, they want rather superficial action very quickly ... they parachute in for three months and deliver some superficial change ... What I think the NHT did was to develop community participation in a very much more systematic and evolutionary way.

They have played a good facilitation role - good at coordination and administration, but they are caught in the cross fire.

They have political awareness and will push issues as far as they can.

Limitations; occasions of need for stronger management

Achieving a balance between non-directive community development skills, and the need to ensure progress is difficult and was achieved with varying success. In the NHAMT, the following problems were mentioned.

It is sometimes difficult to strike a balance between the meetings and the follow through ..., the action that you need to take to implement the decisions made at meetings ... and sometimes probably the balance was a bit wrong.

There is a need for long term planning.

Community participation

There was evidence that a "high level" of community participation was being achieved in some respects. The emphasis on the community's contribution to care was recognized and appreciated.

There has been a lot of commitment; real engagement with the community.

So it was not seen that the community activity was simply lobbying or a pressure group, but that it was integrated into the activities of the establishment.

A more democratic input into services ... one of the great achievements (of the project) is putting residents on the map as providers of health care rather than simply as consumers of it.

Barriers to community participation

Many barriers to community participation have been identified. Particular issues in the NHAMT were:

The relatively long timescale of some aspects of the process:

> Community representatives were frustrated at the time it took to get things done.

> One of the disadvantages of spending a lot of time on the process is that people tend to fall by the wayside ... so the community representatives ... on average (only had) a total of two or three residents when there should have been six.

The difficulties that some members had in comprehending the "system":

> I (a NHAMT member with some experience of the system) find the public health side of it difficult to understand, the various committees, line managers, policies, and things. It is all foreign to me, the various structures, etc. So obviously a person in the community might be lost.

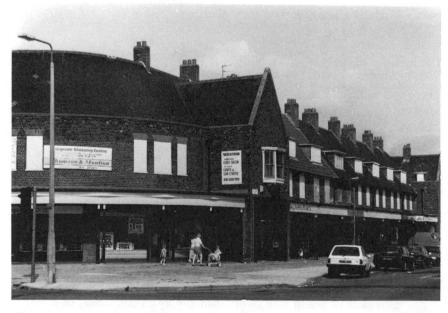

The economic decline of the area has meant addressing the needs of more vulnerable, less mobile people

The implications that some historical and social features of this community had for attempts to promote community involvement:

> We have lost a huge proportion of people ... the economically active have gone elsewhere ... so the vulnerable groups have been left because they are not mobile.

The implication being that "vulnerable" people have further to go before they can participate effectively in this type of activity.

Achievements and benefits of intersectoral working

Trust and familiarity:

> In working at this level you get to know each other and develop a much better understanding and trust; feel more confident.

> You know who you can go to with more ease.

Understanding of other sectors' roles and difficulties:

> Get a good perception about other professional's roles - a good idea of their working, you don't feel yourself so much in isolation.

> It provides a forum where you can get an understanding of the problems facing other agencies, voluntary and statutory.

More honest and open exchange of ideas and concerns:

> To be able to share problems - to be open about difficulties.

> Provides a forum where you can test ideas before they actually happen.

These reports of better understanding and more honest and open exchanges are very important and valuable, and mark a refreshing shift in the style of working.

119

Difficulties experienced with intersectoral co-operation

Participants come with different perceptions:

> It highlighted this problem that we all work to different boundaries, different terminology and therefore confuse each other as well as everyone else.

Pressures of restructuring of organizations:

> Management changes caused by the restructuring of statutory agencies has planning implications ... it is difficult to get a stable environment in which to systematically plan your health services and to take account of the lessons that you are learning locally.

Financial restrictions:

> Working within financial constraints ... with pressures of work, intersectoral working can get pushed down to the bottom of the agenda.

Costs and benefits

Whilst the costs of the NHT staff and other professionals' time was clearly apparent, participants were beginning to recognize the potential for greater efficiency. Measuring the benefit side of the equation however, remains a considerable challenge.

Apparent costs:

> Expensive to put three workers in a small neighbourhood, although ideal.

> In terms of the finances that are available to statutory bodies it could not be replicated across the city.

Potential (financial) benefits:

> (Of intersectoral collaboration) ... complement each other - perhaps save money in the long term.

> This model of working is expensive, but it could be good investment

... because the community provides nine-tenths of health care and with training and support could do it a lot more effectively.

Evolution and sustainability

Problems of uncertainty about the project's future and funding were prominent, and undermined commitment:

Since the needs assessment and survey, (the project has been) drifting.

Coming to the end of the second phase funding and not meeting as regularly as there is no certainty about the future.

... under the impression that the thing was winding up.

The perceived consequences of abrupt project termination were judged as being potentially very serious:

I have a degree of scepticism about time limited pilot models ... people set up a project then pull the plug out by which time they have raised community expectations and involved a lot of peoples' time.

If we were to withdraw it now, we would have a great deal of disenchantment in this area and it would be extraordinarily difficult to get those groups back on board, because there are people who have worked tremendously hard - well over and above what you would expect.

Barriers to overall progress

Economic barriers

Local people were aware of the enormity of economic barriers to major investment and development of the area, and this leads into a measure of conflict between statutory sector and community over priority issues:

The project has tried to highlight their needs, but it can only scratch the surface really. Addressing them would require the sorts of resources they are prepared to put into building the Trident (nuclear submarine).

121

From a community viewpoint, the stress of unemployment should be dealt with. Now for someone like a district nurse or health visitor ... it is very difficult to do anything about that. How do you cure unemployment? You are just dealing with the symptoms.

Boundaries

Statutory sector boundaries provided administrative difficulties. There was also historically some tension between the two principal communities involved, and this suggests that local community boundaries should also be taken into consideration:

> We actually stride two of the community health boundaries and about three of the General Practitioner zones. Our boundaries don't tally with housing, nor with education in any way. So its an absolute nightmare.

> A health action area should have been established for the whole of Norris Green not just a quarter ... the community should have been involved in the setting up of the area.

> Groups in Norris Green need support of the NHAMT. Groups in Croxteth are better organized. They have had more funding from the urban regeneration programme.

The need for greater control

> It is only representatives from agencies attending who have not got any real accountability ... need someone with their hands in the till.

> If the people who engage in the dialogue don't have the final power to make decisions, then things take a long time.

Personal development

In many projects there has been considerable personal development in the form of training (e.g. counselling, assertiveness, public speaking) and members have gained knowledge of the working of other agencies. This personal development is difficult to measure, and to assess the extent to which such changes might have happened anyway. Despite these cautions, the stimulation of the personal development of participants in these projects could potentially be of great importance, and one of the most significant outcomes of the CHAA's work.

Discussion

Resources required to achieve and maintain community participation

The level of community participation varied a lot among the projects, and formally was low in the NHAMT. This was due in part to a perceived lack of clarity about purpose, confusion over the jargon and ideas being used by the statutory sector, and the pace of the process not meeting expectations. If left at this however, our conclusion about the adequacy of community participation would be inappropriately negative and very misleading. Thus, in the case of the NHAMT, community representation overall was considered by respondents to be reasonably good, and this was due to the focus groups and surveys, as well as the practice adopted by the NHT to brief the Norris Green Community Federation and the Croxteth Community Federation. In this, as in so many other activities, the NHT was central to achieving this level of community participation.

Although it is not possible to define clearly the role that the NHT has had in promoting and maintaining community participation, it seems most unlikely that the observed level would have been achieved without the resources of time and organizational effort put in by the NHT. Professionals working in the area do not have the time or flexibility to fulfil this role, and inevitably have to consider the needs of their own agencies. The time, commitment and community development skills of the NHT (or an equivalent) are an important ingredient for community participation, particularly for communities that do not have highly organized and motivated community activists.

Balance of leadership and facilitation

Although in many cases the NHT had a very prominent role in promoting the development of the projects, and in chairing and servicing meetings, the approach (particularly as observed in the NHAMT) has been generally reported as non directive. While this style is generally appropriate in community development, there was a frequently expressed need for clearer leadership in the NHAMT, and this should be taken into consideration in the future development of this project and in setting up locality based primary health care projects elsewhere.

Involvement of other sectors, and intersectoral collaboration

In general, intersectoral working was valued by many members as an opportunity to get to know people working in other agencies and in the community. There was value in knowing their faces, and this eased communication at other times. Some members expressed the view that this was a forum where they could air the real concerns that they felt, which is a considerable achievement. The style of intersectoral working in the NHAMT was found to be most valuable by people whose job already demanded contact with other agencies and the community, for instance in locality planning. On the other hand, some of the other team members saw it as interesting but peripheral, and of secondary importance when there were other demands.

Timescale of process

The resources of skills and personnel required to support community involvement and promote intersectoral working has been mentioned. In addition to the time that this implies, there is also a natural evolution required to build up knowledge, trust and commitment, and this applies both to the community and statutory sectors. It is not possible to be prescriptive about how long it takes, since this will vary depending on the initial level of commitment and experience of those concerned.

Community involvement in policy development

There are examples such as the Supported Independent Living project (a programme of supervised housing for learning impaired adults currently living with carers) where it is reported that carers are getting actively involved in the development of policy, but this was not always the case. In the NHAMT, the extent of community involvement in policy development is so far limited, with the exception of the Multi-Purpose Centre (MPC) at Ellergreen. This centre has been the base for the NHAMT meetings, and the community (led by the local Health Forum) wishes to develop it as a focus for community activity as well as a broad range of services including the health centre, a nursery school and the local government's housing office. There appear to be differing views about the importance of the MPC as the primary policy outcome of the needs assessment process; the community is very committed to the MPC, while the statutory sector (including the health authority) - though supportive - has not seen it as so central.

While respondents felt that the contribution of the community to the focus groups and survey represented influence on policy development, there do not appear to have been any explicit plans for ensuring community involvement in the development of actual policy. This is in part because the project is seen by some as coming to an end, partly due to funding uncertainty, and partly because of some lack of clarity about the objectives of the project.

Most respondents felt that the NHAMT model could be used elsewhere in city, but there were reservations. One of the most important was for better links into planning boundaries of the various organizations involved. In the case of the NHAMT which cut across rather different communities (Croxteth and Norris Green), it was felt that this might have been better avoided. The lesson from this is to use local knowledge in planning the boundaries.

The cost of generalizing the NHT model has been questioned. Undoubtedly, reproducing the staffing level and other expenditures more widely would be expensive, but it is necessary to consider cost effectiveness. Measuring the gains, including the health gains, of the CHAA's activity is going to be extremely difficult, but it would be premature to make judgements on the basis of information relating solely to the cost side of the equation. For example, what are the benefits of the training and personal development of individuals which has been a quite common occurrence in a number of the projects? What has been their health gain? It is also important to consider the cost of intersectoral working. If this is to be the pattern anyway for locality planning - and it is recognized that intersectoral working can be very time consuming - then it is necessary to take into account the potential costs of inefficient or failed activities that founder due to inadequate community support and facilitation.

Conclusion

In the CHAA, the Neighbourhood Health Team has contributed much to the development, facilitation and administration of a broad range of projects, one of which has been studied here. In the absence of these designated community development workers, it is difficult to see who else would have been able to facilitate the setting up and organization of this type of process, and maintain commitment among community and statutory sectors as their own understanding and commitment develops. If community development is regarded as a vital pre-requisite for effective participation in local needs assessment and policy development - as is implied by contemporary local government and health policy - then the time, skills and resources required to achieve this must be allowed for.

Successful collaboration between the statutory sector and the community requires the transcending of traditional "us and them" barriers. This study has identified evidence that the NHT has helped to overcome this barrier, and acted as a "focus for partnership."

References

Ashton, J. (ed.) (1992), *Healthy Cities*, Open University Press, Milton Keynes.

Bjaras, G., Haglund, B. and Rifkin, S. (1991), "A New Approach to Community Participation Assessment", *Health Promotion International*, vol. 6, pp 199-206.

Bruce, N. and Winters, L. (1994), *Evaluation of Croxteth Health Action Area, Liverpool Public Health Observatory, Report no. 17*, PO Box 147, Liverpool L69 3BX.

Cooke, R. (1992), "Community Participation in Healthy Cities, Healthy Cities: reshaping the urban environment, Proceedings of the Second National Conference of Healthy Cities Australia" in Rees, Allan (ed.), *Australian Community Health Association*, 1992.

Habib, J (1993), *Carer's Needs of the CHAA*, Liverpool School of Tropical Medicine.

HMSO, (1992), *The Health of the Nation*.

Hotchkiss, J. (1993), *CHAA: Community Needs Survey and Community Response, Liverpool Public Health Observatory, Report no. 15*.

NHSME, (1992), *Local Voices: The Views of Local People in Purchasing for Health*.

WHO, (1985), *Targets for Health for All*, WHO, Copenhagen.

WHO, (1988), *Improving Urban Health: Guidelines for Rapid Appraisal to Assess Community Health Needs*, WHO, Geneva.

Appendix 10.1
NHAMT - Key informants interviewed

- Priest
- Tenant's association
- Community representative (also chair of NHAMT)
- Community services
- HC project co-ordinator and manager
- Environmental services
- Public health
- Police
- General practitioner
- Locality manager
- Community representative, also from community drug support organization
- (Housing: unavailable due to leave)

Appendix 10.2
Topic headings for semi structured interview
with key informants

Personal

- Role
- Length of involvement
- Who/what represent

Intersectoral working

- Understanding/shared objectives/commitment
- Support from top
- Perceived advantages for self and organization/group
- Were there interests not represented, or duplicated
- Were there persons who made a special contribution to promoting networks/facilitating project
- Explore understanding of stage of project; planning/policy
- Explore understanding of roles of different sectors

Community involvement

- Who was represented
- Leadership/ownership
- Level of attendance and commitment

Needs assessment

- Methods; focus groups/surveys
- Whether critical priorities tackled
- Community-statutory sector conflict on main issues
- Partisan views; evidence that needy groups unrepresented

Policy development

- Community involvement in policy development
- Knowledge and views about funding of, and responsibility for new policy

Overview

- Benefits of community involvement
- Lessons/weaknesses
- Generalizability
- Personal expectations; at beginning, and now
- Will community have (some) control over budgets
- What is needed for continued evolution of the process

11 Liverpool minorities health survey – HIV/AIDS

Femi Oduneye

HIV infection has been described as the greatest new public health challenge this century (Department of Health, 1992). This relative importance resulted in it being included as one of the five key Health of the Nation target areas, despite the comparatively low mortality rate. The problems that HIV infection currently pose or may present in the future is therefore of considerable importance to all sections of the population.

The experience in America has demonstrated that no section of the community should be left behind in the drive to overcome the epidemic. The disproportionately high HIV/AIDS morbidity and mortality within the ethnic minority communities of America, immediately comes to mind and this has been well documented (National Commission of Aids, 1992; New York State Department of Health, 1992; Miller, 1990; Public Health Service, 1990). For example, in 1989 the age - adjusted HIV related death rate among African American males was three times that of white males while African American females were nine times more likely to die from HIV than white females (United States and Prevention Profile, 1991).

Policy documents in England do recognise this and have identified black and racial minority communities as being among the groups that should be specially targeted when planning HIV programmes (Department of Health, 1992; The Health of the Nation, 1992). The prioritization of this group might also have been necessitated by the fact that there is a difference in the uptake of health services by these communities, in addition to language and communication difficulties and cultural/religious differences (Balarajam and Raleigh, 1993).

The need for information

In order to plan and deliver a robust HIV prevention programme within

Liverpool's black and racial minority communities, there was a need for reliable information. This paper describes aspects of the process used to obtain that information.

While epidemiological and demographic data are readily available from OPCS, there was no existing data on the views of these communities, their health promotion needs and level of knowledge and attitude to HIV/AIDS. This data was needed for the planning of an effective health promotion programme, especially when dealing with such a sensitive issue. In order to address this information gap, Liverpool Health Authority, commissioned the survey described here. The aim of the survey was to obtain baseline information from Liverpool's racial minority population which could be used in planning and implementing health promotion and education activities for HIV/AIDS within these communities. This had to be achieved against a historical background of "short-termism" in policy initiatives, and of extensive survey work which had resulted in little concrete benefit to the communities concerned. Thus, for the project to yield meaningful results, there was a need to ensure, in so far as was possible, the following:

1. Community participation at all stages.

2. To recognise the diversity within the racial minority population as a whole and ensure that this was reflected in the methodology.

3. The collection of both qualitative and quantitative data.

4. To develop good and constructive relationships with the community on such a sensitive issue as HIV/AIDS, which would assist future work with these communities.

In 1991, the 1991 Census included, for the first time, a question on ethnicity. Liverpools' ethnic minority population, according to the 1991 Census is 17,052, which amounts to 3.77 per cent of the total population, compared to 5.9 per cent nationally (see Table 11.1) (Liverpool Public Health Annual Report).

The response to the Census based on how individuals view their ethnic group, allows for the non-white population of England and Wales to be divided into nine categories (see Table 11.2). This is an attempt to place into broad categories the diverse range of people that contribute to the non-white population.

Table 11.1
The non-white populations of England and Wales and of Liverpool

	England and Wales	Liverpool
Total population	49,890,000	452,480
Non-white population	2,952,000	17,052
Non-white population (%)	5.9%	3.8%

Source: 1991 Census

Table 11.2
Categories of the non-white population used in the 1991 census, and composition (% of total non-white population)

Ethnic Group	England and Wales (%)	Liverpool (%)
Black Caribbean	16.9	8.9
Black African	7.1	14.5
Black Other	6.0	19.2
Indian	28.1	7.9
Pakistani	15.4	3.7
Bangladeshi	5.5	2.4
Chinese	5.0	19.4
Other Asian	6.5	4.1
Other	9.5	20.1

Source: 1991 Census

There are, however, notable disparities between the above classification and the groupings that exist in reality within the communities, as the latter is usually formed around religions and nationality. Whilst the Census classification has nine categories for the non-white population, there are over 20 community groups representing the interests of these communities (see Table 11.3). This further demonstrates the disparity between the way people group and associate with one another and the attempt nationally to classify these communities.

Table 11.3
The diversity of ethnic minority community groups
within the nine non-white census categories

Census category	Examples of related community groups
Black Caribbean	Merseyside Caribbean Council
Black African	The Ibo Union
	Merseyside Somali Community Association
	Liverpool Somali Association
	Somali Womens Association
	Nigerian National Union
	Ibo Womens Association
Black Other	The Methodist Centre
	Liverpool Black Sisters
Indian	Friends Information Centre
	Hindu Cultural Organisation
	Liverpool Muslim Society
	The Sikh Community Organisation
Pakistan	Liverpool Muslim Society
	Friends Information Centre
	Pakistan Community Association
Bangladeshi	Bangladesh Community Association
	Liverpool Muslim Society
Chinese	Wah Sing Community Association
	See Yip Community Association
	The Chinese Pagoda Community Centre
Other Asian	Hindu Centre
	Liverpool Muslim Society
	Vietnamese Community
Other	Yemeni

Approximately 46 per cent of these ethnic minority communities reside in four electoral wards (Granby, Abercromby, Arundel and Smithdown) while the rest are widely dispersed across the city. These four wards are among the most socially deprived wards in the city as demonstrated by their Jarman score (see Table 11.4). The Jarman scores of the 33 wards in the city range from -9.4 to 56.7 (Preliminary Neighbourhood profile, 1994). Some of the communities also have a considerable percentage of people who do not speak English and may have literacy problems in their own language (Rudat, 1994).

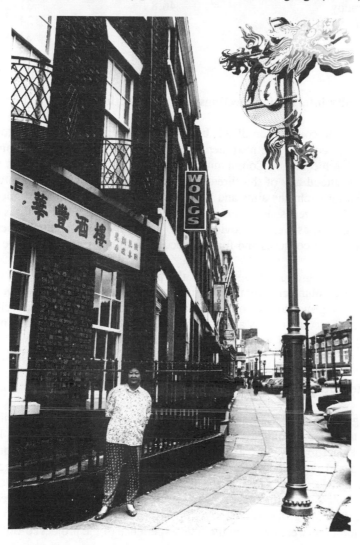

The social organization of ethnic minority communities is often much more complex than suggested by the administrative categories such as those in the census

Table 11.4
Jarman score for the four electoral wards in Liverpool
in which around 46% of the city's non-white population live

Ward	Jarman Score	Rank (1-33)
Abercromby	46.8	31
Arundel	33.7	24
Granby	56.7	33
Smithdown	38.8	28

Community information meetings and consultation

Following the compilation of this background information necessary to place the work in context, the next step was to organise three sets of community information meetings. Community leaders and other key informants where invited to attend any of the three meetings. The aim was to inform people about the research, the aims and what we hoped to achieve. These meetings sought to gain their support and ask for their involvement as members of the steering group, as well as providing an opportunity for community members to express their concerns and for any necessary adjustments to be made to the process.

The steering group was set up for the purpose of nominating and vetting prospective volunteers from the communities taking part in the survey. In addition, the group advised on the suitability of the survey methods, facilitated access to the communities and also reviewed the questionnaire thus making it more responsive to sensitivities within the various groups.

Interview design

In designing the interview schedule, while it was recognized that it might be useful to utilise an already existing questionnaire, the need to have locally relevant questions was of greater importance. Also, qualitative input was required and the difficulty of analyzing and presenting that on a large scale was accepted. The section of the interview designed to assess the level of knowledge by the community was based on a list of questions provided by a local community group as the most important things they would like to know. Other questions were based on the field experience of the project co-ordinator.

Volunteer interviewer training

Because of language barriers and a need for qualitative feedback, bilingual volunteers were recruited from the communities. They were trained in communication skills and interviewing techniques. The training included going though the survey instrument and discussing the rationale for each question. This was necessary as detailed qualitative feed back was expected without undue prompting. The survey interview was adjusted after the pilot study based on the experiences of the volunteers.

Selection of respondents

The sample size was 258, judged adequate to give acceptable statistical precision in responses for the whole group of respondents. The sample however, covered the numerous distinct communities that make up the ethnic minority population. Proportional quotas were then allocated to the various communities using the 1991 Census figures with the proviso that the minimum number of interviewees per community should be ten, so that some feel for circumstances specific to a given community could be gained - at least through the qualitative responses.

Respondents were randomly selected from community group lists, and interviews in places preferred by the respondents, carried including: their homes, community centres, religious centres, libraries and other public facilities. All respondents received £5 in exchange for their participation. A total of 200 interviews were conducted, giving a response rate of 77.5 per cent. Where the selected individual was not available after three visits at different times or refused to be interviewed, they were not replaced.

Interviews were carried out individually, by in small blocks of ten. Each block was followed by a meeting with the project co-ordinator in order to determine difficulties encountered in the field and to maintain uniformity of approach. The project co-ordinator also sat in on a few interviewing sessions. Information packs in relevant languages were handed over to respondents after their interviews. The pack contained information on basic HIV/AIDS awareness, HIV and racism and local services available.

One of the greatest challenges in this study was in collating the results as it involved translating a large amount of qualitative information into quantitative data for summary analysis. An example of the way in which the responses to the open question, "What is HIV?", is shown in Table 11.5.

Table 11.5
An example of the criteria used to classify qualitative
responses to open questions for the purposes of summary
analysis on knowledge of HIV/AIDS

Open question	Coded answers	Criteria used
What is HIV	CORRECT	Identification as a VIRUS and /or an infectious agent
	INCORRECT	Anything other than the above

This basic "definition" of HIV was used in this question for the following reasons:

1. Sections of the community do not speak or read english and therefore may not be able to relay the specific terms for HIV in their language. Since language is a reflection of culture, the concept of a virus if absent from a culture therefore leads to the absence of specific terms for the word virus in that language. Even when new terms are coined they may not be widely understood and usually serve academic purposes. For example, amongst the Yorubas from West Africa, causes of illness are traditionally defined in terms of physical changes and or spiritual or supernatural elements.

2. The main purpose of ascertaining the knowledge of HIV is related to the ability of the individual to identify it as the agent of infection and thereby differentiating it from AIDS which is the resulting syndrome.

Similar concepts informed the definition of the various criteria used in deriving the results, that is:

1. The appreciation of the question/concept in the simplest form.

2. The relevance of the answers to the achievement of the objectives of the survey which is primarily health promotion and education.

Once the analysis is complete the final step in the process will be to draw up recommendations which would then be used by Liverpool Health Authorities in the planning of HIV/AIDS services to ethnic minority communities. We plan to do this through a half day seminar with community leaders and other key informants. It is very important that the community has the opportunity to discuss the results of the survey and provide what they consider to be the most effective way of tackling the issues. The involvement of the community at the beginning of the process gives the project the necessary legitimacy and credibility which will allow the community to treat the results of this work in a more constructive and balanced way.

Conclusion

The process itself has provided some benefits, other than those arising directly from the research and recommendations which follows, and these include:

1. The training of 12 volunteers from the community in communication and research skills, and interviewing techniques. This resulted in them being awarded Introductory Certificates in Community Research by the City of Liverpool Community College.

2. Increased level of awareness of HIV/AIDS issues by interviewees and interviewers.

3. Demonstration of the possibility of involving the community in the design and implementation of a survey of this nature.

4. Development of positive relationship with the community in dealing with a sensitive issue.

5. Though undeniably time consuming, the project has demonstrated the feasibility of gathering qualitative information for planning purposes.

6. The qualitative information will be used in designing training programmes, campaigns and development of resources. For example, a low level of awareness of existing HIV testing services and services for HIV positive people would necessitate development by the relevant agencies of action plans to increase the uptake of their services by members of these communities. The type of information available from this study will be of particular value in that process.

References

Department of Health (1992), *Key Area Handbook HIV and Sexual Health*, HMSO, London.

National Commission on AIDS (1992), "The Challenge of HIV/AIDS in Communities of Color", *National Commission on AIDS*, Washington DC.

New York State Department of Health (1992), *AIDS in New York State*, NYS DOH, Albany, NY 12237.

The Health of the Nation: A strategy for Health in England, (1992), Presented to Parliament by the Secretary of State for Health, HMSO, London.

Balarajam, R. and Raleigh, V.S. (1993), *Ethnicity and Health. A Guide for the NHS*, Department of Health.

Liverpool Public Health Annual Report 1992, Department of Public Health, Liverpool.

Preliminary Neighbourhood Profile - Neighbourhood 9, (1994), Department of Public Health, Liverpool.

Miller, H. (1990), *AIDS: The Second Decade*, National Academy Press, Washington, DC.

Department of Health and Human Services (1990), *Public Health Service: Healthy People 2000: National Health Promotion and Disease Prevention Objectives - Conference Edition*, Washington, DC, DHHS.

Rudat, K. (1994), *Black and Minority Ethnic Groups in England -Health and Lifestyles*, Health Education Authority, London.

Department of Health and Human Sciences (1991), *Health: United States and Prevention Profile*, DHHS Pub, no. 92-1232. Hyattsville, Maryland: Department of Health and Human Sciences 1992.

12 Immigrants and health in Amsterdam: A case study on the translation of research into action

Joop ten Dam

The problem

Practical

Research into initiatives aimed at improving local health, conducted within the framework of the Healthy Cities project (ten Dam, 1995), shows that many health related projects are based on research which examines the health profile of a neighbourhood or district. Translation of this research into actions, however, is not particularly simple. Research does not usually give adequate coverage of the needs and problems which were identified while these should, to a large extent, form the basis of any project. The basis of a project should therefore be formed, not by needs which the professionals assume to exist, but by the actual needs identified by those directly affected by the projects. It is worthwhile (but not often done) to involve at a very early stage, those people who will be directly affected by the project and allow them to provide input in as many aspects as possible of local health initiatives. Useful strategies to achieve this are, for example, to aim at a specific group in a local context, to avoid stigmatization and "blaming the victim" and to involve local volunteers in professional initiatives. In order to correspond to existing wants and needs, it is necessary to agree on a broad definition of health and to work on collaboration between institutions concerned on health related issues (both on implementation and management level). In addition, it is also vital to take account of the generally narrower definition of health. In doing so, clarity is given to inhabitants, to collaborating institutions, and to those providing subsidies. Finally, it is important to make the project itself and the results thereof as transparent as possible.

However there are pitfalls and difficulties in initiating Healthy Cities projects in urban neighbourhoods, especially when low income groups e.g.

immigrants, are involved. Some of the questions which may be posed are:

1.   How to resolve the conflict between "waiting for the people to act" (bottom up) and professional initiatives (top down)?

2.   How to organize collaboration in health related areas between sectors who have not previously worked together?

3.   How to put healthy communities on the political agenda?

4.   How to avoid epidemiological research resulting in no action?

   The Dutch local health project "Immigrants and Health"' is an attempt to find answers to these questions and to bring action and research together.

Theoretical background

Before coming to the health project, we have to analyze some problems of a more theoretical nature. As we found, at times, assumptions and definitions are utilized in Healthy Cities projects which, later, prove to complicate the issues. Here we name four; the broad definition of health as an aspect of medicalization, the relation to everyday life, the neighbourhood concept, and the assumption that everyone is willing to invest in health.

Medicalization Local health policy initiatives and the adoption of a broad definition of health, as is the case in the Healthy Cities project, are aspects of the further deepening of the standard of health in society. If health policy thus far was restricted to the elimination of illnesses and the organization of care, now health itself is also the object of intervention. In his model, Lalonde (1974) shows that not only are individual illnesses and health care the focus of policy but also lifestyle and the social and physical environment. Local health policy is therefore not neutral but may also be seen as a form of medicalization (Parsons, 1951; Freidson, 1970; Zola, 1972; Illich, 1975; Crawford, 1980). Lay people become proto-professionals and the healthy become potential patients. However, health may also be viewed in a positive manner, namely, as an investment for society: health as capital (Bourdieu, 1989). In a society where social mobility exists and where health is a great benefit, it is possible to use health as a stepping stone to a better position in the social structure. The opposite may also be true: poor or neglected health can lead to negative selection, whereby one must take lower status jobs with lower income and responsibility. This process can occur during the course of a lifetime but

140

can also take place from one generation to the next. Excellent health is a prized road to success while poor health can lead to failure (ten Dam, 1995).

Social and cultural environment The social and cultural environment plays an important role in the Healthy Cities project. How people perceive their own health is especially important when discussing increased involvement in health matters. People's social and cultural environments are, however, affected by the economic system. Habermas (1981) calls this the colonization of the life world. The economic process, focused on profit maximization, supplants the communicative process which is focused on communication and mutual agreement. The medicalization of society may be regarded as one of the aspects of this colonization process. In essence, colonization concerns communication being superseded by the rational actions of professionals (Mol and Van Lieshout, 1989). However, the further this process goes, the opportunities to resist medicalization also increase. The system's functioning creates its own counter forces. Thus, new social movements like that in psychiatry, the women's issues and the environment are, according to Habermas, manifestations thereof. Developments are thus not solely one sided as in Foucault's disciplining process: Habermas speaks of increased rationalization and of the increased power of the counter forces. Self organization concerning health matters, such as self help and resistance, is more than a form of proto-professionalization which can be viewed as a higher rung on the ladder of discipline and medicalization. It is also an opportunity to resist that discipline.

Neighbourhood In local health policy "local" is usually understood as "neighbourhood" while "neighbourhood" is taken to mean "community". There are several practical reasons for using the neighbourhood as a focal point. Differences in health are best observed on a local level. In addition, citizens at a local level have the greatest chance of influencing policy: the institutions are closer to the inhabitants, a shared culture exists and it is easier to gain a clear view of the situation. In addition, working on a local level provides greater opportunities to communicate with citizens on health related issues. For various reasons, collaboration on a local level is easier to bring about than at a regional or national level. Hancock pointed out that policy makers on a local level take decisions that often affect their own living and working conditions (Hancock, 1990). A social network approach at neighbourhood level can increase the existing social support and can offer alternatives to the difficulties in reaching lower income groups (Walle-Sevenster and Kok, 1991). Finally, working at a neighbourhood level corresponds to the current tendency to work less with a planned top down approach. Instead of this approach, a more differentiated intervention is adopted whereby those affected by the projects are directly involved (Rijkschroeff, 1989).

There are, however, a number of comments on the manner in which the definition of neighbourhood has been used:

1.   Instead of the commonly shared neighbourhood culture the past 50 years have led to the development of individual private households while, at the same time, the anonymous arrangement of the welfare state has come into existence. People have become decreasingly dependant on each other as they might have once been in times of lesser prosperity. Because of this increased independence, people tend to behave more like individual consumers. Contacts with distant friends have often become more important than contacts with one's own neighbours. Consequently, the solid community culture that once existed now makes way for a more individualistic style of living.

2.   Neighbourhoods are now characterized more by the lifestyle of those who live there rather than a common class or history. Some neighbourhoods are attractive for parents with children while others are more suited to single person households or double income households.

Neighbourhoods have, therefore, become more like arenas than communities. Approaching a neighbourhood with the assumption that it is a community with a shared culture and solidarity will lead to disappointment.[1] A more differentiated approach is necessary.

Health cultures   Often the assumption is made that all people want to live healthy and long lives and will therefore invest greatly in order to achieve this goal. This is, however, a middle class attitude towards health. Using the social theory of Merton (1958), the group grid model of Douglas (1978) and the culture theory of Thompson (et al. 1990) and Engbersen (et al. 1993) a number of different health cultures can be identified. The criteria for differentiating the separate behaviour patterns or strategies are "group" and "grid". The group represents the extent to which someone's life is controlled by the membership to a group. In a strong group there is a great difference between "us" and "them". Group members do not step outside the group. Grid indicates the extent to which ones life is driven by rules. Differentiated roles and a clear hierarchy are associated with a strong grid. With the differentiation between strong/weak grid and strong/weak group, five health cultures can be identified (see Figure 12.1):

142

fatalism (e.g. fetishists), individualism (workaholics, alcoholics or drug addicts), hierarchy (cautious citizens), egalitarianism (uncontrolled labourers), and autonomy (tramps and people with alternative lifestyles). Not every culture is open to a call to improve health. Only the hierarchial culture is really suited. Before the implementation of a local health initiative, the health culture of those affected must be established.

To summarize, from the viewpoint of medicalization it is essential not only to see health promotion as an important and universal objective, but also to have a keen eye on the negative aspects, such as the compulsion the health ideal can impose on people. The connection between health as perceived in everyday life and health promotion is important as well as complicated. It is useful to look at the system influences on the "life world" of people, and at the possible role of self organizations. The neighbourhood approach is equally prominent, but due to changes in urban neighbourhoods it needs to be more differentiated. Lastly, the significance of the different cultures of health for local health initiatives is demonstrated.

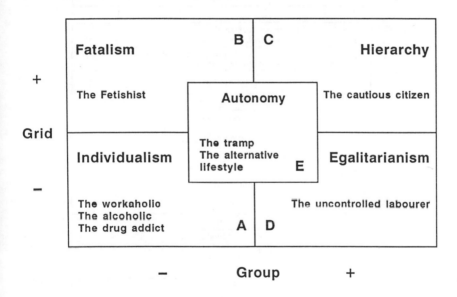

Figure 12.1   Health cultures

The project

This paragraph describes an intervention project that was aimed at improving the health status of Turkish and Moroccan immigrants in an area of north Amsterdam.[2] The project is a part of Health in City Boroughs, the local health policy of the Health Service in Amsterdam. The goal of this project is twofold: an improvement in the health of immigrants, and a policy methods goal: finding ways in which obstacles can be eliminated. The central focus of the project is on a number of conferences held with health care workers and immigrants on the subject of the health problems of immigrants in the neighbourhood and possible solutions to these problems. These conferences are based on research conducted on the neighbourhood's health status, on discussions with health care workers and immigrant associations and on discussions with individual immigrants in the Van der Pek neighbourhood on issues of health, illness and care. The reports of the latter discussions are in the form of so called individual health profiles: brief individual life histories on the themes of health, illness, and care. The research design is shown in Figure 12.2.

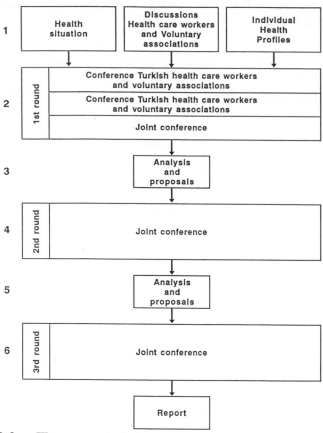

Figure 12.2   The research design

144

The project is situated in the Van der Pek area of Amsterdam, a small neighbourhood of approximately 5000 inhabitants. It is situated north of the city centre, across the IJ river (see Figure 12.3). The neighbourhood was built in the 1920s for labourers in the ship building industry. After this industry disappeared, many labourers were left unemployed, and the housing in this area is no longer up to standard. Residences have low rents and are usually small, have no central heating and are often damp. The original inhabitants have, whenever possible, left the neighbourhood and moved to the suburbs, and Turkish and Moroccan immigrants have since replaced them. The immigrants now make up approximately half of the population of the neighbourhood. As a result, Van der Pek has the highest percentage of immigrants in Amsterdam. The unemployment rate among immigrants is high and their level of education low. As can be observed in Figure 1.3, the general health status of the Van der Pek neighbourhood is poor compared to the average health status for the rest of Amsterdam (Lau-IJzerman et al. 1980; Van der Maas et al. 1987; De Ceuninck van Capelle et al. 1992). The health status was measured using standardized mortality rate, hospitalization rates, and unsuitability for employment.

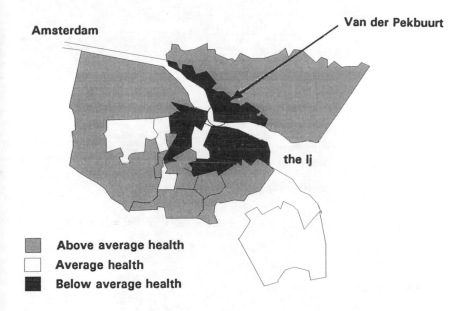

Figure 12.3 Amsterdam and the Van der Pek neighbourhood showing overall health status

145

This is done not on an individual, but on the neighbourhood level, using existing data mainly from various Amsterdam municipal services. The most common health complaints proved to be respiratory illnesses, back problems and afflictions of the digestive system. Health care and social facilities are well represented in the Van der Pek neighbourhood: general practitioners, community services, mental health services, physiotherapists, dentists, pharmacies, social workers, and community workers are all present. In spite of the occasional collaboration, care giving institutions are usually at cross purposes with each other. This is especially the case for initiatives that are geared toward immigrants.

The course of the project: phase I

The delphi approach

Given the goal of the research, the chosen research method is a variation of the so called Delphi method.

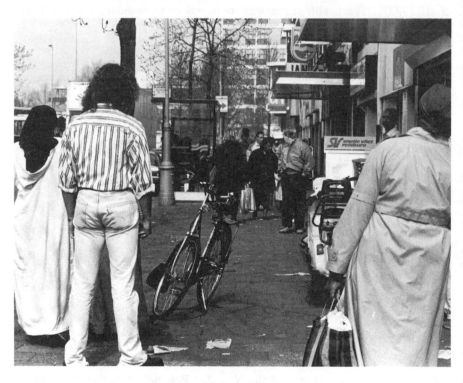

The Van der Pek neighbourhood, Amsterdam   Source: Joop ten Dam

146

This variation can be described as scenario research whereby the goal is "to involve clients, care workers and other directly interested parties in the development of the design and contents of (mental) health care in an open dialogue aimed at consensus" (Rijkschroeff, 1989). The method consists of a number of rounds of discussions. Every round of discussion consists of one or more conferences, whereby as many as possible of the interested parties are represented. Primarily, these conferences are based on individual health profiles which describe personal experiences and expectations concerning health, illness and health care of Turkish and Moroccan inhabitants. In total, three rounds of discussion were held. This research design is not only intended to utilize the knowledge of experts but also to incorporate the experiences of immigrants.

Interviews

Considering that the statistics only give a limited amount of information concerning health, illness, and care, intensive interviews were held with all the concerned care givers and immigrants associations. An important goal of these interviews was to establish how care givers and the associations viewed the question of immigrants and their health status. In addition, existing areas of collaboration were investigated. Finally, these interviews were used to examine to what extent people were willing to invest time and energy in participating in conferences and co-operating with possible intervention projects. In other words, the extent to which those involved were committed to the problem at hand.

Individual health profiles

In order to gain an accurate account of the health problems of immigrants residing in the Van der Pek neighbourhood, individual health profiles of nine inhabitants were constructed using prolonged interviews. The profiles are brief life histories of health, illness and care. In order to avoid a biased picture in the selection of the respondents, variables of native country, gender, age, employment and current health status were matched to those of the local population. The respondents were found through intermediate persons in the Moroccan and Turkish communities. The individual health profiles form the basis of the conferences of the first round of discussions. A (condensed) example of the individual health profiles is given in Table 12.1.

Table 12.1
An example of an individual health profile (condensed)

Woman, married 24 years, employed, residing in The Netherlands since 1975.

The respondent does not have any major health problems. From her mother she learned how to use various herbs to treat different ailments. She only uses things in which she herself believes in "if I have the flu I make a herbal tea and if I have sprained something I use flowers, water and oil. That eases the pain." A large amount of attention is given to the meals, enough iron and vitamins must be present. According to this respondent the first generation of immigrants use the methods which they were taught in their home countries before going to a doctor "upon experiencing pain, the second generation is much quicker in going to a doctor."

She states that especially the first generation is plagued with homesickness, this homesickness brings with it a number of ailments "they pine for ... (the country of origin), but once there, they miss their children". An important problem, especially for the first generation of female immigrants, is the language problem. This brings an extra obstacle to visiting the doctor "they can't explain what is wrong with them anyway."

The use of a husband or child as an interpreter does not automatically mean that they are able to make their complaints understood. An important obstacle is the fact that patients feel that doctors do not have the time or the patience to investigate, together with the patient, what the complaints and causes could be. This is also the case when discussing psychological problems. When the patient has specifically female complaints, embarrassment plays a clear role. This can lead to situations in which the doctor also becomes embarrassed.

The respondent concluded that women usually develop the same complaints as their husbands "This is not surprising: most men belonging to the first generation have been rejected, there is little money, no future prospects and these men are really bored. These feelings are taken out on their wives. Who else should they take it out on?"

Conferences

In total there were three rounds of short conferences of care givers and immigrants associations. The individual health profiles were the main focus of the agenda of the conferences of the first round.[3] The participants were asked if, in their opinion, the health profiles were accurate. The participants were also asked to add any elements they thought were missing. Through the use of the profiles an attempt was made to form a collective definition of the problem. The discussions were recorded on tape and written down verbatim. The texts of these three conferences were distilled to provide the main areas of concern for possible projects. These were then presented to the interested parties for their approval. In order to form project proposals the obstacles which had been named during the conferences were recounted and compared with the obstacles which had been named during the discussions with care givers, the associations, and the people who had given their individual health profiles. Language and cultural differences, lack of knowledge concerning the health care situation in The Netherlands among immigrants, and about immigrants by care givers, as well as lack of knowledge regarding Occupational Disability Insurance and care among general medical practitioners were identified as the main items. The project proposals have therefore been formulated with these obstacles in mind. These proposals were briefly explained at the beginning of the working party of the second round. The participants were then asked to give their reactions to the proposals. Questions regarding the proposals as well as obstacles, possibilities regarding the implementation of the proposals and for financing of the projects were discussed. In addition to the contents of the project proposals, the organizational aspects of the projects were discussed, for instance: who would be named coordinator for the follow up of the proposals; and how politicians should be approached. Following analysis and adjustment by the researchers the revised versions of the proposals were discussed during a third round. A progress report regarding several of the projects was included during this round, since in a number of cases, projects had already been initiated during the summer months. For example, discussions were held regarding the organization of language courses and a request for subsidies was submitted for the project concerning Occupational Disability Insurance groups for immigrants.

The course of the project: phase II

In October 1992, the active intervention of the research team with the project was rounded off with a presentation of the research report titled Healthy Collaboration (ten Dam et al. 1992). The head of the research team has kept in contact with the original initiatives and played a supporting role in most of the meetings later on. In the following December, the report was discussed with the participating institutions. The parties concerned were satisfied with the report and the progress to date. Hope was expressed that the report would not remain only on paper but that actual initiatives in the area of health and the immigrants of the Van der Pek neighbourhood would be encouraged. The board of the Boroughs Council for north Amsterdam will play a vital role.[4] The board had welcomed the initiative at the onset and had promised to provide financial support if a satisfactory proposal were submitted. The Occupational

149

Disability Insurance group for immigrants has since been subsidized and began in February 1993. The project has been given a working title of Health Information Centre. This name can be easily translated into both Turkish and Moroccan.

In the months leading up to the summer of 1993, most of the institutions concerned — the steering committee — developed activities which could be used in the Health Information Centre. In addition, the organizational structure and the finances of the centre were reviewed. The centre should be a collaboration between already existing institutions rather than a new institution. In most cases, the communication between institutions is maintained by an appointed contact person. It is this person's responsibility to inform the directors of all developments. The institutions which are most involved are the Amsterdam Community Health Services, the Health Education Bureau Amsterdam, North Amsterdam Community Development, the Amsterdam General Social Services, Mental Health Institute North Amsterdam, Youth Health Care, and the Amsterdam Municipal Health Service. Several of the existing plans of these institutions may be adjusted to suit the new centre. For example, Youth Health Care plans to give courses concerning children and upbringing. The Health Education Bureau regards the centre as a suitable place to distribute information materials. Community Health Services is searching for a location in North Amsterdam for a "home care bureau".

During the course of the autumn of 1993 and the winter of 1994 the Council of the borough of North Amsterdam kept their promise to financially support the initiative. The sum of 82,000 Hfl. to be used over a two year period would be set aside and a start subsidy given. The collaborating institutions have, as a steering committee, taken an option on a suitable venue. All the participating institutions have put the activities, which will take place in the centre, on paper. The three most important services that the Health Information Centre will provide are: a walk in consultation bureau, activities (such as courses and self help groups) and distributing written information. In this last case, a Gezondheidswijzer (Health Information Centre) may be established. It has been proposed to draw up a contract which the participating organizations must sign in order to give the project a common basis. Lastly, ideas have been developed for the administrative structure of the initiative. It has been proposed to create a foundation with an external chairperson whereby the participating institutions take seats on the board. Discussions have shown there is a significant risk that people will regard this centre as a health care facility. Publicity for the centre must make clear that its responsibilities are to inform and educate on issues of health, illness and care rather than treatment. The steering committee considers it desirable to have a focus which extend beyond the needs of just the immigrants. The most important cause of the poorer health status in the Van der Pek neighbourhood is the lower socio-economic status and only secondly the status of immigrant. Additional policies for the different immigrant populations may also be necessary.

Results

At the time of writing, an elaborated proposal for activities in health related areas in the Van der Pek neighbourhood and its surroundings exists: the Health Information Centre. The centre will be used to work on:

1. Behaviour modification (through the method of health information and education).

2. The improvement of accessibility of care (through information passed on to the health care facilities, education and information, reallocation and renovation of care facilities and representation of patient interests).

3. The improvement of general living conditions in the neighbourhood which influence the health status, for example, the environment and the physical surroundings (through community health work).

This approach is related to the Healthy Cities project in the Dutch Programme for Social Innovation. Important characteristics are the participation of inhabitants, an integral and intersectoral approach and a neighbourhood focus. The planned centre will not be a goal in itself but will be created by restructuring existing branches of various institutions. A growth model will be used: begin small and grow according to the experiences of the centre.

Directly involving the target group with the initiative seems to have given positive results. The input of the immigrants themselves through the individual health profiles ensures that any solutions are closely related to the lifestyles of those affected. Through the use of the individual health profiles associations could be made with the health culture of the immigrants. From the start, the immigrants associations and care givers were involved with designing the initiative. A continuous and open dialogue with politicians was also strived for. Because of this, an uncomplicated transfer can be made from the research (the health situation, the health profiles and discussions with the care givers) to actions (the realization of the centre). The pitfall that after the presentation of the research results nothing more will be undertaken is thereby avoided. In doing so, a strong initiative from below has been brought about which could be reinforced by the researchers. In this way an escape route has been found for a dilemma: directional steering from the top by professionals versus waiting for initiatives from below. Health has become a major issue both in the neighbourhood and in local politics. Because no new (medical) facilities are created and only a reallocation of existing health care and social facilities occurs, the degree of medicalization is minimal. New ways have been found to improve health and care for a specific group.

Notes

1. In this text the notion "neighbourhood" is used in the geographical (and not the relational) sense of the notion "community".

2. The intervention project was carried out by a research team belonging to the section Urban Studies in the department of General Social Sciences of the University of Utrecht. The team was compromised of Ms P. Liem, Ms I. Starmans, and the author, in co-operation with the Municipal Health Service in Amsterdam and the support of the Research consulting bureau of the Social Sciences faculty of the University of Utrecht (ten Dam et al. 1992 and Starmans et al. 1993). The first phase of the project ran from January to October of 1992. The second phase ran from November 1992, and is still in operation.

3. The first round consisted of three conferences: a first with the Turkish (health) care workers and Turkish immigrant associations, the second with the Moroccan workers and associations and the third conference with the Dutch workers. In the second and third rounds these groups were brought together in one single conference.

4. The City Council of Amsterdam is decentralized into 18 Borough Councils.

References

Bourdieu, P. (1989), *Opstellen Over Smaak, Nabitus en Het Veldbegrip (Essays Concerning Taste, Habits and Field Definitions)*, Van Gennep, Amsterdam.
Ceuninck van Capelle, C. de, Herrebrugh I. en E. Jonkers (1992), *Boven

het IJ. *Verkenning van de gezondheidssituatie in Amsterdam-Noord (Above the IJ-river, Introduction to the Health Care Situation in North Amsterdam)*, GG & GD Amsterdam, Amsterdam.

Crawford, R. (1980), "Healthism and the Medicalization of Everyday Life", *International Journal of Health Services*, vol. 10, no. 3, pp. 365-89.

Dam, ten J., Liem, P. en Starmans, I. (1992), *Gezonde Samenwerking,. Een Interventieproject Rond Gezondheid van Migranten in de Van der Pekbuurt, Amsterdam-Noord (Healthy Collaboration, an Intervention Project Concerning the Health of Immigrants in the Van der Pek-Neighbourhood, North Amsterdam)*, Wetenschapswinkel Sociale Wetenschappen, Utrecht.

Dam, ten, J. (1995), *Health in the Local Context*, Forthcoming.

Douglas, M. (1978), *Cultural Bias*, Royal Anthropological Institute, London.

Engbersen, G., Schuyt, K., Timmer, J. en van Waarden, F. (1993), *Cultures of Unemployment. A Comparative Look at Long-Term Unemployment and Urban Poverty*, Westview Press, Boulder.

Freidson, E. (1970), *Profession of Medicine: A Study of the Sociology of Applied Knowledge*, Dodd, Mead and Company, New York.

Habermas, J. (1981), *Theorie des Kommunikativen Handelns. Band 1. Hand lungsrationalitat und Gesellschaftliche Rationalisierung. Band 2. Zur Kritik der funktionalistischen Vernunft (Theory of Communicative Actions. Volume 1: Acting Rationality and Communal Rationalisation. Volume 2: On the Criticism of Functional Rationality)*, Suhrkamp, Frankfurt am Main.

Hancock, T. (1990), "Developing Healthy Public Policies at the Local Level" in Evers, A., Farrant, W. and Trojan, A. (ed.), *Healthy Public Policy at the Local Level*, Campus Verlag, Frankfurt am Main.

llich, I. (1975), *Het Medisch Bedrijf - Een Bedreiging Voor de Gezondheid? (The Medical Institution - A Threat to Health?)*, HetWereldvenster, Baarn, Original: Medical Nemesis, 1974.

Lalonde, L. (1974), *A New Perspective on the Health of Canadians. A Working Document*, Health and Welfare Canada, Ottawa.

Lau-IJzerman, A., Habbema, J.D.F. and van der Maas, P.J. (1980), *Vergelijkend Buurtonderzoek Naar Sterfte, Ziekenhuisopname en Arbeidsongeschiktheid in Amsterdam: Eindrapport (Comparitive Neighbourhood Research of Death, Hospitalisation, and Unsuitability for Employment in Amsterdam, Final Report)*, GG & GD Amsterdam, Amsterdam.

Maas, P.J. van der, Habbema, J.D.F. en van der Bos, G.A.M. (1987), *Vergelijkend Buurtonderzoek Amsterdam II 1977-1983: Naar Sterfte, Ziekenhuisopnamen (Comparitive Neighbourhood Research Amsterdam II*

1977-1983: Into Death and Hospitalisation), UvA, Instituut voor Sociale Geneeskunde, Amsterdam.

Merton, R.K. (1958), "Social Structure and Anomie" in Merton, R.K. (ed.), *Social Theory and Social Structure*, Glencoe Illinois, Second edition.

Mol, A. en van Lieshout, P. (1989), *Ziek Zijn is Het Woord Niet. Medicalisering, Normalisering en de Veranderende Taal van Huisartsgeneeskunde en Geestelijke Gezondheidszorg, 1945-1985 (Being Sick is Not the Term. Medicalisation, Normalisation and the Changing Language of General Medical Practice and Mental Health, 1945-1985)*, SUN, Nijmegen, p. 166.

Parsons, T. (1951), *The Social System*, The Free Press, New York.

Rijkschroeff, R.A.L. (1989), *Ondersteuning van Participatie in de Ggeestelijke Gezondheidszorg (Support of the Participation in Mental Health Care)*, Platform GGZ Amsterdam, Proefschrift Universiteit van Amsterdam, Amsterdam, p. 46.

Starmans, I., Liem, P. en ten Dam, J. (1993), "Migranten en Gezondheid in de Van der Pekbuurt; een Interventieproject (Immigrants and Health; an Intervention Project)" in ten Dam, J. en de Leeuw E. (ed.), *Gezonde Steden en Onderzoek. Reikwijdte, Methoden, Toepassingen (Healthy Cities and Research. Range, methods, and applications)*, Van Gorcum, Assen/Maastricht, pp. 26-32.

Thompson, M., Ellis R. and Wildavsky, A. (1990), *Cultural theory*, Westview Press, Boulder.

Walle-Sevenster, J. de en Kok, J.G. (1991), *Gezondheidsbevordering en Armoede (Health Improvement and Poverty)*, NKB-Uitgeverij, Bleiswijk.

Zola, I. (1972), "Medicine as an Institution of Social Control", *Sociological Review*, vol. 20, no. 4, pp. 487-504.

154

13 Researching need for primary care in an inner city housing estate: A comparison of methods

Carol Duncan, Rachel Jewkes, Peter Whincup, Patrick Towe and Keyvan Zahir

Telling it how it was

Broadwater Farm is a council estate in Tottenham, North London. Completed in 1970, it includes some 1,060 dwellings and over 4,000 residents. The population is ethnically diverse and unemployment is estimated to be 40 per cent. Over the years there have been a remarkable variety of community organizations and self reliant initiatives on the estate, which have led to strong assertions of rights to partnerships with the statutory sectors and community participation in decision making. Nonetheless many researchers have "come and done" surveys since the notorious riots of 1985, leaving little feed back, no sense of ownership and generating considerable resentment amongst residents.

In early 1992 the Director of Public Health was invited by the Residents Association to discuss her annual report. This was the start of a dialogue between the Health Authority and residents, an early offshoot of which was the recognition that a greater understanding of the health needs of the estate was needed, not least to inform primary health care developments. Three years on, a major health needs assessment exercise has been completed, a health promotion programme for the estate is underway and a "breaking of the soil" ceremony has been held to mark the commencement of the estate's new Health Centre. The project has been run collaboratively throughout by residents, two Health Authorities and the Local Authority together with local providers.

This chapter reports on the health needs assessment components of the project. The methods used sought to avoid the mistakes of previous research in the area by incorporating a strong commitment to ownership and participation by local people, acknowledging their own skills and knowledge and their need to have their inputs recognized and valued. There is no consensus in the literature on health needs assessment about the best methods

155

for gathering information for planning health interventions and empowering local people. For this reason the health needs assessment incorporated two contrasting approaches, a questionnaire survey and a series of focus groups and was designed in such a way that comparison of the two methods could be possible. Formulated in this way as methodological research, the needs assessment was funded by the North East Thames Regional Health Authority's locally organized research scheme.

Keeping on course

The aim of the research was to investigate the health of residents, priority areas for interventions and the services required in a new health centre. A bid for funding a primary health care centre was placed during the development of the needs assessment work and the research was to inform this process. Intersectoral partnerships inevitably involve a learning process as trust is built between partners and compromises and adjustments made to working practices. Episodes of uncertainty and vulnerability are unavoidable during these processes and at such times the project mission statement (opposite) became the touchstone and helped keep it on course.

The questionnaire survey

Soon after the first meeting with the residents, staff of the Department of Public Health began to develop a proposal for conducting a household survey of health needs, in co-operation with local people. It was realized early on that the success of the research was as dependent on the building of trust and the breaking down of boundaries as it was on the scientific requirements of good study design and analysis. A committee was therefore set up to steer the household survey, with membership drawn from the Department of Public Health of Haringey Health Authority, the Family Health Service Authority and the London Borough of Haringey's Housing Department. This committee met over many months and identified the major areas of inquiry of the questionnaire and oversaw its development.

The main areas covered in questionnaire were: respondent's views of their home and the estate; their health, lifestyle and use of preventive services; their experiences with and views about general practice; and, services which they wished to see in the new health centre. Questions were also concerned with the social demography of the household. Wherever possible standard validated questions from other sources (the General Household Survey for questions on health and disability, and the 28 item General Health Questionnaire, for questions on mental health status, in particular anxiety and depression) were used.

Broadwater Farm Health Centre, Mission Statement

The Broadwater Farm Residents Association Health Project is a community led initiative developed in partnership with the New River District Health Authority, Haringey Health Care, Enfield and Haringey Family Health Services Authority and Haringey Council.

By continuing this partnership the project will deliver realistic, equitable and holistic health care on the basis of accurately assessed needs and on going community participation. This will be achieved by:

(i)   The provision of health information and advice

(ii)   Establishment of a needs assessment process

(iii)   The development of Primary Health Care facilities on the Farm

It will break down bureaucratic barriers and promote mutual respect, genuine listening, inter-agency networking and co-operative decision making.

As a result both the health and well being of the individual and the whole estate of Broadwater Farm will benefit.

A pilot study of a systematic sample of 100 households was undertaken before the main study. Its results were reviewed by the committee and the residents who had been recruited as interviewers took an active role in defining the options for closed questions and in further refining their role.

A list of households was obtained from the Local Authority Housing Department. The estate residents particularly wanted a survey of every household on the estate and so all occupied ones were included in the main survey, with the exception of those already visited in the pilot study. Twenty one interviewers were recruited from the residents and given special training. Each interviewer was allocated a group of households and asked to make contact with an adult householder in each. They were asked either to complete the questionnaire on the doorstep, or to leave it for self completion and subsequent collection. All questionnaires were anonymized and interviewers were paid for each one completed. The survey was carried out over two months, prior to which a leaflet was distributed to each household explaining the survey and its purpose.

The focus group survey

The focus group research was designed to be based on 12 focus groups which would cover males and females separately for the following six age groups: 13-14 years; 15-16 years; 17-20 years; 21-34 years, 35-55 years; and 60 years old and over. The participants were recruited by local residents, who were not researchers, and financial incentives were offered to all recruiters and to all participants. The recruiters were given stratification requirements for each group, which were designed to secure participants who differed from each other, where appropriate, in ethnicity, marital status, employment, ages of their children, life cycle stage and carers. They were asked to find people who were not related or good friends. In order to determine whether this had been achieved, each participant was also asked to complete a brief questionnaire, which enquired about demographic details, health status and medication use.

The focus groups were carried out over a fortnight in May, mostly in the early evenings, and took place about six months after the pilot of the questionnaire survey and before the main household survey was done. There were three facilitators and five note takers who worked in various combinations in the groups; two of whom came from a market research company (Open Mind) and offered their services for free, whilst the others were from the Departments of Public Health and Health Promotion. Discussions were one to one and a half hours long and were audio taped and transcribed. The analysis was carried out by the researchers from the Public Health Department, each analysed the groups they facilitated and those of the third facilitator for whom they had taken notes. They compiled the analyses together into a final report.

Response rates

In all 980 households were invited to take part in the survey. Of these 30 were found to be unoccupied, while a further 110 were inadequately covered by the interviewers and had to be excluded. This left 840, from which 504 questionnaires were returned - a response rate of 60 per cent, which is very similar to that obtained in other questionnaire surveys of this nature (Camden Healthy Cities Project, 1990). Of the 12 focus groups planned, all were held with the exception of the 17-20 age group due to difficulties in recruiting participants. A mixed gender and age focus group was held instead, and overall 70 participants were involved with reasonably close correspondence to the planned characteristics. Ages ranged from 12 to 85 years and they came from a wide variety of ethnic backgrounds. Some had lived on the estate since it opened whilst others had recently arrived from overseas. They lived in all sections of the estate, in all types of accommodation available. Occupation ranged from those at school to the unemployed, students at college, housewives, voluntary workers, retired people and those in paid employment outside the estate.

How did the two studies compare?

The comparison of the studies is based on the following questions:

1.   Do the two methods identify different problems, or convey a different emphasis, which may have different policy implications?

2.   Does one method help to identify priorities better than the other?

3.   Which is more useful for health promotion and health service development?

4.   Which method best promotes the involvement and empowerment of local people?

5.   Which method better represents the views of those whose need is greatest?

6.   How do the methods compare on time and cost?

Nature and emphasis of the information conveyed

The two studies were conducted and analysed without conferring. As would be expected, the character of the information derived from the two studies was very different. The questionnaire survey provided a quantification of the prevalence of socio-demographic, health and lifestyle characteristics, service use and views about services. In contrast to this the focus groups provided, often passionate, insights into the meaning of social problems such as unemployment for individuals concerned. Residents gave vibrant descriptions of cockroaches in their food, difficulties carrying refuse to the chutes whilst caring for small children, the effects of heating problems on the very young and the very old, and the problems of dog mess in the children's playground. Extracts from some of the transcripts are shown in Table 13.1.

In most cases the contrasting methods did not so much identify different problems as different aspects or facets of the same problem. The additional flexibility of the focus groups did however enable new problems to be raised which had not been included in the questionnaire planning stages, one example of which was the need for low cost entertainment facilities for young people. Both the questionnaire and the focus groups revealed different information on smoking which in their own way had different implications health promotion. The survey revealed substantial inter-ethnic differences in smoking prevalence which potentially could influence the targeting of health promotion programmes, although in practice this might be more difficult. The focus groups provided insight into the subjective experience of smoking, raising some of the barriers to smoking cessation, an understanding of which is vitally important to effective health promotion.

Overall, the two types of survey work proved complimentary and the depth of understanding of need was greatly enhanced by having data collected in these contrasting ways. It appeared that the questionnaire survey generated information on the presence or absence of disease, reflecting a biomedical model of health or "negative health", the focus groups tended to generate data relating to factors which influence the state of well being of people on the estate, or "positive health".

Identifying priorities

Both the questionnaire survey and the focus groups provided information which helped to shape the development of the Primary Care Centre. The demographic information on the estate population, demonstrating its youth and the high proportion of households with children, suggested that antenatal care and child health services were likely to be particularly important in this community. This was borne out by the specific questions about the new Health Centre, which identified child health clinics (including both child development and immunization), antenatal care and also family planning services as being of high priority.

The focus groups provided a similar emphasis on specific services. However, they made concrete suggestions about particular needs, for example a creche for mothers visiting the surgery and a dispensing chemist (the nearest chemist to the estate did not dispense). They also emphasized the importance of same day consultations and of a translation and link worker service, particularly for Turkish and Kurdish residents.

Several problems with accommodation were raised consistently in both the questionnaire survey and the focus groups.

160

Table 13.1
Extracts from the focus group

Topic	Comment
Heating	When I had Tommy it was September and the heating wasn't on ... and I just put on the cooker in the kitchen to keep the baby warm. I used to bath him in the kitchen because the bathroom was too cold.
Cockroaches	They go all in your clothes and in your food, they are everywhere. [They] give you stress ... especially when you wake up in bed and you have got one crawling down your arm.
Refuse disposal	One some of the floors they are a pain to get to, you have to walk all the way round to them, you can't always leave your kids and run round to the chute, its like a half an hour journey, you have to make your kids walk there and come back.
Services to meet needs	Actually having a range of clinics, because if people's you have a toddler and a little one who is due for an injection and it's chucking it down with rain and you live on the 15th floor, the effort is enormous. But to have a place where there can be antenatal, family planning, children's clinics, geriatric, chiropodist, just a range, even once every two weeks or something, it doesn't need everything there all the time, but just catering for people.
Social conditions and	I met somebody the other day who is a good health worker and really is somebody that can make a job out of nothing ... he said to me "I am so depressed" I said "Why?". He said "I can't find anything to do" and he said "what's happening to me is people that I used to go with, when I was bad," (he put it like that) "now come back to me and they are drawing me back into drugs and different things that I hoped I had given up." Because there he was trapped in a no go situation.
Giving up smoking	I don't need to, no I would like to, but I enjoy smoking to be honest.

161

The most serious concerns about accommodation were the high levels of cockroach infestation, levels of noise from neighbours, housing repairs and the difficulty in controlling the heating system. The most serious issues on the estate were dog fouling and rubbish collection. An appreciable proportion of respondents were concerned about security, either in their own homes, or on the wider estate. The most important priorities for expenditure of resources on the estate, upgrading of accommodation and security arrangements, reflected these concerns.

From research to implementation

It is difficult to disentangle the precise influence of the research process from other influences including the publicity received by the project and the very process of intersectoral working. The recommendations of both studies, however, were taken into account in the primary care commissioning process (although the decision to fund the project had been taken before the results were available). A cockroach eradication programme was mounted by the local authority after the completion of the pilot survey and focus groups, but before the results of the full survey was completed. In the focus groups poor relationships between the residents and the police and an impasse over management of the estate community centre were raised as important problems. Through the process of participation in the research projects, residents empowered themselves take initiatives to improve these and resolve longstanding tensions.

Following publicity surrounding the needs assessment work, funding has been received for a health information desk, with volunteers given training and paid for their services. Health promotion programmes were revised to become more culturally sensitive and premises were extended to provide additional services for mothers and babies. A nurse practitioner has been funded by the Department of Health. Relationships have been redefined and a commissioning group with newly elected residents are planning the new health centre. Further focus groups have and will take place to reconfirm how residents want health services to be delivered, how they want health information channelled and how user participation can be improved and maintained. Residents now seek greater opportunity to engage in research implementation. Survey work on the Farm has also been utilized to compare need from a neighbouring area.

Promoting involvement

In addition to the partnership which steered the whole project, both research methods were based on the participation of local residents. They identified the need for a survey and substantially influenced the methods followed and areas to be covered by the questionnaire, including insistence on the use of local interviewers. In contrast to this the focus groups were initiated by the researchers and they dictated the methods, although local people recruited participants. However, the participants in the focus groups were able to determine and control the content of the discussion in a way which is not possible when completing a questionnaire. Possibly for this reason, they perceived themselves to be very directly involved in the research and many reported that the process of discussing their problems had been therapeutic. Both the questionnaires and the focus group results were analysed off the estate and written into reports (Duncan and Jewkes, 1993; Whincup, 1991). It might have been possible to involve residents in both these processes but in the event there was not time to do so. When the focus group report was produced people who had participated in the groups eagerly searched through it to find quotes from them. This process was empowering for them and in a very direct way affirmed their knowledge. When the project started residents believed that they needed a health centre for the estate and they essentially used public health research skills in order to help them most effectively achieve their objective. To this extent the partnership was with a quite unusually empowered Resident's Association. Empowerment on a housing estate, or even within a Resident's Association, is not homogeneous and individuals may be empowered to take action on certain issues but not on others. Whilst not being able to really assess or measure it, we believe that the process of involvement in both research projects was empowering for many of the residents as well as the researchers, in particular in so far as a number of concrete initiatives were seen to follow from the findings.

Representativeness

One important concern in research such as this is the extent to which the methods used reflect the views of those most in need and least empowered to participate in the process. The relatively low response rate on the survey indicated that many on the estate did not express their views. Unfortunately we do not know the demographic characteristics of the non-responders, however, interviewers did report that householders from some ethnic minority groups were less likely to take part. Although attempts were made to gain varied groups of participants for the focus groups it is impossible to really understand the extent to which the views expressed in those discussions reflect those more widely held, or in other circumstances expressed, on the estate. The findings of qualitative research are ultimately not generalizable. It may be that we were unable to reach the most needy on the estate and thus provide for them an opportunity for empowerment through the project. Nonetheless the concrete improvements to the estate which followed from the project will hopefully be enjoyed by all and to that extent what is important is that the needs which were identified and prioritized by participants and incorporated into policy responses should be important respects similar to those of non-participants. Whilst we hope this is so and have seen no evidence to the contrary, we ultimately do not know if this is the case.

Resources

The survey was more time consuming and considerably more expensive than the focus groups, however, caution is needed in comparing the two because the focus groups undoubtable benefitted from the lengthy period of relationship building which had been undertaken as part of the process of questionnaire development and survey planning. Both research projects were influenced by periods in which there were other demands on the researcher's time and seasonal and other factors on the estate. The survey took about 18 months to complete, including the pilot, whilst the focus groups took four months. The cost of the survey was five times that of the focus groups.

Conclusions

The work has undoubtedly mobilized resources, created greater participation and to better effect. It has given the Health Authority greater insights in its understanding of community participation in the process of health improvements. Both methods have enriched thinking on "need" and provided an ongoing partnership with the residents. Health promotion programmes are better informed and planned and both types of survey have influenced the design and layout of the health centre as well as the services to be provided. The results from both surveys have become powerful tools in influencing policy and action. The two methodological approaches to needs assessment were ultimately complementary, with the qualitative methods providing valuable insights into the meaning of quantitative findings - making the numbers come alive.

References

Camden Healthy Cities Project, (1990), *St Pancras Ward Health and Environment Project: Results of a Survey*, Camden Healthy Cities Project.
Duncan, C. and Jewkes, R. (1993), *The Health Needs of Broadwater Farm*

Estate: Part One, Findings of the Focus Group Discussions, New River Health Authority.

Whincup, P. (1994), *The Health Needs of Broadwater Farm Estate: Part Two, Findings of the Questionnaire Survey*, New River Health Authority.

14 Monitoring spatial variations in urban health and the delivery of health services: The role of Geographic Information Systems

Alexander Hirschfield

A Geographic Information System (GIS) is a system of hardware, software and procedures designed to support the capture, management, manipulation, analysis, modelling and display of spatially referenced information.

This paper discusses the role of GIS in monitoring health status in urban areas, in identifying relationships between health and social conditions and in analysing the spatial distribution of health services and the patients who use them.

These applications of GIS are discussed through a series of case studies undertaken in north west England by the Regional Research Laboratory at the University of Liverpool. The research has featured the capture and incorporation, within a GIS, of a wide range of address referenced data sets on health related topics including disease notifications, hospital admissions for acute conditions, information on services provided by General Practitioners and community pharmacies, patient registrations (by age and sex), and domiciliary visits by community nurses.

A common approach running through this research has been the use of GIS to forge links between these data sets and contextual information on infrastructure (e.g. digital street networks and transport routes) land use, and the socio-economic environment (e.g. small area statistics on demography, social conditions and deprivation, residential neighbourhood classifications). This has enabled a number of important issues to be explored including the mapping of catchment areas for different services, the identification of spatial overlaps in service provision and mismatches between the siting of facilities and patient populations.

Attention has been drawn recently to the important contribution which Information Technology (IT) is expected to make to the creation of an internal market within Britain's National Health Service (NHS). Indeed, one commentator notes that "it is not an over statement to say that IT is seen as the means by which a market based system of health care provision in the

United Kingdom can be operationalized" (Wrigley, 1991).

One area in which improvements are urgently needed is in the spatial analysis in the demand for and supply of community based health services. The matching of supply to demand is a process which is largely carried out geographically. However, information systems which currently support health care delivery invariably fail to give adequate recognition to the role of space. There is likely to be increasing demand for IT tools which are not only capable of analysing and displaying map based information, but also which feature basic spatial analysis and interactive graphics techniques. This places geographical information systems (GIS) at centre stage.

Geographic information systems and their uses

GIS systems enable links to be established and spatial relationships to be explored between data derived from different sources. There are numerous ways in which a GIS can be used to display, interrogate, cross reference and analyse spatially referenced data sets. Some of the appropriate applications in the context of health include:

1.   The use of GIS map composition options to produce enhanced maps of a health district's social geography which restrict the shading on the map to areas containing residential development (i.e. exclude open space, agricultural land, industrial development, etc).

2.   The use of grid reference co-ordinate mapping to identify actual catchment areas for health services based on the residential location of registered patients.

3.   The production of detailed social profiles for administrative and user defined areas.

4.   The super-imposition of different maps (i.e. GIS map overlay) to reveal how the location of patients and health services relate to other aspects of the social and physical environment (e.g. service boundaries, the street network, residential neighbourhoods).

5.   The use of GIS map overlay facilities to identify the proximity of health service outlets to each other and to other health and social care services.

6.   The use of more complex GIS functions in conjunction with digital street network data to identify areas and patients falling within

specified travel times to selected facilities.

7.   The linking of neighbourhood classification codes to individual patient registrations to profile the types of residential area from which patients are drawn (referred to as "geodemographic analysis").

Applied research by URPERRL

The Urban Research and Policy Evaluation Regional Research Laboratory (URPERRL) at the University of Liverpool is a research unit specializing in applied urban research and the development of information systems for service delivery planning, particularly in the health field (Hirschfield et al. 1991). In recent years, URPERRL has worked with Directors of Public Health and resource managers in several health authorities to explore the potential of GIS as a planning and policy making tool. Applications range from the analysis of relatively rare conditions (e.g. food poisoning, selected cancers) in Blackpool (Brown et al. 1991; Brown et al. 1995), to a comprehensive study of primary health care provision on the Wirral peninsula (Hirschfield et al. 1993; Hirschfield et al. 1995) and an examination of community pharmacy location in Mersey Region (Hirschfield et al. 1994).

A common methodological approach running through most of this research has involved bringing together spatially referenced information from a variety of sources, enhancing it by various means importing it into a GIS, then cross referencing, analysing and displaying it in ways which provide new and useful insights into the deployment of community based health services. Typically the research has involved analysing the data to produce a visual and statistical profile of services in relation to the population, and of patients in relation to services, in order to address a number of important practical questions. These have been concerned with:

1.   The range of services provided in different locations and their correlation with social and health need.

2.   The size and social composition of catchment areas for different services.

3.   The accessibility of health care facilities to patients.

Some of the questions are strategic and concern the spatial organization of health care facilities and their use. Typical examples might be: What is the geographical distribution of GPs in a health district by size of practice and by range of services provided? Are there differences between the more affluent

169

and poorer areas in the way in which primary health care services are organized? Are the larger group practices concentrated in the more affluent areas? Is the range of services provided by GPs (e.g. minor surgery, well person clinics, child health surveillance) better in the more affluent areas? Is there a relationship between deprivation and the use of health services in the area e.g. take up rates for immunization, hospitalization rates, etc).

The intention in addressing these questions would be to shed some light on broader issues concerned with equity of provision and access to services. Evidence abounds to support the notion of an inverse care law where the availability of health care varies inversely with the health needs of the population (Tudor-Hart, 1975). This can be tested, in part, by measuring the relationship between service provision (i.e. the location of facilities and the range of services offered) and social deprivation.

Other questions may concern the characteristics of patients registered with health care providers, for example, their age, the distance they live from a surgery or clinic and the type of residential neighbourhood in which they live (geodemographic analysis). Questions of interest might include:

1.   In which types of residential neighbourhood do patients registered with selected GPs live? (e.g. underprivileged areas, multi-ethnic areas, council estates with elderly people, affluent suburbs).

2.   Do patients experiencing acute health problems (e.g, asthma) live near to facilities offering treatment?

3.   At what distance from the surgery can be found 80 per cent, 90 per cent or 100 per cent of all registered patients?

4.   What proportion of patients live within 2,4,6,8, or 10 minutes drive time from the surgery?

Data capture

Prior to any analysis, information needs to be imported into the GIS software. There are several methods of data capture; digitising (i.e. tracing and digitally storing) spatial objects such as boundaries, line segments (e.g. streets) or points directly from maps, capturing maps as images using a scanner and/or importing existing digital data sets from other sources.

A limited amount of data preparation is often required before some of these techniques can be implemented. In the health field, this will usually involve appending grid references to postcoded patient records to enable point distribution maps to be produced. This can be achieved by matching the unit postcode of the home address of each patient against the Central Postcode Directory. The latter is a correspondence table between each unit postcode in Britain (around 1.5 million in all) and the National Grid Co-ordinate of the lowest numbered address sharing a given unit postcode. Additional processing is required to calculate the total number of patients or health care facilities in each area (e.g. electoral ward) to derive population based rates for subsequent correlation with area based social indicators.

A wide range of data sets have featured in URPERRL's applied research using GIS. They fall into the four broad categories:

1. Background information on the population's social, economic and health status.

2. Information on the spatial location of health/social care facilities (GPs, clinics, hospitals, residential care, community pharmacies) and the range of services they provide.

3. Postcoded data on patients using health care facilities (GPs surgeries, hospitals).

4. Information on administrative and service boundaries and infrastructure.

Examples of background information include demographic, social, economic and health indicators for small areas (e.g. from the 1991 Population Census), deprivation indices, vital statistics and information on the use of health services (e.g. immunization take up rates). Background data provide a framework for the subsequent examination of patient locations and the deployment of community based health services. They also provide the "raw material" used to construct social profiles for user defined areas within the GIS.

Residential neighbourhood classifications

The use of residential neighbourhood classifications (i.e. "geodemographics") has featured prominently in the research and represents a particularly important contextual data set. The term geodemographics refers to the development and application of residential neighbourhood classifications based on census data (Brown, 1991). Geodemographic classifications are generated using cluster analysis techniques to group together areas which are similar in terms of their demographic, socio-economic and housing composition.

In URPERRL's research, attention has been focussed on the use of the

171

Super Profiles Lifestyle Classification. This distinguishes ten clusters, including different types of deprived, middle income and affluent area. The demographic and social characteristics of each cluster are described in Appendix 14.1. Geodemographic analyzes are useful because they provide GPs and other health care professionals with an indication of how the demographic, economic, ethnic and housing characteristics of the population vary within their catchment area. For example, some areas of public housing might contain an over representation of pensioners living alone, others might comprise large families experiencing over crowding. Both types of neighbourhood may be present within a GPs catchment area, although each will present different demands on health services. This highly differentiated view of the population is more likely to give a better indication of potential work load than scoring systems based on aggregating census and other indicators for relatively large administrative areas such as electoral wards (Jarman, 1983).

The general approach has been to capture, on computer, information on the location of health/social care facilities using address lists supplied by the Family Health Services Authorities and local authority social services departments. Inclusion of the full unit postcode for each address is essential as this is used to generate the grid references and electoral ward codes required for mapping and spatial analysis.

In each of the research projects the initial data bases were extended by incorporating information concerning the range of services provided at each site. For example, the address referenced data base on GPs, used in research undertaken in Wirral, included size of practice (number of GPs) and details of additional services provided at the surgery such as minor surgery, child health surveillance, maternity services, contraception advice/services, asthma clinics (Hirschfield et al. 1995).

Patient data

Information about patients obtained for the Wirral research included those registered with GPs and those admitted to Wirral hospitals for four acute conditions; asthma, diabetes, angina and Ischaemic Heart Disease. This was supplied by the Family Health Services Authority and included the postcode, age and sex of each patient on file.

A number of digital boundary files were created or employed for GIS analysis or mapping purposes. These included boundaries used in the population census (enumeration districts and wards) and service area boundaries adopted by the health and local authorities.

Other useful data sets

Other extremely useful strategic data sets have been made available to URPERRL as a result of the laboratory's close research collaboration with the Merseyside Information Service, a local authority research and intelligence unit sponsored by Merseyside's five metropolitan boroughs, and the Fire Service, Police and Development Corporation. The most important of these was a digital street network covering the whole of Merseyside, known as the Merseyside Address Referencing System (MARS) and boundaries demarcating the residential areas.

The digital street network serves several purposes; it can be used to delineate areas falling within specific travel times of health facilities and it can be overlaid with administrative boundaries and point data depicting health care facility and patient locations to produce a comprehensive spatial picture of service provision. An extract from MARS appears as Figure 14.1.

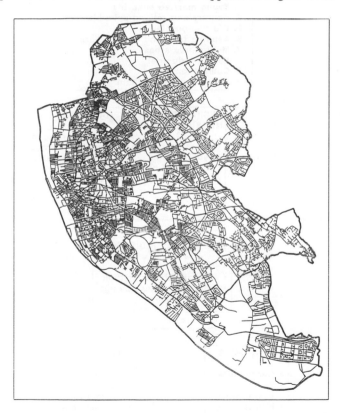

Figure 14.1   **An extract from the Merseyside Address Referencing System, with each line representing one street**

Data consolidation

The analysis of disparate data sets within a GIS, is facilitated considerably if they are organized it into a series topic based files or data modules and accessed through an inter active menu system. A common feature of URPERRL's health services research has been the creation of simple menus for accessing data which will run under "Windows" on a standard PC.

Menu interfaces automate many of the procedures which have to be gone through to call up different data files in order to produce maps. They speed up considerably the whole process of producing maps "interactively" on the computer screen and querying the data which underpin them.

"SUPER PROFILE"
Neighbourhood classification 1981:

1. Affluent minority
2. Metro singles
3. Young married suburbia
4. Country and retiring suburbia
5. Older suburbia
6. Aspiring blue and white collars
7. Multi-ethnic areas
8. Fading industrial
9. Council tenants
10. Underprivileged Britain

GENERAL
PRACTITIONERS

• Practice size
• Additional facilities
 - Child health
 - Minor surgery
 - Maternity
 - Contraception

RESIDENTIAL/
NURSING HOMES

• Client group
• Type of home
• Number of beds

PHARMACIES

• Supplies oxygen
• Needle exchange
• Advice to residential homes
• Patient medication records
• Dispensing volume
• Charged prescriptions
• Non-charged prescriptions

1991 CENSUS INDICATORS

• Population structure
• Household composition
• Long term illness by age
• Unemployment
• Sub-standard housing
• Overcrowding

BOUNDARIES

• Census EDs
• Wards
• L.A. District
• FHSAs
• Service Areas

INFRASTRUCTURE

• Primary roads
• Secondary roads
• Tertiary roads
• Built up area

Figure 14.2   Information modules for the pharmacy location project

The menu system has proven particularly effective in producing user defined maps which cross reference aspects of service provision (e.g. clinics providing family planning services) possible demand (e.g. patients registered with GPs aged 16-20) and the social environment (e.g. areas of deprivation from the super profiles classification). The data modules comprising the GIS menu system for URPERRL's pharmacy location project are shown in Figure 14.2.

Results from selected case studies

The applications of GIS are best illustrated by reference to a series of case studies. There is not the scope, in this paper, to discuss the findings of each project in great detail, although, a few carefully selected examples should serve to illustrate the benefits of adopting a GIS approach.

Enhanced maps

The maps in Figure 14.3 illustrate the use of procedures available within a GIS to produce more refined and meaningful background maps for plotting address referenced patient records and other data sets. Both maps utilize the same data; codes depicting different types of residential area from the super profiles classification. Figure 14.3a is a conventional shaded map in which the entire area of each spatial unit is shaded. In this case the spatial units are Census Enumeration Districts (EDs) containing, on average, 500 persons. In Figure 14.3b, the shading is restricted to those parts of each ED in which there are residential areas. This was achieved by superimposing, upon a conventional shaded map, a digital boundary file depicting all the built up areas on the Wirral. A series of GIS commands was used to eliminate or filter out from the original ED map all non residential areas (e.g. those with commercial or industrial development, public open space, derelict land) to reveal those parts of an ED which contained population. By shading these it was possible to pinpoint, more precisely, the areas where people more likely to have certain social characteristics actually lived.

Locational analyses of patients and health services

In the research on the deployment of community based health services on Wirral, GIS techniques were applied to identify the links and relationships between GP practices and the patients they serve.

175

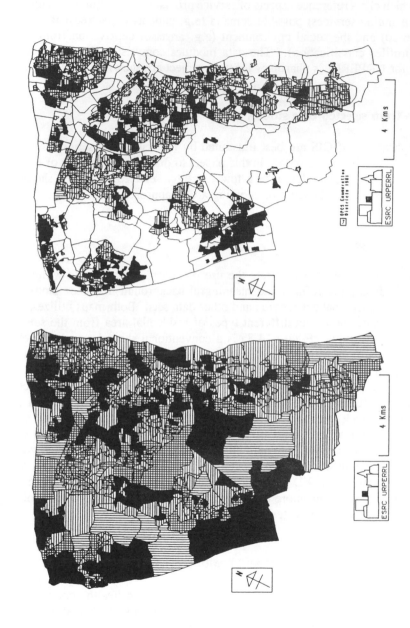

Figure 14.3 Assignment of Wirral enumeration districts to super profile lifestyles for (a) conventional shading of complete enumeration districts and (b) shading restricted to residential areas

To address these issues a study was undertaken focussing on four general practices in contrasting areas of the Wirral; an inner city practice in Birkenhead, a practice on a housing estate in Woodchurch, a practice in the affluent suburb of West Kirby, a fund holding practice in Moreton.

The types of residential neighbourhood from which patients were drawn was examined by counting the number of patients falling into each geodemographic cluster (see Table 14.1).

Table 14.1
**Distribution of number of patients (and %) between super
profile lifestyles by GP practice (Wirral study)**

Super Profile	Practice 1	Practice 2	Practice 3	Practice 4
Affluent minority	140 (4.7)	274 (4.4)	1,533 (35.3)	340 (5.6)
Metro singles	14 (0.5)	119 (1.9)	122 (4.5)	17 (8.0)
Young married suburbia	109 (3.6)	760 (12.1)	197 (4.5)	483 (8.0)
Country and retiring suburbans	44 (1.5)	5 (0.1)	203 (4.7)	109 (1.8)
Older suburbia	163 (5.4)	392 (6.3)	830 (19.1)	937 (15.5)
Aspiring blue and white collars	253 (8.5)	470 (7.5)	688 (15.8)	1,514 (25.1)
Multi-ethnic areas	20 (0.7)	14 (0.2)	4 (0.1)	526 (8.7)
Fading industrial	1,274 (42.6)	108 (1.7)	163 (3.8)	227 (3.8)
Council tenants	516 (17.2)	2,731 (43.6)	568 (13.1)	1,263 (20.9)
The underprivileged	453 (15.1)	1,395 (22.3)	4 (0.1)	623 (10.3)
Unclassified	8 (0.3)	0 (0.0)	34 (0.8)	1 (0.0)
Totals	2,994 (100)	6,268 (100)	4,346 (100)	6,040 (100)

Fifteen per cent of the patients registered with the "inner city" practice (no. 1) and over one-fifth of those attending the Woodchurch estate practice (no.

2) lived in the most seriously deprived residential neighbourhood type "underprivileged Britain." The characteristics of underprivileged Britain included very large families, overcrowded conditions, high levels of unemployment, very low car ownership, very poorly qualified and unskilled labour force. By contrast only a handful of patients registered with the West Kirby practice (no. 3) were drawn from these types of area, although over one-third lived in affluent suburban neighbourhoods.

Another way of analysing grid referenced patient addresses is to identify the number of patients living within selected distances or radii of each surgery. This enables other questions which GPs might want to ask to be addressed, such as how many elderly patients live a relatively long distance from the surgery?, how many live within one kilometre?

The use of GIS functions such as the "buffering" facility (which allows the user to define a buffer zone around a particular site) and the "point in polygon" procedure (which counts the number of points falling within a specified zone or buffer) are appropriate in this context. This analysis revealed that the majority of patients registered with the inner city practice lived within one kilometre of the surgery compared with only one-third of those registered with the suburban practice in affluent West Kirby.

An alternative approach is to identify the distance from the surgery within which 75 per cent, 90 per cent or 100 per cent of all registered patients live (i.e. catchment area analysis). On this test, the West Kirby practice had the largest catchment area, although, the variation between the four case study practices was remarkably small. There was some evidence in Birkenhead that patients under 17 and those aged 65 or over tended to live nearer to the surgery than patients in general (see Table 14.2).

Derivation of travel times

The digital street network for the Wirral was used to calculate the proportion of patients living within selected travel times of each surgery. This involved deriving travel time isochrones (lines delineating the boundary of a given travel time) taking into account average traffic speeds achievable on different classes of road (motorways, A roads, B,C, and local access roads). Using the allocate function in the Arc/Info GIS, sections of the street network (arcs) are examined progressively from the practice origin and assigned to the practice if the upper travel time condition (e.g. four minutes) continues to be satisfied. Sections of the road network that fall within successive time intervals can be identified by assigning them different colours or line thicknesses.

Table 14.2
Distribution of distances (in kilometres) from practice for all patients and by age group (Wirral study)

	Practice 1	Practice 2	Practice 3	Practice 4
All patients	2,994	6,268	4,346	6,040
Minimum distance	0.1	0.1	0.1	0.1
25% closer than	0.4	0.5	0.7	0.6
50% closer than	0.8	0.9	1.4	1.0
75% closer than	1.6	1.4	2.4	1.5
90% closer than	3.5	2.9	3.4	3.2
Maximum distance	11.6	10.3	14.9	13.3
Patients aged <17	558	1,397	789	1,291
Minimum distance	0.1	0.1	0.1	0.1
25% closer than	0.3	0.6	0.8	0.7
50% closer than	0.8	0.9	1.6	1.1
75% closer than	1.4	1.4	2.4	2.1
90% closer than	2.6	2.7	3.5	3.5
Maximum distance	8.4	6.3	12.0	9.4
Patients aged >65	600	1,280	1,111	1,147
Minimum distance	0.1	0.1	0.1	0.1
25% closer than	0.3	0.4	0.6	0.6
50% closer than	0.7	0.6	1.1	0.9
75% closer than	1.3	1.1	2.0	1.2
90% closer than	3.1	3.0	2.9	2.1
Maximum distance	8.4	10.3	14.9	9.5

Thus an impression can be gained of the influence of the road network in shaping accessibility to different practices, and an example is shown in Figure 14.4. This analysis revealed that some locations which were only a short linear distance from the surgery were relatively far away in terms of travel time forming small islands of relatively low accessibility. These can be seen in Figure 14.4 which shows varying degrees of accessibility to the Birkenhead practice. The analysis can be refined further by modelling accessibility by different modes of transport, especially public transport, and by foot.

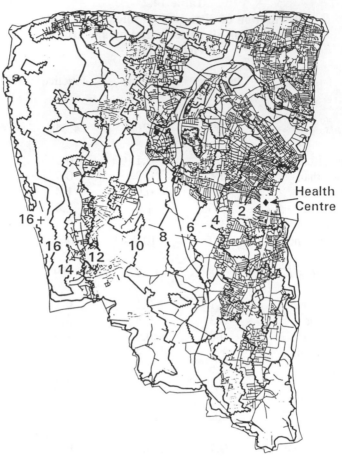

Health
Centre

16+

16

12

14

10

8

6

4

2

Figure 14.4   **Travel time "isochrones" for a health centre in
Birkenhead, Wirral (times in minutes)**

Morbidity patterns and service provision

Further analyses were undertaken of data relating to in patient admissions to
Wirral hospitals for acute conditions. A key objective in this part of the study
was to determine whether patients suffering from certain illnesses lived near
to GPs offering treatment. The GIS was used to plot the residential location
of patients admitted to hospital with asthma and that of GP surgeries operating
asthma clinics. Close scrutiny of the resultant map suggested that GPs
running asthma clinics were generally not located in the neighbourhoods in
which the admitted asthma patients tended to live. The identification of these

180

disparities has led subsequently to the prioritization of asthma services by GPs in several under served areas.

The location of community pharmacies

In URPERRL'S most recent health related research project, GIS techniques have been used to study the location of community pharmacies in Mersey Region. Information has been assembled on the 513 community pharmacies currently in the Region, together with some historic data on the location of pharmacies in 1981 and 1986. This is had been augmented with data on social conditions, health status, health care facilities, infrastructure and transport.

GIS functions have been applied to calculate the straight line distances between each pharmacy and those between individual pharmacies and the nearest GP surgery based on the grid references of each location. These results provided useful information on the density of provision. For example, more than half of the pharmacies in Mersey Region (58.7 per cent) were within 500 metres of another pharmacy indicating high level of provision in urban areas. The analysis revealed a strong tendency for pharmacies to cluster around GP surgeries and health centres; nearly 51 per cent of pharmacies were located within 200 metres of the closest surgery although only four per cent were more than one kilometre from a GP, (see Table 14.3).

It may be convenient, for a local population, to have a pharmacy near to their doctor's premises in order to have prescriptions dispensed. This proposition would have to be tested by further studies as would the possibility that the advisory role of pharmacies, and those providing extra services, may better serve the resident population by becoming more widely dispersed.

A GIS can cross reference different types of information and to produce detailed maps for a given area. This has been used, for example to show the location of pharmacies classified by the additional services which they provide (e.g. oxygen supply and delivery, needle exchange schemes, advice to residential homes) in relation to GP surgeries by size of practice, the major roads, and affluent and underprivileged residential neighbourhoods.

Conclusions

GIS undoubtedly has a role to play in the analysis and display of information on health services and the patients who use them.

The advantages which it offers over traditional methods of data analysis are considerable; in particular the ability to utilize digital street networks to derive improved measures of accessibility to health facilities.

Table 14.3
Number of pharmacies within selected distance bands
of the nearest GP surgery for Mersey region and
for Cheshire and Liverpool FHSA's

Mersey Regional Health Authority

Distance (metres)	No. of pharmacies	Percentage of total
< =200	261	50.88%
201-400	108	21.05%
401-600	74	14.42%
601-800	26	4.07%
801-1000	23	4.09%
>1000	23	4.45%

Cheshire FHSA

Distance (metres)	No. of pharmacies	Percentage of total
< =200	95	51.63%
201-400	36	19.56%
401-600	17	9.20%
601-800	9	4.89%
801-1000	12	6.52%
>1000	15	8.15%

Liverpool FHSA

Distance (metres)	No. of pharmacies	Percentage of total
< =200	59	48.36%
201-400	26	21.31%
401-600	29	23.77%
601-800	5	4.09%
801-1000	3	2.45%
>1000	0	0%

URPERRL's research in this area has had two main outcomes; first, the identification of spatial disparities in the demand for and supply of services, leading, in some cases, to the prioritization of services in under served areas and second, the successful transfer of GIS technology to health care planners. As a result of this work, GIS now plays a key role in the purchasing decisions of health care planners in several health authorities in north west England. For example, the GIS techniques developed by URPERRL have been used by North West Regional Health Authority to inform decisions on where to locate a new regional oncology centre for northwest England (Todd et al. 1994).

The specific techniques used by URPERRL in north west England, can easily be applied to other areas of Britain given the national coverage and availability of the key data sets. These include FHSA patient registrations, digital street networks (some available on a non commercial basis for research purposes) and the super profiles geodemographic classification which has recently been acquired by the Department of Health.

In general, GIS offer considerable potential for service delivery analysis and planning anywhere in the world. However, the ease with which GIS applications can be developed will depend upon the availability of information on population, patients and health services and the extent to which such information is geographically referenced and in machine readable form.

References

Brown, P.J.B. (1991), "Exploring Geodemographics" in Masser, I. and Blakemore, M. (eds.), *Handling Geographic Information: Methodology and Potential Applications*, Longman, London, pp. 221-58.

Brown, P.J.B., Hirschfield, A. and Batey, P.W.J. (1991), "Applications of Geodemographic Methods in the Analysis of Health Condition Incidence Data, Papers in Regional Science", *Journal of the Regional Science Association International*, vol. 70, no. 3, pp. 329-44.

Brown, P.J.B., Hirschfield, A. and Marsden, J. (1995), "Analyzing Spatial Patterns of Disease: Some Issues in the Mapping of Incidence Data for Relatively Rare Conditions" in de Lepper, M.J.C., Scholten, H.J. and Stern, R.M. (eds.), *The Added Value of Geographical Information Systems in Public and Environmental Health*, Dordrecht: Kluwer Academic Publishers and Copenhagen, WHO European Office, pp. 145-63.

Hirschfield, A., Brown, P.J.B. and Bundred, P. (1993), "Doctors, Patients and GIS", *Mapping Awareness*, vol. 7, no. 9, pp. 9-12.

Hirschfield, A., Brown, P.J.B. and Bundred, P. (1995), "The Spatial Analysis of Community Health Services on Wirral Using Geographic Information Systems", *Journal of the Operational Research Society*, vol. 46, pp. 147-59.

Hirschfield, A., Brown, P.J.B. and Marsden, J. (1991), "Database Development for Decision Support and Policy Evaluation" in Worral, L. (ed.), *Spatial Analysis and Spatial Policy Using Geographic Information Systems*, Belhaven, London, pp. 152-87.

Hirschfield, A., Wolfson, D. and Swetman, S. (1994), "The Location of Community Pharmacies: A Rational Approach Using Geographic Information Systems", *International Journal of Pharmacy Practice A 3*, vol. 1, pp. 42-52.

Jarman, B. (1983), "Identification of Underprivileged Areas", *British Medical Journal*, vol. 286, pp. 1705-9.

Todd, P., Bundred, P. and Brown, P.J.B. (1994), "The Demography of Demand for Oncology Services: A Health Care Planning GIS Application", *Proceedings of the AGI94 Conference*, Birmingham, pp. 17.1.1-17.1.8.

Tudor-Hart, J. (1975), "The Inverse Care Law" in Cox, C. and Mead (eds), *A Sociology of Medical Practice*, Collier-Macmillan, London, pp. 189-206.

Wrigley, N. (1991), "Market-Based Systems of Health-Care Provision, the NHS Bill and Geographical Information Systems", *Environment and Planning A*, vol. 23, pp. 5-8.

Appendix 14.1

The 1981 super profile geodemographic classification: description of the 10 "lifestyle" clusters

Lifestyle A: Affluent Minority GB Population in 1981: 4.77m (8.9%)
This most affluent of the lifestyles is characterised by large, detached, owner occupied housing which accommodates highly qualified multi-car owning, professional worker households with few children, in low density, suburban and semi rural areas from which the majority of workers commute by car and train to office jobs.

Lifestyle B: Metro Singles GB Population in 1981: 1.87m (3.48%)
Typified by young single, well qualified, professional and other white collar workers, with some single elderly, living in small, furnished and unfurnished rented flats, often lacking in basic amenities, in areas of ethnically mixed population with a high residential turnover, well served by rail and tube, resulting in an unusually low level of car ownership and use for work travel.

Lifestyle C: Young Married Suburbia GB Population in 1981: S.26m (9.82%)
Young married couples with younger children, with very few older and elderly people, in households of well qualified, professional and other white collar workers, owning their own detached and semi detached houses in "leafy" suburban estates, virtually all owning one or more cars, one of which is likely to be used for the journey to work.

Lifestyle D: Country and Retiring Suburbans GB Population in 1981: 4.63m (8.64%)
Rural areas which are mainly associated with farming but also popular locations, some urban or semi urban, for retirement and holiday homes, providing spacious out of town accommodation for multi-car owning and car commuting managerial households and tied properties for agricultural workers.

Lifestyle E: Older Suburbia GB Population in 1981: 4.39m (8.20%)
Stable suburban areas populated largely by smaller households of retired and elderly in their own semi detached housing, together with some managerial and other white collar workers, some working part time, with average car ownership, low unemployment and close to average performance with respect to many other indicators.

Lifestyle F: Aspiring Blue and White Collars GB Populationin 1981: 8.60m (16.05%)

A lifestyle distinguished from Older suburbia (Lifestyle E) by its much younger age structure and the presence of families with young children living in owner occupied semi detached property, including families of those in the armed forces, more working wives and skilled manual workers, many using a car for the work journey from the car owning majority of households.

Lifestyle G: Multi-Ethnic Areas GB Population in 1981: 3.83m (7.16%)

Areas in which large ethnic families with young children are most evident, living in overcrowded rented property, in generally poor condition, some occupied by students and single workers, high unemployment and most households without a car, but those in employment working in the manufacturing and transport sectors in semi and unskilled jobs to which many commute by rail and tube.

Lifestyle H: Fading Industrial GB Population in 1981: 5.S5m (10.36%)

Generally typical national age structure with rather more older people, living in poorest quality unimproved terraced property accommodating a largely semi and unskilled blue collar labour force in older industrial and mining areas, with a level of male unemployment a little above average, and many of those working travelling to work on foot.

Lifestyle I: Council Tenants GB Population in 1981: 8.44m (15.75)

In common with Lifestylef, a very high proportion of council rented property, mostly in the form of flats in a good state of repair, but having a much older age structure than] with more singly female pensioners, no overcrowding and a rather lower but still relatively high level of unemployment amongst its blue collar work force, which includes many part timers, and most of whom rely upon foot and bus travel to reach their manufacturing jobs.

Lifestyle J: Underprivileged Britain GB Population in 1981: 5.80m (10.83%)

This lifestyle accounts for those areas in which the worst conditions of social stress and deprivation are concentrated. It is characterised by very large families, including young children, living in cramped and overcrowded conditions in council flats that are in generally good condition, but with the highest levels of unemployment amongst a very poorly qualified, unskilled labour force, with very low car ownership, those in employment thus reliant upon the bus for the work journey.

15 Assessment of health in cities by employing a Geographical Information System: Its contribution to the health policy development

Keiko Nakamura, Takehito Takano, Sachiko Takeuchi and Atsuko Tanaka

Contemporary urban society is undergoing rapid change, and an understanding of the interaction between health and the environment, social, economic and physical, is crucial if we are to be prepared for the future of life in the city. How can we best describe the health effects of rapid environmental changes in a particular area of the city, and relate these to the process of developing new urban policy? How can we assess whether a proposed plan for the city, be it a local initiative or an integrated plan for the whole urban area, will satisfy the needs of residents and be effective in improving the health of the community or city? These are among the questions that research should be able to answer, because substantial and concrete information are expected by, among others, the citizens who wish to make their city healthier place in which to live.

We have developed a method of evaluating health in cities, which we have termed "image diagnosis", based on a Geographical Information System (GIS). Adequate and valid information is important for citizens as well as policy makers if they are to choose the most effective and efficient strategy for the city. The method we have developed includes the following three processes:

1. To elucidate health and environmental conditions in a city from a wide range of aspects.

2. To demonstrate by using visual (graphical) presentation health and environmental conditions identified by the use of multi-variate statistical procedures.

3. To give visual (graphical) images of the interaction between health and the environment in cities which can supply information about how a combination of city environments will affect people's health.

In this paper we will describe how information analyzed and presented in these ways has been used in collaboration with citizens and the city authorities to develop plans for improving health.

Information for the city and its people

The city of Tokyo is a self governing unit of 12 million residents, occupying an area of 2,182 square kilometres. In addition to the metropolitan government, which has its own assembly and governor elected by all voters in Tokyo, it is divided into 64 municipalities which consist of 23 wards, 26 cities, 7 towns and 8 villages.

The Tokyo Citizens' Council for Health Promotion is a core organization for the whole of the 12 million population of the city. The Governor of the Tokyo Metropolis is the president of the Citizens' Council, and it consists of 467 members representing citizens, the metropolitan government, municipal governments, the private sector, non-governmental organizations, and the academic community (Tokyo Citizens' Council for Health Promotion, 1993; Takano, 1995). Good information has played an important part in helping the many and varied members of the Tokyo Citizens' Council for Health Promotion, as well as some of the 12 million people living in Tokyo, understand what is necessary to build a strategy for a healthy city. It has been particularly valuable to work in a team representing three key interests, those of citizens, administrators, and researchers (Nakamura and Takano, 1992).

Making health visible - the development of image diagnosis

Making the health conditions in a city more visible to citizens by providing up to date multi-faceted information is important. One method we have adopted for this is through GIS, using an approach which combines the following:

1. Graphical designation (within the software) of the particular study areas required.

2. Compilation of the data needed from a wide range of sources, and the computation of essential indicators.

3. Computation of summary indicators to produce variables which represent different aspects of health and environmental conditions, using multi-variate statistical procedures.

4.   Mapping of these indicators and variables.

5.   Analysis of the relationships between health and the environment.

6.   Formulation of models for predicting patterns of health in the city.

All of these are applicable to communities of various sizes.   We have applied this method to greater Tokyo area, to individual municipalities in Tokyo metropolitan area, and to other cities in Japan where people are interested in developing a healthy city approach.

Mapping of health and environmental indicators in the greater Tokyo area

Our first studies were of health and environmental conditions in the greater Tokyo area (Takano and Nakamura, 1990), including an area falling within a 50 km radius of central Tokyo. This area consists of the Tokyo metropolis, excluding the islands area; the southern part of Saitama Prefecture; the bay areas and the west part of Chiba Prefecture; and Kanagawa Prefecture, excluding the south west and south east parts. This area represents three per cent of the total land in Japan, yet houses 23 per cent of the total population. It consists of 197 different municipalities in which each municipality has is own assembly and mayor elected by its citizens. We divided the area into 83 districts to make our Healthy City Tokyo Map. The criterion for this division was population size, with each of our new "districts" having a population of approximately 250,000. We compiled data from about 100 different sources, then calculated more than 600 indicators pertaining to health and environment. The information we used included not only existing official statistics such as census, vital statistics, and business establishment census, but also both governmental and non-governmental community based information such as emergency calls to each fire station, statistics on welfare assistance, land use, statistics on waste disposal, and road surveys in each municipality (Nakamura and Takano, 1992). The main categories are shown in Table 15.1. These indicators were then presented in mapped form, and some 220 out of the total of 600 figures were compiled in a book entitled "Baseline Data for Healthy City Tokyo" (Gyosei, 1990). Figures 15.1 shows an example of this mapping.

Studying the complex associations between health and the environment

Associations between health and the environment are generally complex, and need to be understood from a review of many aspects of the environment.

Table 15.1

**Main categories of information used for image
diagnosis of greater Tokyo area**

- age-adjusted death rates and infant mortality
- age-specific death rate
- age-adjusted death rates by causes of death
- population and land
- housing, and number and composition of households
- structure of the labour force
- industrial structure
- roads and vehicles
- medical expenditure, medical care facilities, emergency care, and care workers
- volume of waste
- welfare assistance
- income
- municipal expenditure

Although we had developed some 600 indicators which may have some bearing on health, it is obviously very difficult to interpret in any meaningful way differences in various combinations of these many indicators.

It is much more useful to identify indicators of health and of health determinants which can usefully represent the different aspects of each. This was done using correlation matrices in order to study the strengths of associations between different indicators. We first selected 27 health indicators (representing levels of health) and 107 health determinant indicators. These indicators were selected so as to explain more than 80 per cent of the variance of the full set of indicators: selected indicators were therefore regarded as representative of the complete set of indicators.

Health determinant indicators were categorized into demography; amenity; infrastructure; education; working conditions and health care services (Takeuchi et al. 1995). We then performed a principal factor analysis which essentially yields a smaller number of factors characterising the key issues held within a much larger number of indicators. These factors were then rotated using the varimax operation, which identified 5 health variables, 3 demographic variables, 3 amenity variables, 4 infrastructure variables, 4 educational variables, 5 local economic activity variables, and 4 health care and welfare service variables.

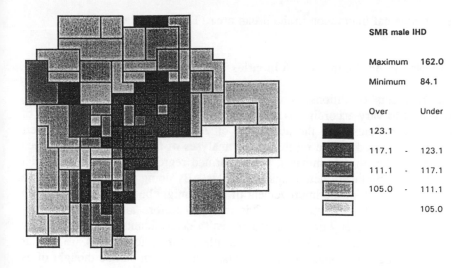

SMR male IHD

| | Maximum | 162.0 |
| | Minimum | 84.1 |

	Over	Under
	123.1	
	117.1	- 123.1
	111.1	- 117.1
	105.0	- 111.1
		105.0

Figure 15.1   Pattern of male ischemic heart disease deaths within 50 km radius of the centre of Tokyo. Standardized mortality ratios (SMR) adjusted to the national death rates in 1985 were calculated. Number of deaths in years from 1983 to 1987 were used for standardisation. Each "unit" has a population of about 250,000 and the darker tones indicate higher death rates

Mapping of these health and health determinant variables were also performed by the GIS programme. These maps, presenting these key variables, facilitated the understanding of comprehensive features of health and environmental conditions which is so important if the wide range of influences on health are to be considered, and were far more practical than trying to interpret 600 different maps.

The next stage in this investigation was to look at the associations between health levels and health determinants. Pearson correlation co-efficients were calculated for the associations between health level indicators and health determinant variables as well as between health level variables (factors obtained by a principal factor analysis) and health determinant variables. Individual health indicators as well as health level variables had significant positive or negative relationships with several health determinant variables. For example, male Standardised Mortality Ratio (SMR) correlated significantly with 1 demographic variable, 2 infrastructure variable, 2 amenity variables, 1 education variable, 2 working conditions variables, and 1 health care services variable. These results showed the structure of health and

191

environmental interaction in the urban area (Takeuchi et al. 1995).

Models for predicting health in cities

Environmental conditions, as represented by the health determinant variables, will tend to vary according to the degree of urbanization, implementation of new city policies, and the actions of citizens, including changes in their lifestyles. Based on the results of our analyses of the relationships between health and health determinants, we performed regression analysis to predict health level by health determinant variables. By doing this, it is possible to show how much of the improvement of health might be expected for a given change in health determinants. This model therefore allows us to predict health levels of a city under particular health determinants conditions on the assumption that the relation between health and its determinants are similar within the densely populated urban areas. This in turn can be thought of as the product of certain policy options. In this way, citizens, administrators, and policy makers are able to consider the likely changes in people's health when that city adopts a particular strategy for development, including the development of health services.

Health and environmental conditions in smaller areas

In order to develop effective action at the local level, it has been useful to develop our image diagnosis method for smaller areas of the city. We have already compiled various indicators which would be appropriate for the development of healthy city projects in individual wards and cities, including population, morbidity, work force, land use, industry, and health infrastructure.

Monitoring health in smaller areas requires locally available and appropriate data: mortality statistics, although available and relatively valid, are not a practical option as the number of deaths in individual areas is usually too small. Morbidity statistics however, are available for these smaller areas. Morbidity rates, based on statements of medical care remuneration can be obtained and in Japan have a high reliability, since there is a compulsory medical care insurance programme to which all residents in Japan are required to subscribe. Using statements of medical care remuneration, we will be able to get a clearer picture of morbidity distribution between these smaller areas (Nakamura and Takano, 1992). Analysis in smaller areas improves visibility of health in cities by revealing the health status of individual communities and by highlighting situations which need to be changed. It therefore facilitates the awareness of municipal governments and citizens to these issues and encourages their activities in creating a healthy city.

Evaluation using health promotion activity indicators

The monitoring of health promotion activity using indicators which measure a broad range of lifestyle and environmental features and characteristics is also important. Some examples of the indicators which we have used are: per capita alcohol consumption; coping health behaviours in response to conditions such as chest pain, for instance whether they visit the hospital emergency room or visit their family doctor, or care for themselves; specific percentage of current smokers and per capita cigarette consumption; number of voluntary community care workers; number of facilities available for community group meetings; number of sports facilities for the public; number of well maintained public gardens; number of facilities with disabled person access; facilities for safe open play space for children; information regarding garbage recycling; and changes in people's attitude toward health (Nakamura and Takano, 1992).

In instances where there was a lack of locally based health promotion activity indicators, co-operative efforts were made on the part of researchers, citizens, and municipal administrators to collect the needed information, which was then incorporated into our analysis. This type of joint effort is essential for the success of any healthy city project.

Conclusions

In the process of linking research results to the policy development for Tokyo Healthy City, Committees of the Tokyo Citizens' Council for Health Promotion have worked well to facilitate intersectoral communication. The Drafting Committee of the Action Plan consisting of researchers, administrators and citizens, have been working out a draft for "Towards Healthy City Tokyo - Our Action Plan for Health Promotion". The research and investigation committee has conducted empirical research to study key strategies for developing group self help health promotion activities, for improving family health, and so on. This process has helped translate research results into action which encourages community health promotion.

Our experience has shown that in order to effectively use research results effectively in developing a policy for a healthy city, the following conditions are necessary:

1. Joint efforts which involve citizens, administrators and academics to carry out research revealing actual health needs and the quality of the

environmental.

2.   The development of well designed, easy to handle analytic tools to evaluate health in a city.

3.   Explanation of academic results to the general public.

4.   Joint work to develop a policy for a city.

5.   Joint endeavours to take actions in the actual community.

Image diagnosis is considered to be a useful tool in helping people to recognize the effects of the urban environment on health. The range of information used, as well as the modelling of health outcomes, encourages people to communicate with each other, and to understand better the implications that various policy options may have for health in the city. An important product of this approach is that it also supports citizens' participation in the process of urban policy development.

References

"Baseline Data for Healthy City Tokyo" (1990), Gyosei, Tokyo.
Nakamura, K. and Takano, T. (1992), "Image Diagnosis of Health in Cities: Tokyo Healthy City" in Takano, T., Ishidate, K. and Nagasaki, M. (eds.), *Formulation and Development of Research Base for Healthy Cities*, Kyoiku Syoseki, Tokyo.
Takano, T. (1995), "Tokyo Citizens' Council for Health Promotion and Its Action Plan", *Public Health Medicine*, vol. 17, no. 1, pp. 11-4.
Takano, T. and Nakamura, K (1990), *Baseline Data for Healthy City Tokyo*, Gyosei, Tokyo. (in Japanese/English)
Takeuchi, S., Takano, T. and Nakamura, K. (1995), "Health and its Determining Factors in the Tokyo Megacity", *Health Policy*, vol. 33, no. 1, pp. 1-14.
Tokyo Citizens' Council for Health Promotion, (1993), "Towards Healthy City Tokyo - Our Action Plan for Healthy Promotion", *Tokyo Citizens' Council for Health Promotion*, Tokyo. (in Japanese)

Section 4 Towards participative evaluation

In the last section we looked at some of the contemporary experience of assessing community need, and noted the potential value of participation in that process. We have seen a variety of research methods, and observed that there is not a single best method: in any given situation, variety gives added richness and can contribute to validity. This variety in methods has implications for greater demands on already limited resources, as does the background community development work that can help the research component to succeed as a participative and collaborative venture. In this section, we move on a step to the experience of evaluating the process of community health development. In doing so, we should keep in mind the resource needs.

In evaluation, at least part of the research task moves away from being a vehicle to express the needs of the community, and with this shift the tension between research and action re-emerges. This is an immensely complex matter, and one that we will explore through the remaining papers of this book, and in the discussion in section eight. One of the distinctions that emerges, or at least is a feature of contemporary practice, is that between evaluation as a participative exercise assessing how well the programme has met the goals set by the participants, and evaluation which is more external and at its baldest seeks to test (for example) whether a given programme has improved population health in a cost effective way.

This distinction is complicated by the fact that it is in part a product of differing goals on the part of citizens and community development workers on the one hand, and policy makers and service funders on the other. By and large, the research community has been allied with the latter grouping. Ultimately, we will explore whether these two viewpoints can be brought closer together, because, if they can, this offers a more constructive and realistic approach to evaluation of some of the most crucial questions. In order to arrive at that point in the debate however, it is valuable to look first at the existing experience of process evaluation reported in this section, and of strategies for change presented in section five.

In search of an appropriate model for evaluation

In the first paper, Ainé Kennedy describes how she and her colleagues working on the Drumchapel Community Health Project in Glasgow sought and developed a varied model of evaluation that could meet their needs, one that would embody the fundamental principles that they were working to promote: empowerment, participation and collaboration. One particularly important principle is that evaluation should be pluralistic, reflecting the fact that there is no single outcome but many different outcomes for all the various interests involved. One response to this need was to use a "portfolio" of methods including a questionnaire survey, focus groups, video, art and drama. While this flexibility and complexity may have been desirable in terms of the aims, the consequent lack of structure and direction was found to be uncomfortable and sometimes paralysing, but this is something that must be accepted and adapted to. Among the achievements of this work has been the loss of fear of evaluation among people associated with the project, but the conflict between time spent on evaluation versus time spent sustaining practice in the community remained.

Evaluation of lifestyle based community health promotion programmes

The other three papers in this section take as their starting points programmes closely related to lifestyles. The first, by Lenneke Vaandrager, reports on the experience of evaluating participation within a community nutrition project involving collaboration between a number of European cities. An important observation in that study was that the process of trying to define and measure the level of participation required was more important than the ability to "objectively" measure levels of participation. The other two papers by Linda Ewles (Bristol) and Martine Standish (Sheffield), are about work that was based in the Health Education Authority's "Look After Your Heart" programme. All three projects are however, in terms of implementation, firmly rooted in the principles of Health for All, and have much in common with the Glasgow experience.

All of the papers in this section are quite personal, some presented from the viewpoint of the researcher, some from that of the community development or health promotion worker. There is a good deal of sharp observation about methods, strengths and weaknesses that should be of value to others. There is also something else which arises from the experience of these authors, and that is the uncertainty and tension that pervades the evaluation activity. The choice of title for Martine Standish's account, "A view from the tightrope", well illustrates the balancing act that she and her colleagues are engaged in.

To a degree, this tension is a product of the stage of development of this research, and can be expected to change over time. The research is innovative and interdisciplinary, without the security of a long established theoretical base and the structures, funding, institutional and other manifestations of support that are afforded to research operating in more traditional settings. As we have also seen this evaluation work is caught between the hostility, or at least scepticism, of both the community practitioners and the scientists. There are signs that this can be, and is being, resolved. The value of this evaluation is beginning to be appreciated by those involved, although it seems that the conflict it presents in terms of taking time away from "getting on with what needs doing" is still a problem. This situation will remain a barrier until the resources for carrying out appropriate evaluation are acknowledged and allowed for in terms of budgets, staff and time.

16 Measuring health for all – a feasibility study in a Glasgow community

Ainé Kennedy

As a community health worker and manager of a "Health for All" project in Glasgow, I have for many years been frustrated by the apparent inability of the research world to get to grips with what we do. The difficulties in evaluating community health work in any meaningful way have often led to accusations that the work is "unscientific" and/or been used as an excuse to withdraw funding (Smithies and Adams, 1993). Community health practitioners of whatever discipline tend to be suspicious of the world of research, mis-trust evaluation techniques which they often see as irrelevant and inappropriate indicators of the work that they do and the two camps of researchers/evaluators and practitioners can become increasingly polarised with little or no opportunity for mutual exchange of ideas and skills.

All too often projects are moulded to fit evaluation techniques rather than the other way around and the effect of the "let's measure what's easy approach" can be to lose the essence of a project which has at its core processes such as empowerment and participation. My profession of health promotion has been particularly hard hit in this respect because of its proximity to medicine which tends to favour positivistic, reductionist, approaches to evaluation with their emphasis on easily measurable outcomes - often called "hard" research. The current climate of "Health for All" and "Healthy Cities" offers an opportunity to remedy this situation by prompting a call for research which will not only clarify the campaign's core principles of participation, collaboration and empowerment but also demonstrate these principles in the research process itself, (WHO, 1988; Kelly, 1990; Hancock, 1993; Smithies and Adams, 1993).

In the two year pilot phase of the Drumchapel Healthy Cities Project, now the Drumchapel Community Health Project, we were particularly keen to come up with appropriate ways of evaluating our activities. Being well aware of the obstacles to successful evaluation of community health work, we were determined to try out a number of methods until we found those that provided the best "fit" with our requirements i.e. it was as important to pilot the evaluation methods as to pilot the practice. Our requirements were that the evaluation methods chosen should be: capable of reflecting the essence of what the project is about, namely participation, empowerment and collaboration and that the evaluation process itself should reflect these principles i.e. be empowering, participative and collaborative.

This paper describes how we got on and considers some of the implications for the wider Health for All and Healthy Cities movement.

Participatory evaluation and health for all

Given its commitment to values such as participation and empowerment it is particularly important for Health for All initiatives not to fall into the trap of allowing evaluation to be seen purely as a funders' tool. Why should evaluation be exempt from the requirement to reflect the same values that underpin the rest of the practice? Evaluation is integral to mature, reflective practice - not something separate to be carried out by mysterious "experts" with different values and a different world view to the subjects. Doing our own evaluation in Drumchapel made us realise just how much informal evaluation we do "on the hoof" all the time. It's impossible to be effective otherwise.

Our search for appropriate methods and approaches took us to the so called "softer" research tradition drawn from the fields of anthropology, education and the social sciences. There, we came across descriptions of process or illuminative evaluation (Parlett and Hamilton, 1977) which attempts to shed some light on the "hows" and "whys" of a project's activities rather than focusing exclusively on what has been achieved.

> Good evaluation assesses what has been achieved against what was intended and explains why this happened in order to derive some lessons for future work. It is about measuring change and making changes to approach more nearly the core purpose of the work (Graessle and Kingsley, 1986).

The concept of pluralism also made a lot of sense. Pluralism represents the notion that there are different groups within a project with different perceptions as to what the project is about and consequently different criteria of success. Pluralistic evaluation attempts to incorporate these various perceptions and criteria into the evaluation process. It goes some way towards compensating for the deficiencies of traditional evaluative research which often fails to recognize that, "Success is a pluralistic notion ... not a unitary measure" (Smith and Cantley, 1985).

Participatory evaluation is evaluation carried out by or with the participants in a project rather than on them. It "aims at removing the dichotomy between the producer and the consumer of knowledge - between creating and using knowledge" (Starrin and Svensson, 1991). Consequently, it challenges in a very fundamental way, many of the premises on which scientific inquiry is traditionally based e.g. the neutrality and objectivity of the researcher and their complete control of the research process. The role of the researcher in participatory research "is not as a producer of expert knowledge but as a facilitator whose task is to support the development of the community's own knowledge" (Smithies and Adams, 1993).

Participatory research has also been called co-operative inquiry and is one of a number of approaches to research in the social sciences which has been termed "new paradigm" or "post-positivist" (Reason and Rowan, 1981), because of the challenge it poses to traditional scientific assumptions.

The following "Ladder of Participation" (Arnstein, 1969; Elden, 1981) describes the various key stages in the research process and illustrates that there is a continuum of participation for each stage. It is a useful tool for assessing the level of participation in any research or evaluation exercise.

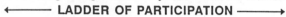

←——— **LADDER OF PARTICIPATION** ———→

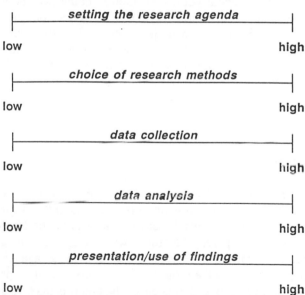

setting the research agenda

low   high

choice of research methods

low   high

data collection

low   high

data analysis

low   high

presentation/use of findings

low   high

Research is participatory when those directly affected by it influence each of these four decisions (I added data collection) and help carry them out. For participation to be meaningful and consequential I assume it must involve more than merely being consulted but not necessarily as much as exercising

201

control. It means here having enough involvement and influence to impact on the decision and in carrying it out (Elden, 1981).

If evaluation aims to be empowering, participative and collaborative, it is perhaps most important to get stage one of the research right. Getting all the participants in a project together with any other parties with an interest in the evaluation to discuss answers to questions such as: Who/what is the evaluation for? What should we be measuring and how? Who do we want to do the evaluation? Where do we find the time and resources? ... is vital and can be very illuminating. It reveals the different constituent groups within a project and their various values and ideologies which is a key component of participatory and pluralistic evaluation. In my experience of participatory research, this is the stage with the greatest empowering potential and the one that lends itself most easily to a high degree of participation. Subsequent research stages require more specialized skills and knowledge thus making time for training and support imperative. This is not something that is generally acknowledged in the literature about participatory research. Data analysis is a particularly challenging stage to make into any kind of appealing, collective activity but probably becomes easier with greater experience in this approach.

At the risk of stating the obvious, it's important to be very clear, and honest, from the outset about your motivation in doing evaluation. For my part as a participant in the project, I wanted to reflect on and record the practice and achievements of the project with a view to improving it and enabling both ourselves and others to learn from it. Other potential consumers of evaluation might have very different requirements. Alan Beattie (1991) talks about a portfolio approach to evaluation which uses a variety of different types of measurement to try to accommodate the different audience's requirements of evaluation.

Project structure and participants

The Drumchapel Healthy Cities project, (now the Drumchapel Community Health project) had a relatively complex structure due to its role as a catalyst and resource for community health activity and a pilot for Health for All. During its two year pilot phase, the project was managed by and accountable to a local executive group with representation from all the agencies who had put money or staff time into the project as well as community representation. Figure 16.1 which was devised during the evaluation process by a small group of project participants, illustrates the organizational structure of the project. The executive group (now called the management group) is seen as the forum for inter-agency collaboration on health at a strategic or policy making level for the locality whereas the working group and topic specific community health forums such as the Women's Health Network are the focus for collaboration at an operational level. The working group grew out of the informal network of social workers, community workers, health visitors and health promotion staff who worked together on a variety of health issues prior to the project's formal existence.

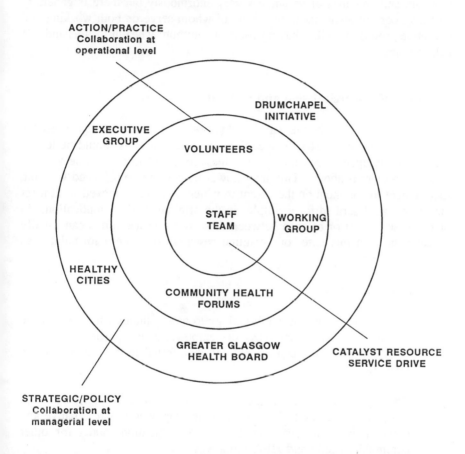

Figure 16.1 Organizational structure of the Drumchapel healthy cities project

The diagram to illustrate project structure is circular because a more conventional linear diagram reflecting a hierarchical structure was not felt to be appropriate. The circle is meant to give the impression of a stone being dropped into a pond with the ripples spreading outwards into different levels of activity relating to health in Drumchapel. The project is designed to support and facilitate the process of local politicians, local people and staff at a number of levels within a variety of organizations incorporating HFA principles into their practice and policy. The training, support and deployment of community health volunteers (lay health workers) is central to the project's activities and the main vehicle for empowered participation. The numbers and activities of volunteers vary enormously but there is generally an active core of about six to ten some of whom serve on both working and executive groups as well as having roles in community health forums and self help groups.

Evolution of research design and method

In participatory research, the way in which research aims and objectives are formulated is critical. Strictly speaking, the research aims should be left as simple and as open as possible so that they do not reflect only one view of what the project is about. This may however, need to be balanced with the requirement to comment on the extent to which a project achieved what it set out to do - as described for example, in the original funding application. In practice, some sort of balance between these two considerations can usually be achieved. In this case, our original research aims were formulated as follows:

Original research aims

1.   To pilot an evaluation methodology to assess the extent to which the Health for All principles of empowerment, participation and collaboration have been upheld and manifested in the practice of the DHCP.

2.   To pilot a research methodology which in itself reflects these principles - the research process being empowering,participative and collaborative - to serve as a potential evaluation model for other community health and HFA initiatives.

With increased knowledge of and confidence in the participatory and pluralistic approach, I would have been less prescriptive at the outset about the criteria to be used for evaluation. I also learned that the above aims were somewhat over ambitious given the time and resources available and consequently formulated the following simpler, more modest objectives.

Subsequent research aims

1.   To explore a variety of approaches to the evaluation of the DHCP.

2.   To seek the views of a range of participants as to indicators of the project's success.

3.   To assess the feasibility of reflecting the HFA principles of participation, empowerment and collaboration in the research process itself.

   In reality, the research design was sufficiently flexible to accommodate both sets of aims which was important since funding had been awarded on the basis of the original aims.

A portfolio of methods

A summary of the key elements of the evaluation process, their time scale and the numbers who participated is outlined below.

Questionnaire - November 1991

To collect baseline data on attitudes to evaluation among project participants. 19 questionnaires were completed representing the views of 5 working group members, 5 project staff, 3 executive group members and 6 volunteers.

Training workshops - December 1991

Exploring issues in evaluation and looking at some qualitative and ethnographic techniques.   16 people attended, again with various types of involvement in the project.

Series of three group meetings - April-June 1992

1.   To put evaluation back on the project's agenda.

2.   To act as a mechanism for participation.

3.   To identify participants' perceptions of the main achievements of the project and the areas which need improvement.

4.   To look at participants' different criteria for identifying something as

an achievement.

5.   To explore ways of measuring the work of the project.

Total attendance was 20 made up of 9 volunteers, 5 project staff, 3 working group members and 3 executive group members. The sessions each lasted for about two hours, attendance at each meeting was 14, 13 and 9 respectively with volunteers in the majority at each meeting.

Focus group discussions - April-September 1992

Interviews with representatives of various groups within the project, including:

1.   Community Health Volunteers (three meetings, total attendance, eight).

2.   Management group (seven participants).

3.   Women's Health Network (six participants).

4.   Mental Health Action Group (four participants).

5.   Project staff (four participants).

These sessions had a very simple, informal structure of reviewing the progress of the group against its initial objectives, its composition, achievements, obstacles to success, what individual members got out of their involvement and anything else the group wished to raise. Attempts were made to incorporate analysis of minutes into this exercise but this proved relatively unpopular as it was seen as a rather tedious and time consuming task.

The production of a video - April-July 1992

On the Kendoon community health profile - this was seen as a participatory approach to community health needs assessment. A director with community development as well as video making skills was appointed to ensure a high degree of participation by volunteers in every level of production.

Unstructured individual interviews - April-December 1992

With "key informants" to explore their role in and perceptions of the project and the effect of their involvement on their practice and perceptions. A total of 14 interviews took place - 3 with executive group members, 3 with health visiting and health promotion staff seconded to the project, 3 with other project staff, 1 with a working group member and 4 with community health volunteers.

Note that some volunteers and project staff are also members of working and management groups hence the apparent under representation of the former.

Case studies - May-June 1992

With volunteers using the following format as a guide:

1.   Who am I ? (thumb-nail sketch of age, gender, family circumstances)

2.   How/why did I get involved with the DHCP?

3.   What do I do as a volunteer?

4.   What have I got out of my involvement with the project?

A publicity survey - June 1992

Into the profile of the project in the community carried out by volunteers with limited professional guidance.

Follow up questionnaire - January 1993

To ascertain level of participation in evaluation and any change in attitude to research/evaluation. 13 participants took part including 3 management group members, 2 members of project staff, 2 working group members and 6 volunteers. Unfortunately, due to the fluctuating membership of the project, only seven out of 13 respondents remembered completing the original questionnaire. This reflects one of the key difficulties of carrying out "before and after type evaluation" with a constantly changing group of people. Nonetheless, there was a good response rate to the questionnaire which elicited a lot of interesting information and, as the only opportunity to contribute views anonymously, seemed to enable participants to be open about their fears and misgivings in relation to evaluation. It was also extremely efficient from the point of view of the researcher's time.

Art and drama

Were also used throughout the evaluation process in various ways. One volunteer wrote a play about her perceptions of the project which has been performed by volunteers at open days and other occasions. It has recently has been incorporated into a second video about the project ("Drumming Up Health - Power and Participation for Health in a Glasgow Community"). The volunteers have become increasingly skilled at compiling exhibitions to accompany presentations on various aspects of the project's work. Perhaps the most significant art project was the creation of the project's tree. In this exercise, a tree was chosen to symbolize the unfolding life of the project and participants were asked to consider:

1. What are the roots of the tree i.e. where has the project come from?

2. What is its trunk - central philosophy/core values?

3. What are its branches and the leaves on each branch - how would you group its principal activities?

One of the community health volunteers painted the end result - an eight foot high tree in coloured chalk on cardboard which has since gone on to become such a strong symbol of the project and its history that it has been made into a mosaic in the foyer of Drumchapel's new health centre -where the project is now based.

Reflection on method

The most popular methods of evaluation were those that were creative, informal and unintimidating and which allowed different groups within the project to exchange views. The evaluation group meetings and exercises such as the creation of the project tree were excellent ways of helping participants to see and appreciate the project as a whole rather than just from their own vantage point. "I found it a valuable experience being involved in the evaluation process. It furthered my understanding of the project" (working group member).

I had originally hoped to establish some kind of evaluation sub-group with a representative from each component part of the project to share responsibility for the evaluation but this did not come off due to competing demands on participants' time and perhaps a lack of confidence in their evaluation skills.

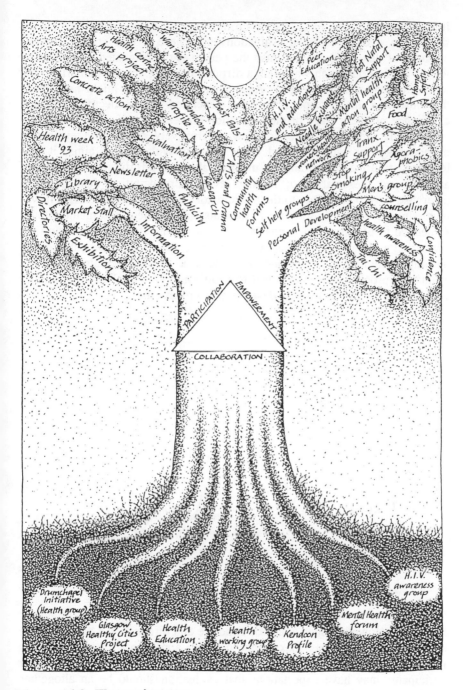

Figure 16.2 The project tree

In the absence of this ideal, the group meetings were the central vehicle for sharing an overview of the evaluation and where it was going. As the manager of this project, I was also the person with designated responsibility for the evaluation which was often a difficult juggling act, particularly at the writing up and analysis stages. An evaluation sub-group might have made this more of a shared responsibility and generated more collective skills and experience of every stage of the evaluation process.

Given that what we were doing was effectively piloting an evaluation methodology for ourselves and other projects with similar aims, it was legitimate to use a whole range of methods although this did make the task of analysis and presentation of findings even more daunting than it would otherwise have been. Due to the participatory nature of the exercise, it was impossible to be too prescriptive at the outset about focus and methodology. I intended to use group meetings as a way of getting started, negotiating the evaluation agenda in more detail and deciding on methods. The initial group meetings provided a focus and a framework for the remainder of the evaluation process which continued to evolve as we went along in a manner very similar to the community development process itself.

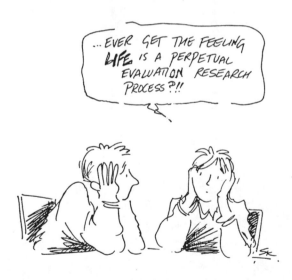

The importance of flexibility in the research design cannot be under estimated. However, such a lack of structure and direction can be paralysing at times to the researcher inexperienced in this approach. Research funders may also be unhappy about the lack of a specified design. Even project participants may have expectations that evaluation should be an altogether simpler process. Smith and Cantley (1985) write about the ways in which they dealt with the expectation of research which would simply answer the straight forward question - "Has the impact of this day hospital upon the community proved beneficial?"

> ... we learned that a particular mode of health service "evaluation" is so deeply embedded in administrative and professional (and some academic) practice that any study which departs from this mode has to treat the term "evaluation" with considerable caution. So in as much as "evaluative" research rests on a presumed rational relationship between means and ends in service provision and on a requirement to specify in advance of the research the service objectives etc, then this study was not an evaluative study but rather a study of some of the problems associated with evaluative research.

They went on to formulate their research questions based on three presumptions which also apply in this context:

1. That a controlled experiment is not possible (even if it were desirable).

2. That there are a range of views about the right criteria of "success".

3. That the nature of the service to be evaluated often remains, initially unestablished.

Much evaluation has been criticized for failing to take account of the "messiness" of the real world. Innovative, pioneering work is particularly difficult to evaluate because it is so fluid and volatile and its activities are difficult to categorize using pre-existing classifications. Evaluation which attempts to do justice to the reality of such projects can also appear messy and unfocused - especially at first, - and this can make the researcher uncomfortable. It is tempting to try to create order prematurely but this temptation must be resisted in favour of having faith in the inductive process inherent in good, qualitative research. There were times when this research felt uncomfortably unstructured and lacking in a clear direction but that, I believe, is the nature of participatory, qualitative research.

The research process as empowering, participative and collaborative

Participation in research may be empowering if participants are given a real say in identifying what matters, what should be measured, how it is measured and how it is presented, and by being encouraged to become actively involved in as many of these stages as possible. Ownership and control issues are fundamental in all types of research but never more so than when the research explicitly aims to be intrinsically empowering, participative and collaborative.

The initial training sessions and subsequent series of evaluation meetings were intended to address the above issues. These meetings were an opportunity to de-mystify the evaluation process and generate a shared sense of ownership of it. The fact that the researcher/evaluator was herself a participant, rather than an outside "expert", in itself made evaluation more feasible for project participants to take on. It also helped to reassure participants that evaluation could be relevant to and in the interests of the project.

The initial questionnaire on attitudes to evaluation revealed a lot of negative feelings among all groups with the exception of the executive group. When asked how words like evaluation or research made respondents feel, common answers were, "depressed", "uneasy", "threatened", "as if every achievement is being measure like a statistic."

One interpretation given of the word evaluation was, "Experimentation. People assessing people/projects. You don't normally see the results."

A lot of work had to be done at the outset, therefore, to present evaluation as something that was valuable to the project and capable of measuring its complexities sensitively. The challenge for the researcher was to find methods of evaluation that were intrinsically useful and/or enjoyable. The potential for evaluation to be seen as relevant, useful, enjoyable and feasible for project participants is a lot greater if the methodologies used are not restricted to formal exercises involving painstaking analysis and resulting in written reports. In order for evaluation to be a participative activity, it is important that a range of approaches are adopted to maximize the chance of appealing to as many project participants as possible. Videos, exhibitions and drama are imaginative and attractive alternatives to the written word and also have the benefit of being more attractive to the ultimate consumers of evaluation. Many people are happy to watch a play or a video where they would be less likely to read a report. And putting together a video or performing a play tends to be a collective activity in a way that writing a report is not. Inevitably, a report is usually required as well but we would certainly recommend a "portfolio" of evaluation including alternatives to the written word, to other projects with similar aims.

Using a variety of methods and data sources is also an important feature of pluralistic evaluation as described by Smith and Cantley (1985). They describe the importance of methodological triangulation, not solely to avoid the danger of being "method bound" as a result of being dependent on a single data source but also because:

> ... each data source tends to be interest bound(as tied to the interests of one group rather more than to the interests of another) and also

ideology bound(as reflecting one group's perspectives on desirable modes of operation and "success" rather more than the perspectives of other groups). The constant use of as many different kinds of data as possible ensures as far as possible, that the research reflects the full range of interests, ideologies, interpretations and achievements abroad within the agency (Smith and Cantley, 1985).

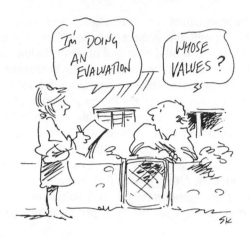

The evaluation process was immensely useful to participants in developing new insights into the project, clarifying and refining its organizational structure and direction and identifying weaknesses as well as strategies to rectify them. The before and after questionnaires demonstrated a significant shift in attitudes to evaluation with the original fear factor almost completely absent and a very high value being placed on evaluation across all categories of participants. The only concern repeatedly expressed was that the time spent on evaluation should not be to the detriment of sustaining the practice. "It (evaluation) should not become the be all and end all" (Community Health Volunteer and Management group member).

In terms of getting a pluralistic perspective on the project, although all groups participated in the evaluation in some capacity, the levels of commitment and involvement varied from one group to another. Perhaps inevitably, those who formed the day to day "core" of the project, namely staff and volunteers, had a higher degree of investment and involvement in the process than those who were further removed from mainstream activities with other jobs and other priorities. Certainly, the executive group were the most challenging group to target and evaluation had to be addressed specifically to them as a group or on an individual basis in order to be successful. This is partly explicable in terms of the competing demands on executive members' time but also might reveal an assumption that what is being evaluated does not include them.

The fundamental question of "who is the evaluation for?" was explored at the outset of the evaluation process and the most common answers were "Everyone involved in the project, volunteers, staff, working and executive members, community health forum members", "Funders", 'Managers", "the Drumchapel Community", "the Health Board", "others wanting to set up similar projects."

Respondents to questionnaires on evaluation were very clear that the evaluation should be serving the project not the other way around. In the words of one respondent, "It should be a tool of contribution not judgement." If participants can be assured that the purpose of the evaluation is to improve the project, then the likelihood of their co-operating is a lot higher.

It is difficult to demonstrate definitively the empowering effect of this style of evaluation on participants ... or at least this research failed to do so. However, insofar as empowerment involves an increase in knowledge and skills and the opportunity to use both of these, I would argue that this evaluation was intrinsically empowering. Comments from participants regarding evaluation such as, "It makes me feel part of the project and lets me know what is working out" (community health volunteer) and, "I am more aware of the need to consult a wide range of people in evaluation.

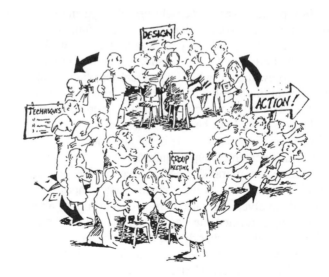

Evaluation is only relevant if all connected with the project feel they have been involved in it" (working group member), are testimony to the positive consequences for participants of being involved in the evaluation process. I am also confident that the experience will have enhanced their potential to contribute to the project in the future.

Conclusion and recommendations

"We need not more highly trained and sophisticated researchers operating with ever more esoteric techniques, but whole neighbourhoods, communities and nations of researchers".

One of the reasons that participatory evaluation is still relatively rare is because it demands a synthesis of skills from the fields of community development practice and research. More opportunities should be made available for people to acquire both sets of skills by means of secondments from one field to another, joint training opportunities and publications and the development of more of an outreach policy on the part of academic or research institutions.

No real progress towards a more appropriate research for Health for All is possible without compromise. Both the research world and the world of community health or Health for All practice need to move towards more of a shared position where there are trade offs on both sides. There needs to be more honesty about the limitation of research and an acknowledgement that there is no such thing as the perfect research design or complete freedom from bias and subjectivity. The scientific mystique which can lead to academic elitism and scientific sterility needs to be abandoned in favour of a more accessible, meaningful and collective way of creating knowledge.

For their part, community health workers need to grasp the nettle of research and evaluation; to see the latter as an integral part of practice and acquire new skills accordingly. There has been something of an unfortunate tradition within community development work that places a greater value on the practice than on the recording, reflecting and disseminating of that practice - a kind of inverted snobbery that makes it very difficult to make realistic amounts of time available for evaluation. In my opinion, this is the mark of immature practice and it is an attitude that must change if we are not to be endlessly reinventing the wheel in community health work.

There is no denying that good evaluation takes a great deal of time and this must be taken into account in forward planning and even in the drawing up of job specifications for staff. Pilot projects in particular, should have a budget for research and evaluation to employ researchers to carry out particular pieces of work and to cover the costs of printing reports and compiling videos and exhibitions. It is also useful to invite someone from a local college or university to provide access to research support, advice and training - perhaps in the context of an advisory or management group. The importance of support and training should not be under estimated as participatory research can rapidly become a disempowering experience if participants are not given adequate support and preparation. Academic institutions are often happy to play this role in exchange for perhaps taking students on placement or presentations to students on the work of the project.

As the manager of this project, I feel that it is now in a much stronger position to fight its corner as a result of this experiment in participatory and pluralistic evaluation. We can now make demands on the research establishment using the right terminology and secure in the knowledge that research methods do exist which are consistent with the values underpinning our community development and HFA practice. It is no small triumph that evaluation is not a dirty word for us as it unfortunately still is for many community health initiatives. Not only that, but participants put an extremely high value on evaluation and report having had a very positive experience of it which has actively contributed to the development of the project and the furtherance of its objectives.

Certainly, this evaluation has been one small step in the right direction but to use the terminology of Baum (1988) and Smithies and Adams (1993) who refer to walking a tight rope between the conflicting demands of service delivery, health bureaucracy and ivory tower academe, more tight rope walkers are required!

> We see before us a vision where much new and valuable knowledge can be developed by people themselves taking part in the process of creating it. Knowledge generation becomes everyone's concern. And through the process of creating knowledge comes active involvement in health, empowerment and social, environmental or behavioural change" (Starrin and Svensson, 1991).

More information on the Drumchapel Healthy Cities Project and the findings of the evaluation described in this chapter are contained in the report, "Practising Health for All in a Glasgow Housing Scheme." This report and the videos referred to in this chapter are available from:

The Drumchapel Community Health Project, Drumchapel Health Centre, 80-90 Kinfauns Drive, Glasgow G15 7TX, Scotland

Acknowledgements

Cartoons by Simon Kneebone from "Everyday Evaluation on the Run" by Yoland Wadsworth

References

Arnstein, S.R. (1969), "A Ladder of Citizen Participation", *AIP Journal of American Institute of Planners*, vol. 35, pp. 216-24.

Beattie, A. (1991), "The Evaluation of Community Development Initiatives in Health Promotion - A Review of Current Strategies", *Community Development and Health Education vol. 1, Occasional Papers*, Health Education Unit, Open University.

Elden, M. (1981), "Sharing the Research Work: Participative Research and its Role Demands" in Reason, P. and Rowan, J. (eds.), *Human Inquiry*, John Wiley & Sons, p. 258.

Graessle, L. and Kingsley, S. (1986), *Measuring Change*, Making Changes London Community Health Resource.

Hall, B. (1975), "Research, Commitment and Action: The Role of Participatory Research", *International Review of Education*, vol. 30, pp. 289-99

Hancock, T. (1993), "The Healthy City from Concept to Application; Implications for Research" in Davies, J. and Kelly, M. (eds.), *Healthy Cities: Research and Practice*, Routledge.

Kelly, M. (1990), "The Role of Research in the New Public Health", *Critical Public Health*, no. 3.

Parlett, M. and Hamilton, D. (1977), "Evaluation as Illumination - A new Approach to the Study of Innovatory Programmes" in Hamilton, D. et al. (eds.), *Beyond the Numbers Game*, Macmillan.

Reason, P. and Rowan, J. (1981), *Human Inquiry, A Sourcebook of New Paradigm Research*, Wiley.

Smith, G. and Cantley, C. (1985), *Assessing Health Care*, Open University Press, pp. 173, 33-4.

Smithies, J. and Adams, L. (1993), "Walking the Tightrope - Issues in Evaluation and Community Participation for Health for All" in Davies, J. and Kelly, M. (eds.) op. cit., p. 96.

Starrin, B. and Svensson, P.G. (1991), "Participatory Research, A Complementary Research Approach in Public Health", *European Journal of Public Health 1991*, vol. 1, pp. 29-35.

WHO, (1988), *Research Policies for Health for All Regional Office for Europe*, Copenhagen.

17 Action research to support the healthy cities "SUPER" project: A nutrition promotion project in six cities in Europe

Lenneke Vaandrager and Maria A. Koelen

In most societies, eating is an enjoyable experience associated with social contact and the taste of good food. Scientific knowledge about nutrition has grown to the point where the contribution to health of various nutrients and amounts of food is reasonably well understood (James, 1988). Cannon (1992) argues that the general agreement can be expressed as follows:

> During the last half century, Western diets have become unbalanced. They now contain too much fat ... and not enough fibre ... the best diet to reduce the risk of heart attacks ... other western diseases ... is also the best diet to promote general good health.

Although the role of diet and illness is widely recognized there is relatively less understanding of the factors which influence how people choose, use, and change their food habits (Abel and McQueen, 1994). The range of requirements is narrow, the ways in which they are met in different societies is hugely diverse. Whilst it is easily seen that the direct consequences of food intake are biological - food meets the energy and nutrient needs of the body - it is also apparent that the nature of that food intake is shaped by social, religious, economic and political processes (Fieldhouse, 1986). Food habits are often inculcated early in life and are on the whole stable and long lasting but, they are nevertheless subject to change. Such change may be induced by educational programmes based on the idea that poorly balanced nutrition is due to a lack of knowledge. However, knowledge is just one aspect of nutrition behaviour; personal taste, cultural traditions, patterns of social behaviour, the foodstuffs available in supermarkets, the menus in cafeterias, restaurants and fast food outlets also have an important effect on food choice. Furthermore, the development of food processing technology has influenced agricultural production and food availability and therefore nutrition patterns, more than any deliberate education campaign on nutrition (WHO, 1993).

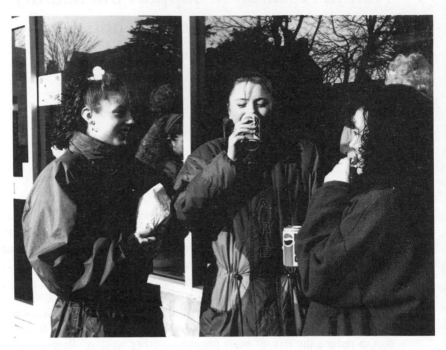

Knowledge is just one aspect of what determines nutritional behaviour

The complexity, the interrelationships and the uncertainty about explanations of eating behaviour does not mean that one should wait until this behaviour is fully understood mainly because viewpoints and research insights will never stop developing. As long as uncertainties are made explicit, action in the quest for positive health does not demand full certainty (Koelen and Vaandrager, 1994). Furthermore, a strategy for improving public health nutrition should be based on a broader perspective incorporating changes in the physical and social environment of the individual. This is not a vision which only concerns improving nutrition but is a basic starting point for health promotion in general (Ashton and Seymour, 1988).

The SUPER-project

The SUPER-project or the nutrition MCAP (Multi-City Action Plan), is a six country project with a focus on improving diets. The basic assumption of this project is that a health promotion approach is necessary for achieving healthy nutrition behaviour since it depends on much more than individual knowledge

(Vaandrager et al. 1993a). Six European cities are participating: Liverpool (U.K.), Valencia (Spain), Horsens (Denmark), Rennes (France), Amadora (Portugal) and Eindhoven (The Netherlands)[1], all of which are members of the Healthy Cities Project of the World Health Organisation. In general, WHO documents (Ottawa Charter for Health Promotion, 1986; WHO, 1993) have defined health promotion as including several key characteristics: the process of enabling people to increase control over and to improve their health, action to build a healthy public policy, the creation of supportive environments, the strengthening of community action for better health, the development of personal skills for health and the reorientation of health care.

The SUPER-project tries to put these characteristics of health promotion in practice in the field of nutrition. It was decided to start on a small scale, therefore each city identified two geographically defined pilot areas. Partnership is developed between the community, the local government, the commercial sector, the health and social professions and community structures (schools, neighbourhood organizations). Working committees with representatives of these sectors have been established which exchange information and try to achieve joint agreement on priorities, targets and plans. Efforts are made to focus on possible adjustments in the physical and social environment of the individual and to make these environments supportive for change. Therefore, activities are organized within supermarkets (which can be made supportive environments since choice for food is often made at point of purchase) and other settings such as schools, neighbourhood centres, restaurants, local festivities, etc.

Research focus within the SUPER-project

The participating cities agreed to link research to the project since the approach was relatively new for Europe and an aim of the project was to develop models of good practice (Vaandrager et al. 1991). Initially the role of research was mainly thought to be important for two aspects: planning of the interventions and evaluation of the effects. It was decided to work with a three year plan. This started with a preliminary study to document frequencies of food consumption, nutrition knowledge and attitudes of inhabitants of the project areas (see for example Vaandrager et al. 1992) and to carry out an inventory in supermarkets to explore the selling policies of local supermarkets. The findings were translated into an intervention and finally the preliminary study would be repeated to be able to show the effects. Each step would take a year, so it would become a three year project.

During the development of the project it became more and more clear that working according the principles of health promotion also has implications for research. The goal of providing support for intersectoral and community

221

participation assumes a learning process. This process requires collaborative problem posing and analysis as pre-requisites to problem solving (Harris, 1992). A classical model of research in which it is up to the behavioral scientist to discover the basic facts and relationships, and that it is up to others to somehow make use of what has been discovered, was therefore too restricted. Both for the advancement of science and the improvement of human welfare strategies, it was recognized that research and action within health promotion should be closely linked.

This experience is not unexpected since all the characteristics of the Ottawa Charter are active concepts. Change or innovation is a main component of all of them (McQueen and Noack, 1988). To be able to develop a process of change, resulting in organizational learning over a considerable period of time, the researcher should stimulate and guide this process. The researcher cannot simply stand aside and just report research findings to the decision makers. The researcher acts less as a disciplinary expert and more as a coach in team building and in seeing to it that as much of the relevant expertize as possible from all over the organization is mobilized (Foote Whyte, 1991). It means organizing ourselves for innovation more effectively (Engel and Salomon, 1994). By working this way, the researcher is constantly challenged by events and by ideas, information, and arguments put forward by the project participants. If the advance of science is a learning process, clearly this continuous learning can be very efficient.

From practical experience within the SUPER-project it was learned that building up and understanding participation processes is very relevant for project outcome and progress. At the beginning of the project representatives of each city were convinced that intersectoral and community participation should play an important role in the SUPER-project but gradually it has become clear that it is experienced as a difficult part of the project. During the annual business meetings of the SUPER-project the issue of involving institutions and volunteers has always been mentioned as a difficult task (see for example Vaandrager et al. 1993b). This is why it was decided to study possible research techniques to support community participation and use them to guide the process of change. This paper focuses on participation within the SUPER-project and the role research can play in guiding and stimulating this process.

Intersectoral collaboration and community participation

Communities can be considered as systems of power and influence with formal and informal functions for maintenance: management of conflict and competition, the allocation of resources, and the formation of public policy. The distribution of information is central to these maintenance functions which are carried out through the interaction of sub-systems including mass media and other institutions, organizations, and groups (Finnegan et al. 1993).

Intersectoral collaboration and participation has received such wide attention because the literature suggests it offers a strategy which can potentially reach more people and allows community members involvement in the programme. Furthermore, it is assumed that it can be more effective in terms of health gain, and that there will be better use of existing resources and opportunities. Finally, it is assumed to be a more sustainable approach. This means that the desired outcomes are continued, made routine, and diffused and that a community can build on this experience.

To achieve participation, initiatives must seem meaningful and reasonable to the participants of interest. It must make sense in terms of community culture (Cook et al. 1988). Differences in the cultural orientations of the different actors can be a primary barrier to communication and collaboration. An important part of a cultural system is its members "valued ideas" that dictate how things should be done.

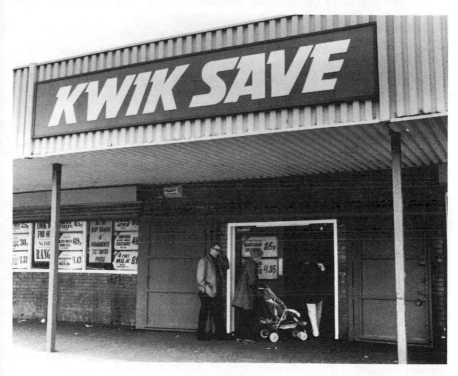

In many poorer communities supermarkets may provide only limited access to healthy food

Furthermore, there must be understanding of each other's major goals (Disogra et al. 1990) and participants should be convinced that their combined efforts become more than the sum of their individual contributions (Koelen and Brouwers, 1990).

Within the SUPER-project several methods have been used for this preliminary work. For example the Valencian Institute of Public Health used the Rapid Appraisal of Agricultural Knowledge Systems method (RAAKS) (Engel and Salomon, 1994) which is designed to identify key actors, their goals and objectives and opportunities for participation structures (Boonekamp, 1993).

Since intersectoral and community participation is a dynamic process it is difficult to have one universal definition of participation and it is also not possible to develop a universal model for managing participation. Rifkin (et al. 1988) suggest the following definition for community participation:

> Community participation is a social process whereby specific groups with shared needs living in a defined geographic area actively pursue identification of their needs, take decisions and establish mechanisms to meet their needs.

Although this definition covers many elements of what participation could be, one could wonder, especially in the European situation, if people living in a geographical defined area have "shared needs". A definition of participation can also change over time. It is important therefore, in a situation were people are working together, that all participants clarify in the beginning of the process what they consider as "participation", who they think should be involved and why, and that the actors keep reflecting on what they are doing during the process. The researcher can play an important role in guiding and stimulating this process.

The participation measurement tool

Community activation, as a health promotion strategy, includes organized efforts to increase community awareness and consensus about health and in this case nutritional problems, co-ordinated planning of prevention and environmental change programmes, interorganizational allocation of resources, and citizen involvement in these processes. The aim of the SUPER-project is to work according this approach. Often the management and responsibilities lie with representatives from different sectors and volunteers who become involved.

Researchers have tried to measure participation as if it were some monolithic phenomenon, not taking into account the wide range of settings in which participation occurred, nor the wide varieties of forms of participation. Therefore impact has most often been assessed by the numbers of participants taking part in programme activities. Other quantitative indicators which researchers have used are:

1. The target groups which are reached.

2. A count of opportunities to set up activities.

3. Percentage of inhabitants which are members/users of the community organizations.

4. Number of collaboration structures.

5. Number of members, member growth and number of people attending meetings.

6. Number of tasks of each participant.

7. Amount of time people spend on the programme.

8. Number of trained people within the project.

9. Number of contacts between the groups etc.

This kind of quantitative data however, although of some value, does not reveal what has happened, how the process took place and how it can be improved. Often less emphasis is placed on analyzing the process of programme development and implementation, particularly where this process has involved community organization activities. As a result, the factors affecting programme development and implementation and its relationship to outcomes remain poorly understood.

Qualitative indicators can be important to understand and discuss community participation. Rifkin and colleagues (1988; Bjärås et al. 1991) have developed a method, using a pentagram model, for assessing community participation in health programmes. Rifkin studied many projects which aimed at involving different sectors and the public. She found that the following indicators for participation play an important role:

1. Needs assessment - how are needs identified?

2. Leadership - which groups are represented?

3. Organization - how are goals achieved?

4. Resource mobilization.

5. Management - how does the organization achieve its goals?

These indicators can be used as a basis for measuring participation at a different time in the same programme, by different assessors of the same programme or by different participants in the same programme. To find a point which can be used for comparison at a later time can be very useful. Therefore, she developed a continuum with wide participation at one end and narrow participation at the other. On the continuum a point can be marked which most closely describes participation in the assessed programme at a given time. The five indicators are visualized in a pentagram model as referred to as "a spiderweb".

Development of the participation measurement tool for the SUPER-project

Within the SUPER-project the participation measurement model of Rifkin was applied and adapted to the specific situation of the SUPER-project. To decide where to plot on a five point scale for the indicators of needs assessment, leadership, organization, resource mobilization and management, questions were chosen from the original model (Rifkin et al. 1988). These questions are guidelines for evaluators to enable them to develop their own questions for each specific programme.

The participation measurement tool was used for the first time at the annual business meeting of the SUPER-project in Liverpool in 1993 (Vaandrager et al. 1993). The aims were threefold:

1. To test whether tool was suitable for internal evaluation and stimulating the discussion.

2. To examine how intersectoral and community participation has been applied in the different project cities and how this can be improved.

3. To motivate project cities to use this tool in their own cities.

It was decided to define narrow participation as: "mainly professionals are in charge" and wide participation as "views, objectives and needs of all different participants (inhabitants, professionals, commercial people, voluntary groups etc.) are represented."

226

The representatives of each city were asked to go through the questions and choose the position on the continuums of the indicators. They were then asked to do the same exercise for the desired situation. To clarify their choice the representatives worked in groups and afterwards the spiderwebs were presented and discussed in the general meeting. Space does not permit description here of the results of the spider webs for each city. Furthermore, this tool is not meant to describe the actual situations in reality, but more perceived realities. Since being an "insider" influences the judgement, the configuration will vary according who does the observing. The outcomes are consequently less important than the actual process of using the tool as a reflection and agenda setting instrument. To illustrate this with an example the application and outcomes of the measurement in Eindhoven are briefly described. This exercise was carried out locally one month after the Liverpool business meeting. The functionality of the tool will then be discussed in more detail.

Assessment of participation in Eindhoven

All members of the local steering group in Eindhoven (supermarket managers, a dietician, social and community workers, health workers, educational staff and volunteers) received a questionnaire beforehand with questions on all the indicators. Discussion took place in three small working groups to fill in the spiderweb and finally each group presented the outcomes of the discussion and the choice of the scores.

The main questions which arose during the discussions were very basic questions going back to the start: What are our objectives? Who do we want to involve and why? Another point put forward was that, although there are many organizations involved in the steering group of the project, no written commitments to participate in the project were obtained. The representatives of the organizations involved, felt that they needed more support from their superiors to justify their time spent on the project.

Furthermore, in general it became clear that the persons concerned were satisfied with the working strategy of the project but they felt that more effort should be made to get local inhabitants involved. Not everybody had this opinion because a social worker questioned the reasons for community participation. He was afraid that professionals were motivating local inhabitants to collaborate that they would not feel responsible any more. The group did not agree with this viewpoint: in particular the people from the neighbourhood centre disagreed because they said that many activities would not be successful without involvement from the community. As a pre-requisite though, the group concluded that if people want to get involved they should have training and proper guidance.

It was also suggested that schools, which until that time had hardly participated, should be more involved in the project. Experience had shown that if activities were concrete, then it was much easier to involve volunteers in the organization than if plans were still very vague.

All these arguments resulted in a spiderweb at the time of the meeting where needs assessment, management, organization and resource mobilization were assigned a value of three and leadership a value of two. The "desired" spiderweb for the future indicated that organization and management should achieve a value of five and leadership a value of four, while no changes for the indicators needs assessment and resource mobilization were expected (see Figure 17.1).

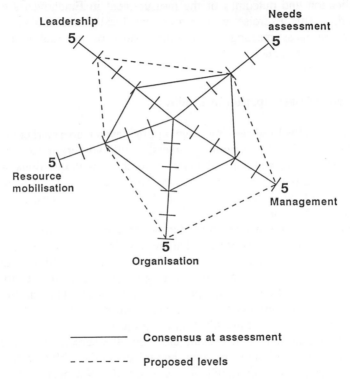

— — — — — — Consensus at assessment

- - - - - - Proposed levels

Figure 17.1   Outcome of participation measurement, showing the consensus at the time of assessment and the proposed values

As a strategy to achieve the proposed levels of participation, it was decided that the Municipal Health Service would write a policy document, based on the results of the assessment, clearly stating objectives and the roles of the different participants and the aim of this collaboration. This document has been produced and discussed with all the participants so that the final issue has been approved by everyone. The document will be offered to managers of the organizations involved and the politicians of Eindhoven.

Discussion and conclusion

Active participation has the pre-requisite that relevant social actors must be willing to get involved (Engel and Salomon, 1994). Therefore, the goals for the combined approach of the possible participants have to be identified and explored. Among the participants there should be a clear understanding of each others' motivations and ability to promote mutual benefits. Moreover, it is necessary to determine their opportunities or "space" for participation and their experience of working in this way. Even though a person or organization has been identified as an essential partner they must be able to carry out the responsibilities within the structure in which they work. For example in Eindhoven, the dieticians of the home nursing service were not allowed to participate because they had to focus their attention on patients with specific dietary needs (e.g. diabetes). In addition to this space for participation, people need to know what it means to work together and what they can expect. Volunteers, and others, may require training, and may need to get acquainted with the decision making structures.

The participation measurement tool helps to clarify whether working strategies are in agreement with what the participants have in mind. It is important to also make the choice of the indicators and the definition of narrow and wide participation a collaborative process. This became clear during the presentation of the spiderwebs at the business meeting. It was questioned why these indicators were the most important and whether additional indicators should be included. Furthermore, some participants experienced difficulties with the definitions and proposed alternatives. Clearly all these remarks were helpful and showed that development and application of these type of techniques require involvement from the beginning. The tool is useful to identify steps forward, the input, requirements and responsibilities of the participants.

By applying this tool at intervals during the course of a programme, it can visualize the process, development and agenda setting.

What is interesting is the discussion stimulated by using the tool. Representatives reflected on their own activities, management and organization and had to make clear what they were doing and why. This implicitly meant that they had to clarify their goals and objectives and think about future strategies, one of the aims of this exercise!

Health promotion approaches need innovative research techniques and an adapted view of science and validity. This view has been applied to the SUPER-project and therefore participatory research techniques have been used. The necessity for good criteria to judge information has also been stressed in this paper. The participation measurement tool is an example of peer and participant checking and the policy document prepared by the Municipal Health Services is an example of a report with working hypotheses, a contextual description and visualization. To stand back and critically assess the nature and status of partnership can help to improve the participation process.

Final remarks

The main concern in society today is change. Research needs to anticipate change, adapt to new needs, and create timely solutions. Although researchers always seek valid research outcomes, one approach or type of research on its own can hardly be called valid; validity is an outcome of different views of scientists, policy makers, practioneers and so on. Research discussions and facts are constructed by human beings together. Therefore, applied social research should stimulate this discussion so that it leads to a more holistic approach and that is what health promotion is about. Within the SUPER-project we have learned much about the advantages of this research approach and it has helped to build a variety of health promoting networks.

References

Abel, T. and McQueen, D.V. (1994), "Determinants of Selected Unhealthy Eating Behaviours Among Male and Female Adults", *European Journal of Public Health*, vol. 4, pp. 27-32.

Ashton, J. and Seymour, H. (1988), *The New Public Health*, Open University Press, Milton Keynes.

Boonekamp, G. (1993), *The Knowledge and Information System of the Food Sector in the Region of Valencia*, IVESP, Valencia.

Bjärås, G., Haglund, B.J.A. and Rifkin, S.B. (1991), "A New Approach to Community Assessment", *Health Promotion International*, vol. 6, no. 3, pp. 199-206.

Cannon, G. (1992), *Food and Hhealth: The Experts Agree*, Consumers' Association, London, p. 11.

Cook, H.L., Goeppinger, J., Brunk, S.E., Price, L.J., Whitehead T.L., and Sauter, S.V.H. (1988), "A Re-examination of Community Participation in Health: Lessons from Three Community Health Projects", *Family and Community Health*, vol. 11, no. 2, p. 1-13.

Disogra, L., Glanz K., and Rogers, T. (1990), "Working with Community Organizations for Nutrition Intervention", *Health Education Research*, vol. 5, no. 4, pp. 459-65.

Engel, P. and Salomon, P. (1994), *RAAKS: A Participatory Action-Research Approach to Facilitating Social Learning for Sustainable Development, Paper presented at the International Symposium on Systems-Oriented Research in Agriculture and Rural Development, Montpellier, France, 21-25 November 1994, Department of Communication and Innovation Studies*, Agricultural University, Wageningen, The Netherlands.

Fieldhouse, P. (1986), *Food and Nutrition: Customs and Culture*, Croom Helm, London.

Finnegan, J.R., Viswanath, K., Kahn, E. and Hannan P. (1993), "Exposure to Sources of Heart Disease Prevention Information: Community Type and Social Group Differences", *Journalism Quarterly*, vol. 70, no. 3, pp. 569-84.

Foote Whyte, W. (1991), *Participatory Action Research*, Sage Publications, London.

Harris, E.M. (1992), "Accessing Community Development Research Methodologies", *Revue Canadienne de Santé Publique*, vol. 83, supplement no. 1, pp. S62-6.

James, W.P.T. (1988), *Healthy Nutrition. Preventing Nutrition-Related Diseases in Europe*, WHO Regional Office for Europe.

Koelen, M.A. and Brouwers, T. (1990), "Knowledge Systems and Public Health, Knowledge in Society", *International Journal Knowledge Transfer*, vol. 3, no. 3, pp. 50-7.

Koelen, M.A. and Vaandrager, H.W. (1994), *Health Promotion Requires Innovative Research Techniques, A paper presented at the Health in Cities Conference in Liverpool, 20-24 March 1994, Department of Communication and Innovation Studies*, Agricultural University, Wageningen, The Netherlands.

McQueen, D. and Noack, H. (1988), "Health Promotion Indicators: Current Status, Issues and Problems", *Health Promotion*, vol. 3, no. 1, pp. 117-25.

Ottawa Charter for Health Promotion (1986), *Health Promotion*, vol. 1, no. 4, pp. iii-v.

Rifkin, S.B., Muller, F. and Bichmann, W. (1988), "Primary Health Care: On Measuring Participation", *Social Science and Medicine*, vol. 26, pp. 931-40.

Vaandrager, H.W., Ashton, J., Colomèr, C., and Koelen, M. (1991), *SUPER, The European Food and Shopping Research*, Department of Extension Science, Wageningen, The Netherlands.

Vaandrager, H.W., Ashton, J. and Colomèr, C. (1992), "Inequalities in Nutritional Choice: A Baseline Study from Valencia", *Health Promotion Int.*, vol. 7, no. 2, pp. 109-18.

Vaandrager, H.W., Koelen, M.A., Ashton, J.R. and Colomer Revuelta, C. (1993a), "A Four-Step Health Promotion Approach For Changing Dietary Patterns in Europe", *European Journal of Public Health*, vol. 3, pp. 193-9.

Vaandrager, L., Koelen, M. and Ashton, J. (1993b), *Report of the Third MCAP Nutrition Business Meeting of the European Food and Shopping Research Network (SUPER), Department of Communication and Innovation Studies*, Wageningen, Agricultural University, The Netherlands.

WHO (1993), *Health for All Targets: The Health Policy for Europe, Updated edition September 1991*, Copenhagen, WHO Regional Office for Europe.

18 The health education authority/Look After Your Heart–Avon localities project: A community heart disease prevention project on the Bournville estate, Weston-Super-Mare, Avon, 1991–93

Linda Ewles, Ursula Miles and Gill Velleman

Look After Your Heart-Avon (LAYH-Avon) is a multi-agency heart disease prevention programme, started in 1987. Members include the NHS (Health Authorities and NHS trusts) and local authorities.

In 1990, LAYH-Avon received a Health Education Authority (HEA) award of £50,000 per year for three years for a community development project focused on two geographical localities, one of which was the Bournville estate in Weston-super-Mare. "The Bournville", as it is known, consists almost entirely of post war council housing and has an estimated population of about 4,500. It was chosen specifically for the project because it was an area of high health need, with its residents particularly at risk of heart disease.

Profile of the Bournville estate in 1991

Weston-super-Mare is an old established seaside resort in the county of Avon whose current population of 45,000 is expanding rapidly, making it one of the fastest growing towns in the West Country. The Bournville estate, or "The Bournville" as it is known to its residents, is peculiarly isolated from the rest of the town. It is the largest council estate in the area, bounded on two sides by railway lines and on the third by a new retail park. Though relatively close to both the town centre and sea front, these boundaries serve effectively to isolate the estate.

The Bournville consists almost entirely of a complex mix of post war council housing: bungalows, semi detached houses, maisonettes, low rise flats and two seven storey tower blocks. In 1991, there were 1,732 dwellings owned by Woodspring Council (including 228 sheltered accommodations) with an estimated population of 4,500. There was a reasonable standard of housing provision and maintenance. Many houses had sizeable gardens and the large central green area together with several open spaces and playing

233

fields made for a generally pleasant environment.

The area contained 8 small shops, a run down public house, a rarely used community hall, youth club, 2 churches, a branch surgery, 2 primary and 2 infants schools. There was no land devoted to industrial use.

There was a high proportion of senior citizens and young families on the estate. 54 per cent of families with children under five were on income support and 31 per cent of their wage earners were unemployed. Unemployment on the estate, among all ages, was the highest in Woodspring district. Employment was often seasonal in the hotel or catering trade for men and low paid for women in the small industrial units just off the estate. Major private employers had recently cut back drastically on their local workforce. Few people travelled further afield than Weston for their work where the local authority and newly opened Weston General Hospital were the major employers.

There was no health centre on the estate and only one lock up GPs branch surgery which opened for only four hours per day. Problems of heart disease, stroke and respiratory illness were confirmed by GPs as the major killers on the estate. Major problems in child health were asthma and hearing problems, specifically "glue ear".

Opportunities for exercise on the estate were very limited, with no indoor facilities and few outdoors. Diet on the estate was obviously a major health issue, defined by what was on offer at the local shops, what residents were used to eating and what they could afford. Two fish and chip shops offered the only take away food outlets and the one small grocers stocked a very limited range of food.

The older Bournville residents generally found it an extremely pleasant place to live. They had their own social networks, day centre and luncheon club, church over 50s ladies' groups and coffee mornings, bingo sessions and outings. Their housing was good and the estate was relatively crime free.

The experience of many of the younger residents could hardly have been more different, as their level of community activity was virtually non-existent. On an estate with over 700 children under the age of 11 years there were no playgroups, no mums and toddler groups, no after school clubs, no nurseries and outdoor play provision of one rusty climbing frame and two swings. The youth club was under used mainly because of the remoteness of its position from the centre of the estate.

Apart from a housing office, none of the local authority departments had a presence on the estate providing face to face services for their clients. There was no health centre or drop in centre for social services or health visitors.

Early comments from the project worker illustrated some of the key issues apparent at the start of the project:

Bournville is going to be a tough nut to crack - let alone understand! Lack of organized groups makes contact with residents difficult. It will be important to proceed slowly without making hasty judgements, to doubt much of what is said by "outsiders", to work through what few groups there are if possible initially rather than taking a hasty initiative that may prove counter productive (February 1991).

I feel that unless some of the fundamental health problems are addressed by the provision of extra resources ... as a matter of urgency other health promotion ... is going to be superfluous. As the headmistress said when I mentioned healthy eating promotion - I'd just like to promote eating! (April 1991).

Involvement with groups of residents is still proving very difficult due to their almost complete absence! (April 1991).

A community development approach

We realized that going into a community such as this with an imposed agenda of lifestyle issues (smoking, diet, exercise and so on) would not be successful, because other issues were much more pressing in people's lives. We started by identifying the issues which were important to the residents themselves, such as developing play facilities for the children. The approach we used was "community empowerment" which means that the project worker worked with individuals and especially groups to: develop perceptions of positive self worth and a belief that harmful or stressful circumstances can be changed; mobilize people in community groups to strengthen social networks and the community capacity to collaborate and solve health problems; promote actual improvements in environmental or health conditions and enable people to experience a sense of community and gaining control over their own destiny, which is in itself health enhancing.

There are many examples of how this approach has led to practical measures which have improved the quality of life and health of Bournville people, and some of these are described. There is also some evidence that local people have started to consider the more "traditional" risk factors to health, such as smoking, when they feel their immediate pressures such as coping with young children in inadequate accommodation on a low income are being addressed, and social networks are in place to help.

What were the project's aims in Bournville?

The project had clear aims which were important in guiding the development and evaluation of the work. It is of interest, however, that these aims evolved somewhat as the true nature of the task became better understood. The modified aims became incorporated into the criteria used for assessing the progress and outcomes of the work. The initial aims and objectives were as follows:

Aims

1. To contribute to a positive change in the subjective health status of the Bournville population and to a reduction in morbidity and mortality from CHD.

2. To develop models of community involvement in CHD prevention.

Objectives

To work with the Bournville community to:

1. Develop positive changes in knowledge, skills and behaviour in relation to the CHD risk factors of diet, exercise, smoking and stress.

2. Develop support structures for individuals and groups who wish to make lifestyle changes.

3. Develop opportunities and facilities to make "healthier choices easier choices" in the localities.

4. Develop appropriate methods of involving communities in CHD prevention.

Project activities

The project's achievements after three years can be clustered under five headings: mothers and children; communication; the community centre and locality centre; environment and facilities; other achievements.

For mothers and children

One of the key early findings of the project was that there were high numbers of mothers with young children on the estate, who were often single, lonely and isolated. There were no play facilities, groups, clubs or social networks for younger residents.

Smilers

This group for women with young children grew to a regular group of about 30 women, soon run by members themselves. There were many benefits: social networks, outings, mutual babysitting, children's discos, a sponsored children's walk, and successful campaigns on traffic hazards and housing issues. It was also observed that most of the smokers in the group gave up cigarettes.

Tiny toes

This group for women with babies and toddlers was started by a health visitor with support from the project worker, and grew into three self run groups involving about 80 people a week. One group was established at the hostel for homeless families on the estate. Activities have included health promotion talks, alternative therapies during no smoking week, taking part in a TV health programme and outings. Several members of this group have also stopped smoking, and there have been other benefits too such as that commented on by one of the health visitors:

> We started a mother and toddler group - this has gone from strength to strength. We have far more coming to the clinic now, average 25-30 a week, and we find that mothers are coming to have informal chats with us more frequently.

Junior activities club

Established with the county council community leisure department, this group is based at the community centre and provides after school activities for 5-11 year olds.

Summer play scheme

The scheme was set up as a collaborative venture with the project workers and council community leisure department, community association, health visitors and churches. After the first scheme in 1991, it went from strength to strength, attracting around 200 5-11 year olds each summer with the help of 50 volunteers. It also included health activities on exercise, healthy eating and safety.

Case study: getting a play park on the Bournville estate

Local people had identified the lack of play facilities for children as a priority for action. This case study shows how the project worker was influential in securing play park facilities in the centre of the estate by working with local people and councillors. It illustrates the way the project worker worked with local people, providing support and "know how" but basically aiming to empower local people, so that they acquired the skills and confidence to make changes.

Speaking at community health council resulting in bad press

The project worker spoke at a Community Health Council meeting where he reported on the lack of play facilities. Unknown to him there was a reporter at the meeting who published front page headlines about this "Deprived Estate" and said that lack of play facilities had a detrimental effect on children. A local resident read this and contacted the Social Services Department, who advised her to contact the project worker.

Meeting local residents

The project worker visited the local resident and her family of four children, who remarked about their mother that "she's never done anything like this before". The project worker suggested that a petition was one way to raise awareness in the council. He got the petition forms produced at the LAYH-Avon office and these were given to the resident. Together with her sister and friends, she collected 1,500 signatures over the next ten days.

Lobbying the council

The project worker phoned up the town clerk to ask who the petition should be presented to and was told to take it to the Parks Department. Because the project worker was familiar with the working of the council he knew it must go to the leader of the council and have the press present. Before the relevant meeting he primed three local ward councillors to speak in favour of the petition and invited the press; he had met the three councillors during the early stages of the project and saw it as vital to gain the support of elected representatives.

The council meeting - local resident speaking up

At the meeting the town clerk asked if anyone wanted to speak on behalf of the petition. When no one spoke he said it would be filed with the others.

238

At this point the local resident who had got the petition together stood up and said "No - I've worked my arse off over this". The matter, instead of vanishing, was referred to the chief officers in marketing and leisure.

The wait - keeping it on the agenda

Over the next few months, the project worker phoned every four to six weeks to find out what was happening. A new assistant director at the council came to have a look at the lack of facilities and the project worker showed him around. He reported back that it should be the number one priority and at the next meeting it was voted that £35,000 from the £100,000 budget for play facilities should go to the Bournville.

Publicising success ... and the future ... then a fortuitous meeting

The project worker publicized the proposal in the Bournville Broadcaster, saw the Parks Department Director to review progress and talked to the Deputy Head of Community Leisure. The latter indicated that although he hoped that the scheme would go ahead there were budget cuts and smaller schemes in other parts of Avon were going ahead first. This was very disappointing for people who had worked on the petitions. Then by chance the project worker found out that the committee were meeting that evening; then again by chance he met the local ward councillor, told him the news and asked if he would speak up at the meeting.

More meetings

The ward councillor spoke up at the meeting with a good speech which got the backing of other councillors. The recommendation was to have another look at the proposal, and it was subsequently voted through.

From plans to reality

The plans were brought to the community centre in October and the local resident who organized the petition and her friends attended. She became a founder member of the Park Users Group. The play park opened about two years after the start of the project.

Communication - the Bournville Broadcaster

A communication network which reaches everyone on the estate was vital to the success of establishing estate activities and encouraging a sense of community "belonging".

The Bournville Broadcaster is a community newspaper established jointly with the council community leisure department in 1991, with copies distributed to every household on the estate with the help of volunteers. In 1993 its production transferred from the LAYH-Avon office to a local secondary school, with 50 students involved in writing, editing and producing it, with help from the school technician, and material costs met by LAYH-Avon.

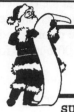

BOURNVILLE BROADCASTER

Issue No : 5
November/December '92

SURVEY RESULTS INSIDE!! ➥ ➥

Broadcaster Briefing

Watch out for the big day on 23rd November when work is due to start on the new play park at Coniston Crescent. Congratulations to Sandra Disney, sisters and friends who collected the original petition and showed that if you're determined enough you can get things done.

Lots of people have been talking to us about their memories of Bournville in days gone by, particularly **wartime stories.** It would be a shame to lose all this, so in January we'll be getting hold of a **tape recorder** and a local historian and sitting everyone down to chat over many cups of tea. If you're interested in **Bournville Bygones** give us a ring.

Tel: (0934) 642195

Anyone out there interested in **amateur dramatics/ possible Christmas pantomime** next year? There's a nice stage waiting to be used in the Community Centre - again give us a ring.

Any budding **DJ's** out there who'd like to get **kiddies discos** off the ground in the Community Centre with their own equipment and won't charge an arm and leg for it.

Bournville Food Co-op - banding together to buy cheaply in bulk is a good idea in these recession days. Anyone interested??

The new locality project building has **good disabled access** and **toilet facilities** - any disabled groups or individuals wishing to use it socially or educationally get in touch .

Trades Directory we are going to compile a list of local people with skills who'd like to offer their services to others who may have need of them - gardening, carpentry, plumbing, building, walking the dog or whatever - if you're in need or would like to put your name on the list let us know.

Rock 'n' Roll any bands out there who'd like to put on a fundraising benefit for the Broadcaster get in touch. We'll sort the venue out, let's keep music live on the Bournville!

Roadsign to Bournville

Why is there only one roadsign to Bournville?
Because, like the databanks of a computer
The engine room of a liner
The archives in a solicitors
The kitchen in a hotel
The essential factors are always tucked away out of sight!

Alan J. Savage

Tribute to Councillor Albert Watts

It was with great sadness that we learned of the death of Albert on the 13th October 1992.

Many tributes have been made since and the Bournville Broadcaster must add our regards.

With the support of the Community Centre, Albert has enabled the Broadcaster to establish itself into a reputable Community newspaper, overseen an increase in community activities, catering for a wide cross section of residents, such as play-schemes for children to tea dances for seniors.

A strong supporter of community work principles, it is without doubt that many new projects are a success today thanks to Albert.

Our thoughts and condolences are with Mrs Watts.
◆◆◆

Produced with the support of
LAYH-Avon,
Avon Community Leisure
Department &
South Weston
Community Association.

Next Issue No: 6
January/February 1993
Deadline : 22nd January

An example of the Bournville Broadcaster

The Broadcaster is an invaluable channel for publicising activities, making suggestions and gingering up support for new things. The Broadcaster had a key communications role for Tiny Toes (mother and young child group), over 50s Keep Fit group, children's discos (attracting about 80 children), a community cafe, a learning difficulties social club, an estate survey, a local history group, a women's self defence group, and a computer festival organized by local women for around 500 people.

The community centre and locality centre

When the project started, there was an under used community centre and no other focal point for estate activity.

At the beginning of the project, there were only four activities a week taking place at the community centre. By the end of 1993, there were 18 activities a week. New events at the centre included Smilers (for women with young children), summer play scheme activities, an over 50s keep fit class, the Bournville beanfeast (a fun healthy eating event for children in 1991), an accident prevention event, aerobics class, karate club, tea dances, children's discos and a local history group.

Turning to the locality centre, at the start of the project there were plans for a multi-purpose health and social services building on the outskirts of the estate. The project worker helped other local workers to lobby successfully for this building to be established in the centre of the estate (next to the community centre), and it opened in 1992. Since then, many activities focusing on health and social well being take place there: child health clinics; social work; counselling for alcohol and drug problems by the local voluntary drug and alcohol agency; sessions with a community psychiatric nurse; a milk token exchange scheme; a parents contact service with the local secondary school; a post natal support group; an older women's health group; a stop smoking group.

Environment and facilities

Some of the most marked changes over the three years of the project were environmental. Parts of the estate changed from bleak, rundown, under used spaces to areas buzzing with activity. There were also a number of campaigns to improve safety. In all these changes, the project worker played a significant role in drawing attention to needs, and working with local people to mobilize support and lobby for changes.

Key developments were that in 1992 the locality centre was built in the middle of the estate, and play parks established. In 1993, the following changes took place: the pub had new landlords, a "face lift" on its exterior and activities attracting a range of people; new street signs and local council

241

notice board were put up; Bournville Infants School had a new playground, using the children's own designs and a small grant from LAYH-Avon; there was a new pelican crossing, traffic hazard lights and road markings and there were plans for a new GP/primary health care facility.

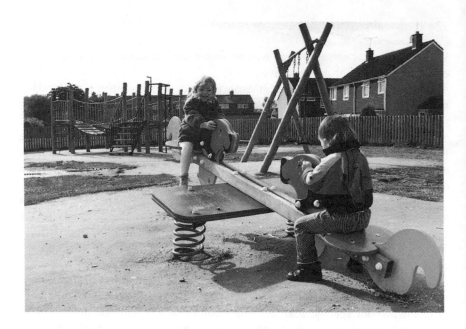

The new play park on the Bournville estate (Source LAYH-Avon)

Other achievements

In many other ways, the project worker played a significant role in drawing attention to needs, and working with local people to mobilize support and lobby for changes. Further examples are a needle exchange scheme set up at the estate chemist shop, after concern from residents about discarded needles left lying around, and a needle injury to a young child which led to a petition with around 1,000 signatures.

At the pub, new activities included fund raising events, a "Drinkwise" event, and promotion of low alcohol drinks.

A better range of "healthy" food became available at one of the local shops.

A women's self defence group became established with the help of the WEA, focusing on techniques of self defence, assertiveness and stress release.

The project worker also ran regular sessions at the locality centre from 1992 at which people discussed particular difficulties; about seven or eight people a week received help in this way.

Evaluation

Development of evaluation strategy

We were aware of the relative lack of suitable guidelines on how to evaluate community development activity. The evaluation strategy that developed had to be carefully adapted to the nature of the work, and to the limited time available. It was not possible within these constraints, nor appropriate, to undertake a quantitative assessment of population behaviour or attitude change, nor a rigorous and detailed analysis of changes in community structures and organization. Because the evaluation was to be carried out at regular intervals as part of the routine work of the project staff, it needed to be simple to use and not make excessive demands on their time. Our approach, put simply, was one of self evaluation which aimed to chart changes in a systematic way.

The initial project objectives have been set out above. We also had an initial list of "outcome headings" under which progress could be assessed. These were: participation of the target population in health related action; perceived changes in attitude and knowledge of the target population; changes in demand for health related services and facilities; perceived changes in behaviour of target population; changes in the availability of support for people wanting to change lifestyle; changes in the provision of facilities and resources to enable lifestyle changes; physical changes to the environment; changes in the knowledge/skills/attitude and practices of local health and allied workers; changes in relevant policy and procedures by local statutory and voluntary organizations; dissemination of good practice and unexpected outcomes which do not fall into any of the above categories.

This provided a useful and manageable tool for evaluation - a framework for recording the activities of project workers on a monthly basis - and yielded a rich picture of the kinds of changes that were taking place, as well as considerable detail on particular activities that were undertaken.

Although this approach provided a robust framework for charting these changes, it was apparent part way through the work on the Bournville that the initial framing of the objectives was too narrowly focused on behavioural risk factors. It did not take sufficient account of the kind of pressures that were present and characteristics of individuals on the estate which made lifestyle changes virtually impossible to achieve. It was at this stage that increasing attention was paid to the issue of people's lack of control over the forces affecting their day to day life.

We therefore decided to include the notion of empowerment into the overall aims and objectives of the project, and to include information about changes in the outcomes data. This has worked quite well, and some interesting material has emerged concerning the changes in lifestyle undertaken by people taking part in group and campaigning activities which in themselves have not been directly related to heart health issues. An "Outcome Measures Checklist" evolved, under which processes and outcomes were assessed by the workers. This is shown in Appendix 18.1.

Some of the key issues we encountered

The activities of the project were varied and complex. At the end, we reviewed our experience, and this is a summary of key issues which emerged for us.

We found that it was absolutely vital to address the expressed needs of the community first. A holistic approach was necessary, taking account of the underlying determinants of health (deprivation, lack of self esteem and self empowerment) as well as the less obvious possible risk factors (stress) and the obvious ones (smoking, diet, lack of exercise). Initially, there was some interest in exercise, but smoking was only addressed when people raised it much later.

The project worker formed huge networks, involving local newspaper reporters, teachers, pharmacists, community police, health visitors, GP practice staff, social workers, publicans, housing officers and others who all contributed to better conditions of living on the Bournville. A local newsletter, the Bournville Broadcaster, produced by a secondary school, was a very useful means of communication, advertising new activities, raising issues and gingering up support for changes.

Initially, the project worker found it much easier to link with women than men on the estate. Almost all networks and activities were for women, and it proved difficult to involve men on the Bournville.

We found that there is an issue of divided loyalties and an inescapable tension when the project challenges the provision of services which are provided by LAYH-Avon member agencies themselves.

It took much longer than we had expected (about 15 months) to set the project up, which included agreeing the proposal with all the agencies involved, applying for the HEA award, and appointing the project worker.

Working with a community development approach was a new experience for some people in LAYH-Avon. Those involved in managing the project learnt that they needed to be flexible, adapting to the difficulties of identifying clear work boundaries, and balancing a "heart health" agenda with the community's "bottom up" agenda which does not directly address traditional risk factors.

We discovered that the amount of time needed to deal with issues of management and evaluation was very much greater than we had anticipated.

We developed a system of "charting changes" using an "outcomes checklist", and found it a useful way of evaluating the impact of the project. It was streamlined to become a not too time consuming part of the project worker's normal reporting mechanism.

Unlike similar projects, we did not set up a steering group, and never found it necessary. The project worker linked in with local people over a range of specific issues as diverse as play facilities, production of the Bournville Broadcaster, and needle exchange schemes. The local community did not perceive the work as "a project" at all. On the estate, there was no identifiable LAYH-Avon programme or project, but a range of locally owned initiatives.

Who is the project not reaching?

We are aware that the changes we observed and recorded relate to a proportion of Bournville residents, not to all of them. Throughout the project, we were concerned about those who were not being reached. As the project worker expressed it in his report of October 1991:

> ... when I came here there were virtually no organized groups to work through, now there will soon be quite a few. So if there are, say, 15 different groups by Spring 1992 each attended by 20 people on average then I shall have the opportunity to get through to 15 x 20 = 300 people. However my feeling at the moment is "What about the other 4,700?". The silent majority who are totally unmoved or unaffected by the apparently frenetic amount of community development activity being acted out on their behalf but whom it totally by-passes ... shouldn't we be aiming at a rather higher strike rate? ... community health work might afford the opportunity to reach beyond the confines of small groups and really touch the lives of the majority of people in an area, given people's concern about their own, their children's or family's health ... I haven't quite got around to cracking yet, but at heart I feel I'm asking the right question!

We have counted numbers of people who became involved in activities, wherever possible, and recorded the changes (such as the new play park) which would affect many others. But we have no objective measurement of how many people were affected by the project, or to what extent. To assess the degree of community penetration, or the "ripple" effect of the work, was impossible, given the resources available. We accept that this is a limitation of the evaluation we undertook, and it is a challenging objective for other projects.

The essence of community health

While there have undoubtedly been limitations as well as strengths, the essence of what appears to be of greatest value about this work, at least for those residents known to have been involved and benefitted, is perhaps best expressed by a final comment from the project worker:

> What we've seen is health in its broadest sense, not meaning absence of illness but a positive and vibrant contribution of active local participation in decisions which affect them. Now we find a whole number of people who've been active in these campaigns looking at their personal health. They're now saying " feel a lot better about life on the Bournville - it's a good place to live, it's a happening place to live, maybe I'll make some changes in my own personal life around issues such as smoking, drink, diet and exercise.

> They feel that life's worthwhile, they want to live life to the full. They want them and their children to have a good time. The Bournville is now a happy place, and as a result of that they've made changes. They'd never have made them if a health promotion official, however well meaning, badgered them into changing their lifestyle when they still didn't feel good about where they live. So we see the two as very much coming together.

> If you help a community to change and people are active in the community they will then go on to make those changes in their particular lifestyles which can help them to live longer and happier lives. One won't work without the other, and that's the lesson of our experience here on the Bournville.

Acknowledgements

Full and summary reports of the project are available from LAYH-Avon, Bristol Area Specialist Health Promotion Service, Frenchay Healthcare NHS Trust Headquarters, Beckspool Road, Frenchay, Bristol BS16 1ND. We wish to acknowledge, with thanks, the Health Education Authority and the Tavistock Institute of Human Relations in supporting this project.

Appendix 18.1
The outcome measures checklist used in the
LAYH-Avon community project

Participation of the target population in health related action

Numbers and characteristics (age range, sex etc.) of people who attend groups, community activities etc.

Perceived changes in knowledge, attitude and behaviour of target population:

Changes in attitude towards participation in group and community activities, changes in belief in ability to have control and influence over one's own life, belief in the power of group action, changes in subjective experience of belonging to a community. Also includes reports of change in the capacity of local groups to identify problems and collaborate to solve these.

Changes in demand for health related services

Changes in demand or requests for community related services and facilities (for example from FHSA audit of CHD screening or noting the requests for "talks" or training).

Changes in the availability of support, facilities and resources for people wanting to change lifestyle:

Changes in group and community activities, informal social and support networks within the community.

Other physical changes to the environment

Changes such as permanent play facilities.

Changes in the knowledge, attitude, skills and practices of local health and allied workers

Changes in attitudes towards local residents to exercise choise and control over the services they receive, or changes in ways of working.

Changes in relevant policy and procedures by local statutory and voluntary

Changes that enable local people to have more say in decisions about local services, changes in

247

organizations	health and health authority policy and procedure.
Dissemination of good practice	What information was sent out and why, talks, presentations, papers written etc, and any evidence that good practice of others has been affected.
Unexpected outcomes which do not fall into any of the above categories	Any other outcomes, for example issues regarding consultation, image of LAYH-Avon programme.

19 A view from the tightrope: A working attempt to integrate research and evaluation with community development

Martine Standish

How far is it possible for the evaluation of a community development project, aimed at promoting heart health, to put the philosophy of community development into practice and maximize community participation? This paper is a personal consideration of the evaluation of the Heart of our City project, at a point two-thirds of the way through a planned six year programme.

The project's evaluation was designed to compliment a community development approach. The evaluation was to assess changes in heart health, assess the effectiveness of a variety of community development interventions and it was hoped, help identify a replicable model of heart health promotion. The Heart Health survey described here was designed as only one key element of the evaluation, providing evidence of changes in heart health knowledge and behaviour. This paper examines some of the problems encountered in undertaking an evaluation of heart health promotion in the community, and reflects on the level of community involvement achieved in the evaluation of the project.

Heart of our City is a community development heart health project based in four wards in North East Sheffield. The area is multi-racial, and like many other inner city areas, scores highly on socio-economic deprivation indicators. Heart of our City is a demonstration project for Healthy Sheffield, and so is closely linked to the Healthy Cities movement and the principles of Health for All. It is committed to reducing health inequalities, promoting partnership and developing community principles and practice.

The project was launched in 1990, with a planned six year programme of intervention, research and evaluation. For the first three years, it was funded by the Health Education Authority's Look After Your Heart (LAYH) programme, Sheffield and Trent Regional Health Authorities, and Sheffield City Council.

Resolving differing approaches to coronary heart disease prevention

The Heart of Our City (HOOC) project aims to promote heart health. Coronary Heart Disease (CHD) presents particular challenges to epidemiology. The purported causes of CHD are multiple, posing complex questions about interactive effects. Moreover, studies of "risk factors" for heart disease and heart attack show that taken together these factors explain only some of the variance in morbidity and mortality (Williams and Popay, 1994). Epidemiology has difficulty in dealing with behaviourial and social factors such as class, diet and stress because they do not easily reduce to simple measurable variables (ibid.).

However, in the UK CHD rates show major variations between different regions, social class and ethnic groups, and these are widening (Marmot and McDowell, 1986). These differences cannot be attributed solely to medical care: health behaviours, material conditions, factors operating early in life and psycho-social factors (including the experience of relative deprivation) are all likely to play a part in generating socio-economic variations in CHD (Marmot, 1994).

The majority of attempts to prevent heart disease are concerned with reducing the known risk factors for the disease, but Hunt has argued that none of the criteria for effective campaigns aimed at the prevention of disease are fulfilled in the case of CHD. "The medical condition is not well defined; the cause is not known; appropriate interventions are not yet clear; and compliance with control strategies is not likely to be substantial" (Hunt, 1994).

She suggests that the predominant focus on individual behaviour (in terms of smoking, diet and exercise, as set out in the Health of the Nation) as the major cause of death from heart disease cannot be supported by scientific evidence. The idea that the particular behaviour of individuals leads to disease, and that the solution lies in individual change is however, easy to grasp, and reflects the dominant medical model (Hunt, 1994).

Behaviours which are considered to be risk factors are not isolated activities but are rooted in the social, psychological and physical environment of community life. Hunt (1994) suggests that:

> The link between certain factors associated with the risk of developing heart disease and death from heart disease is composed of a separated set of possibilities. There are several stages leading up to death: predisposing factors, present from before or soon after birth, such as family history or infections in infancy; factors which increase susceptibility, such as economic and social strain, stress, smoking; factors which may precipitate a heart attack, such as accumulated stress, unemployment, a traumatic event; and factors which increase the

likelihood of dying from a heart attack, such as social isolation, financial problems and the speed of treatment.

The project has attempted to reconcile those two differing analyses of the causes of heart disease. It has tried to carry out development work which will impact on the four groups of factors outlined by Hunt; at the same time it has been important for the project to carry out, and be seen to carry out, activities which impact upon the individual risk factors. The project's community development approach offered scope for working on a broad range of social and environmental issues; individual risk factors presented a tighter focus for work.

Evaluating the project

The challenge for the project was to initiate community development which would effectively tackle the interrelating factors underlying heart disease, but also to carry out an evaluation which was compatible with community development. This raised a number of issues.

Firstly, there is a degree of tension inherent in setting up a community development project with a pre-established health agenda. This did not present major problems in terms of activities if a broad analysis of the roots of CHD was taken. Most community identified health needs could be related to CHD in some way. The evaluation, however, had to consider what brought about changes in heart health specifically.

Secondly, there were the familiar dilemmas of developing research methods which were reliable and valid but also embraced the tenets of community development - which Baum (1988) likened to "walking a tightrope". The evaluation had to address Healthy Sheffield's principles of equity, empowerment and participation. This meant devising methods which allowed local people to participate in the process. The evaluation needed to be valid and useful to local people and communities, and also have scientific credibility in the eyes of the project's funders and the research community.

Thirdly, there was the question of how to evaluate the community's health when the dominant health outcome measures focus on individuals. The prevailing bio-medical model of public health research leads to a bias towards physical health problems, neglecting social and mental issues, and a tendency to investigate personal behaviour at the expense of socio-economic and environmental factors (Whitehead, 1993). Our tools for measuring the well being of communities are still woefully inadequate. The project's emphasis on one disease exacerbated this difficulty.

Fourthly, there was the problem of evaluating the impact on CHD itself. A time limited project could not wait to evaluate long term changes in

251

morbidity and mortality from CHD in the area. The evaluation had, instead, to rely on proxy indicators of improved heart health - changes in knowledge, attitudes and health related behaviour in relation to the most widely agreed risk factors.

The evaluation of the project as a whole has a number of elements: the Heart Health surveys, which will be described in more detail below; detailed process evaluation of the project's activities; a survey of GP's and health professionals; shopping basket surveys; and other elements still in development. Local people were not involved in the initial design of the evaluation, but have contributed to its development since.

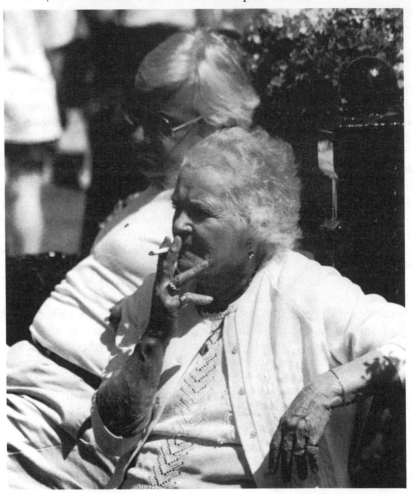

It was recognized that focusing only on heart disease risk factors would not work, and a broader community development approach was also needed

The heart health survey

The Heart Health survey was designed as a way of assessing changes in heart health encouraged by the project which would also involve local people. It forms a major element of the project's evaluation. The survey provides socio-economic information on the local population, and monitors change (over a six year period) in knowledge of CHD risk factors, health related behaviours, measures of health status/well being, perceptions of the causes of illness, use of health services and opinions about other local services. As the survey is not yet completed, discussion will focus on the process rather than the findings.

The survey was designed to assist the community development process, involving local people as far as possible to ensure diffusion of information relating to heart health. Local people were recruited as interviewers to collect data, and have also been involved, to varying extents, in data handling and dissemination.

The longitudinal survey makes use of two complementary samples - a snowball sample and a random cluster sample. Together these provide both representation of minority groups and a representative population sample. Data has been collected in face to face interviews using a structured questionnaire.

The Heart Health survey is a longitudinal, time series study which has two aims. Firstly, to collect systematic and detailed data on issues pertinent to heart health, identifying areas of need on which to base future project activities; and secondly to provide information over time as part of the evaluation of the project. The success of the project in promoting heart health can be assessed by a continuing spread of awareness, discussion, information seeking and behaviourial, social and organizational change throughout the designated area, over that period of time.

The idea of a control group was rejected in the project's evaluation proposal, as it was considered that the evidence from previous large scale intervention studies showed that this was neither feasible nor appropriate in the "real world" situation. The problems which would arise in trying to find a suitable control area are obvious (Thomas and Munro, 1994) and have been reported recently with respect to a similar community development project in Wales (Nutbeam, 1993). The lack of a control group, however, makes it difficult to attribute changes to the activities of the project. This problem has been overcome, to some extent, by drawing comparisons with data from the Trent Health and Lifestyle Survey (1992 and 1994).

Longitudinal studies present a variety of particular problems (Hakim, 1987). One of these is that changes in research staff are more likely. In recent years there has been a shift away from funding long term research programmes to short term projects (Whitehead, 1993). This has been parallelled by NHS changes which have laid a strong emphasis on effective purchasing for health gain (Hunter, 1994), fuelling a desire for rapid results on the part of the Health Service funders. For the HOOC project, funding uncertainties (only three of the six years funding for the programme was initially secured) contributed to breaks in researcher continuity. As the survey had a clear plan, this was not disastrous, but it did lower the level of support available to ensure community participation in the process. The project began with a full time researcher, who recruited and supported the local interviewers. When she left, the post could only be offered for a few months. The new researcher had to work to a very tight time table, and was less able to provide training and support to local people in more than interviewing.

Other practical problems for longitudinal studies include sample attrition and the possibility of the research being overtaken by events in a variety of ways (Hakim, 1987). While attrition has not been a major problem for the project to date, the high level of interest in CHD research and the speed of the NHS changes have made six years seem a very long time.

The samples

The survey samples were drawn up in two ways, using snowball and random cluster techniques. This combination enabled the project to reach the traditionally less well represented members of the local communities.

The snowball sample

Ten local people were recruited as interviewers to undertake data collection. They were seen as key change agents in a diffusion model (Rogers, 1983; Parcel, 1990), which would ensure a spread of information relating to heart health in the local communities. The interviewers were carefully chosen to reflect the diverse ethnic, age and geographical communities in the area. Each of the ten interviewers were asked initially to interview 12 people they knew - friends, relatives, neighbours - giving a total of 120 interviews. Each of these 120 interviewees were then asked to name five other people who would be willing to be interviewed, giving a potential maximum of 720. Interviewers were advised to attempt to interview equal numbers of male and female respondents, and respondents of differing ages.

By relying on the social network of the interviewers, it was possible to include respondents in the survey who may not otherwise have been sampled by more traditional techniques. This is particularly important when working in an area with a high proportion of residents from black and minority ethnic communities. Thus while not "representative" in the technical sense, this technique did encourage representation.

This approach allows for a more equal relationship between interviewer and interviewee. It takes the Acker (et al. 1982) caution that "the researcher's goal is always to gather information, and the danger always exists of manipulating friendships to that end" and turns it on its head, by formalizing the use of friendship. It is also particularly suited to community development, allowing local people to develop skills to work with their own communities.

The random cluster sample

A variety of procedures for rapid epidemiological survey have been developed for sampling large populations, which avoid the necessity of drawing large and costly random samples. Random cluster sampling is one such technique. In this case, 30 residential streets are chosen, at random, in the project area. Ten interviews are completed on each street starting at a random point, generating a sample of 300. The random samples provide a comparison with the snowball sample, and a means of checking on the penetration of the project - assessing how effective the diffusion technique has proved.

This sampling technique had the advantage being very simple to operate. It maximized the use of interviewer time as there was a system for selecting another house if it proved impossible to carry out an interview, and repeat visits were rarely necessary. A possible bias could be introduced by going on to another house in this way, as those at work or absent for other reasons may tend to be missed out. This problem was ameliorated by carrying out interviews at different times of day. Census statistics also provide a means of checking the sample in relation to the total population of the area. One major disadvantage of the method used however, was the difficulty of matching interviewer and interviewee as peers which sometimes caused problems with gaining trust and agreement to interview, and in the quality of rapport established. The definition of peer can be problematic (Scott, 1984), and in this case simply living in the same broad geographical area was no guarantee of a sharing of understanding or identity.

Benefits and problems for local interviewers

The involvement of local interviewers has been an exciting element of the project, but the difficulties which Smithies and Adams (1993) identify for the overall evaluation of community participation also apply to working with locally recruited interviewers. Opposing interests may be involved, work is developmental, change is constant, process needs evaluation as much as outcomes and methods should mirror the community development approach, but they don't always succeed.

There have been major benefits arising from the involvement of local interviewers. For the evaluation to fulfil a community development function, "the community must be involved in all stages of the exercise (design, fieldwork, analysis and follow up) and hence a sense of ownership of both the process and the outcomes" (Hawtain et al. 1994). The interviewers recruited reflected the social diversity of the project area, and brought a range of skills to the evaluation. Several of the interviewers could speak languages other than English. The interviewers all received training and during data collection periods, attended weekly support meetings. (This helped meet one of Baum's (1988) criteria for sound and meaningful research - a supportive research team).

During work on the baseline element of the survey, the interviewers were involved at most stages. While the priorities for research were not set by the community, and the evaluation therefore fails to meet Whitehead's (1993) criteria for ownership, local interviewers suggested changes to the questionnaire. One was involved in coding, and several others assisted with data input. This was seen as a positive experience as most had not worked on a computer before. The interviewers were also involved in dissemination.

The interviewers themselves felt that they gained from the process, as these comments show:

> I gained much confidence in myself. I learnt tolerance of people and understanding.

> I also particularly enjoyed interviewing people in my area. I feel now ... that this area is a lot friendlier than I previously thought and I know more people in the area.

> ... The coding of the data provided me with an added dimension to my involvement in the research and allowed me to follow the process one step further ... I eagerly await the research results and look forward to a role in dissemination of the findings.

The skills and knowledge developed as an interviewer helped the individuals to find employment (a potentially important individual health benefit), but it also meant that the investment in training by the project had to be a continuous one.

The longitudinal study was to take place over six years. "Change is constant" not just in terms of professional input, but also in terms of local involvement. For the second (snowball) survey, five of the original ten interviewers were available, and five more were trained. For the third (random) survey, 8 interviewers were used, 4 experienced and 4 new to the work.

There were particular problems, related to racism, in using the same local interviewers for both the snowball and the random samples. The snowball samples presented few problems for any of the interviewers. After completing the initial snowball sample all interviewers were given the option to continue working on the random sample. Several interviewers from ethnic minority groups decided not to continue because they felt "they were not quite sure what they would be letting themselves in for if they knocked on strangers' doors." Those that did continue did on some occasions suffer direct racial abuse. Some felt unable to complete their quota of interviews as a result of less overt racism. "The roads to which I was allocated for interviews on were mostly populated by English people. When I went there, most people wouldn't agree to an interview ... That is why I gave up working there." A white interviewer commented, "I guess the worst was listening to the racism of a few of the white people ..." However, the study also benefited from the willingness of some of the interviewers from black and minority ethnic groups to continue, despite potential dangers. In some cases, for instance, interviewers were able to exchange interviewees so that interviews in the random sample could be conducted in the appropriate language. Developing participatory research in multi-racial inner city areas demands a balance between "expert assistance from outside agencies and the enthusiastic, insider understanding of the community itself" (Hawtain, et al. 1994), combined with a recognition of the potential conflicts of interest within the community.

Data collection

Data has been collected by face to face interview in people's homes using a structured questionnaire, designed to gather information on a variety of heart health and general health issues. Where possible, questions of known validity and reliability were used, and included both open ended and pre-coded questions. Areas covered included socio-demographic information, health related behaviours, knowledge on CHD risk factors, perceptions of causes of illness, assessment of health problems, use of health services, use of and opinion of local food shops and leisure facilities, and concerns about the local area.

The main criticisms of the questionnaire have been the absence of a recognized health status or general well being index, and the use of questions which do not match those commonly used elsewhere (Thomas and Munro, 1994). Well being indicators remain controversial. Hunt (et al. 1988) argued that there are serious conceptual and methodological obstacles to building positive health indicators because of the paucity of language to express positive health and because of problems of reliability. There will always be a tension between including questions which ensure comparability with other studies and ensuring that the questions asked are useful and appropriate to the particular study in hand. The questionnaire design has attempted to achieve a balance between questions which relate to individual health related beliefs and behaviours, and questions which give a sense of the community in which the individual functions, in an interview which should take no more than one hour.

The survey structure and data analysis

Initially it was envisaged that, following a baseline interview of both samples, re-interviews would take place each year. In practice, this proved unworkable for a number of reasons. At different stages of the project the balance has shifted between maximizing community participation - and working slowly - and producing faster "results" with less community involvement. The baseline surveys had a higher level of involvement and took longer than planned. A break in research funding caused further delays.

The pattern on interviews has been:

1991   Baseline - snowball sample and random cluster.

1993   Repeat interview - snowball sample.

1994   Repeat interview - random cluster.

Both sampling methods will be used again before the end of the project in 1996.

The structure of the survey - alternating snowball and random samples - has meant that data analysis has become increasingly complex as the project has progressed.

In practice this detracted from community participation in that the researcher had to spend more time on analysis and therefore had less time available to support interviewers in working directly on the data; particularly as this coincided with a change of researcher.

The increasingly complex findings also became more of a challenge to present, both to professional and to community audiences.

Dissemination

The project has retained a commitment to effective local dissemination of findings. Reports from the first and second stages of the Heart Health Survey were made available nationally and supported by conference presentations, but particular attention has been paid to local needs. The local interviewers have been enthusiastic in assisting with dissemination, summaries of findings have been distributed through the project's newsletter, and local media coverage has been good.

FOOD SHOPPING

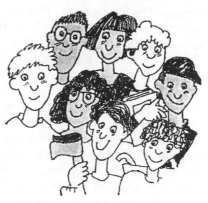

Local food shops are an important service within a local community. About half of the respondents use their local shops for their main food shopping.

Most people said that their local shops are good but they were concerned that:

- the shops are expensive,

- that the choice and variety of foods is limited.

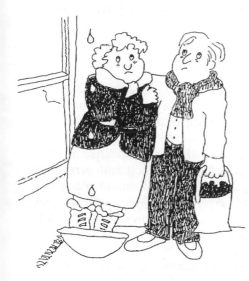

HOUSING AND HEATING

Despite the fact that most homes had central heating, **2/3 of people said they could not heat their home as well as they would like.**

Most of these people found it was too costly to heat their home adequately and many suffered from inefficient heating systems or drafty homes.

An excerpt from the project newsletter

In a further initiative to aid dissemination, funding from the Health Education Authority was provided for a research assistant who was employed with a brief to investigate community interest in information, and carry out small scale analysis of the data responses, drawing out information local people felt would be useful. She developed a variety of techniques to stimulate initial discussion and to feedback findings in different ways, including some suitable for those with literacy problems. This piece of work was particularly appreciated by local groups. One outcome was a display which illustrated the findings for particular sections of the community, for instance, how the Pakistani population had responded.

This approach to dissemination has helped develop a sense of local ownership of the project's findings. It is still debatable whether, given a free choice, the community would have chosen to investigate their knowledge and behaviour with coronary heart disease as a focus. For the project's local steering group their inability to influence funding decisions emphasizes their lack of real power to direct the project. They were not involved in the initial decisions which established the project and the evaluation or the balance of investment in each. They would clearly wish priority to be given to extending the life and activities of the project, rather than carrying out surveys. For them, it is answering real needs, which may have little to do with heart health. However, if the evaluation shows that answering their needs also improves heart health, they would probably agree that it had been worthwhile.

Conclusion

The Heart of our City evaluation was intended to enbed the reflective cycle in the project's activities. The Heart Health survey has helped provide new ideas for interventions as well as indicating changes taking place in the community. It is also important that "the research process itself should be less opaque and more open to scrutiny" (Bell and Roberts, 1984). A community development project largely funded by the health service has a wide range of stakeholders to satisfy and it can feel uncomfortable remaining genuinely open to scrutiny by an array of different interest groups. Moreover, coronary heart disease prevention is a controversial arena. A large number of research and medical interests are involved, and any evaluation findings are likely to be hotly debated.

The design of the Heart Health survey has been an innovative attempt to measure community indicators of heart health. It has employed a variety of approaches to give a rounded picture of changes brought about by the project. Interim findings indicate that there have been changes in knowledge of heart health issues, and some changes in behaviour, particularly in relation to diet and physical activity. It also seems, as might have been predicted, that the changes are greater in members of the snowball sample, who have a clearer association with the project.

There are a variety of answers to the question of how far the project's evaluation has contributed to community participation. In some ways, is has succeeded admirably. The local interviewers have been enthusiastic partners in the process and there has been a high level of participation by members of traditionally marginalized groups. But it falls short of complete participation. The original agenda was set outside the community. The levels of participation have shifted subtly up and down during the life of the project. The project has retained a firm commitment to the principle of participation, but the resources required to support it have varied. External funding and interest has had an effect and so too has the degree of skills, time and experience within the project and amongst the local interviewers. It seems unlikely, in the final year of the project, that local interviewers will be involved in data analysis, because the task of comparing data generated by the stages of the survey has become so complex. Local dissemination remains a priority, however. Overall, it seems that true participation is still such an alien concept to statutory agencies, and to local communities themselves - that it needs constant nurturing.

Acknowledgements

Much of it is based on the work and writing of those most closely associated with the evaluation of the project in its first three years - Emma Witney, Diane Moody and Sonya Hunt.

References

Acker, J., Barry, K. and Esseveld, J. (1982), "Issues in Feminist Research: An Account of an Effort to Practice What we Preach", Department of Sociology, University of Lund, Sweden (unpublished paper).

Baum, F. (1988), "Community Based Research for Promoting the New Public Health", *Health Promotion*, vol. 3, no. 3.

Bell, C. and Roberts, H. (1984), *Social Researching: Politics, Problems, Practice*, Routledge, London.

Cox, B., Huppert, F. and Whichelow, M. (1993), *The Health and Lifestyle Survey: Seven Years On*, Dartmouth Publishing Co. Limited, Aldershot.

Hawtain, M., Hughes, G. and Percy-Smith, J. (1994), *Community Profiling: Auditing Social Needs*, O.U. Press, Buckingham.

Hakim, C. (1987), *Research Design: Strategies and Choices in the Design of Social Research*, Routledge, London.

Heart of our City (1991), *Heart Health Survey (1991), A Study of Heart*

Health Issues and Needs in North East Sheffield.

Heart of our City (1993), *The Second Heart Heath Survey (1993), A Study of Heart Health Issues and Needs in North East Sheffield: Eighteen Months on.*

Heart of our City (1994), "The Third Health Survey (1994) A Study of Heart Health Issues and Needs in North East Sheffield: 3 Years On." (unpublished)

Heart of our City (1990), "Project Proposal." (unpublished)

Hunt, S.M. (1994), "Cold Hearts and Coronaries", *Health Matters*, no. 19, p. 17.

Hunt, S.M. (1988), "Subjective Health Indicators and Health Promotion", *Health Promotion*, vol. 3, no. i, pp. 23-4.

Hunter, D. (1994), "Social Research and Health Policy in the Aftermath of the NHS Reforms" in Popay, J. and Wiliams, G. (ed.), *Researching the People's Health*, Routledge, London.

Marmot, M. (1994), *The Magnitude of Social Variations in CHD: What are the Possible Explanations? Paper presented to Social Variations in CHD: Possibilities for Action Conference, held by the National Forum for Coronary Heart Disease Prevention.*

Marmot, M. and McDowall, M. (1986), "Mortality Decline and Widening Social Inequalities", *Lancet*, vol. ii, pp. 274-6.

Nutbeam, D. (1993), "Maintaining Evaluation Design in Long Term Community Based Health Programmes: Heartbeat Wales Case Study", *Journal of Epidemiology and Community Health*, vol. 2, pp. 127-33.

Parcel, G. (1990), "Beyond Demonstration: Diffusion of Health Promotion Innovations" in Bracht, N. (ed.), *Health Promotion at the Community Level*, Sage, Newbury Park, London.

Rogers, E.M. (1983), *Diffusion of Innovations* (3rd ed), Free Press, New York.

Scott, S. (1984), "The Personable and the Powerful: Gender and Status in Sociology Research" in Bell, C. and Roberts, H. in *Social Researching: Politics, Problems, Practice*, Routledge and Kegan Paul, London.

Smithies, J. and Adams, L. (1993), "Walking the Tightrope: Issues in Evaluation and Community Participation for Health for All" in Davies, J. and Kelly, M. (ed.), *Healthy Cities Research and Practice*, Routledge, London.

Thomas, K. and Munro, J. (1994), "Heart of our City: Review of Evaluation and Recommendations for Future Evaluation." (unpublished)

Whitehead, M. (1993), "The Ownership of Research" in Davies, J. and Kelly, M. (ed.), *Healthy Cities Research and Practice*, Routledge, London, p. 84.

Williams, G. and Popay, J. (1994), "Researching the People's Health: Dilemmas and Opportunities for Social Scientists", *Researching the People's Health*, Routledge, London.

Section 5 Strategies for change

Change is a norm in contemporary urban society and social science has provided many models of the change process from the historical materialism of Marxism, through the social evolutionism of neo-Darwinists to more recent developmental models, models of the diffusion of innovation and systems analysis. While all of these models are informative none truly reflect the complexity of the change process. What is clear is that all change involves learning in which research has a part to play. That learning is also based on experience. Experience as the result of taking action, reflecting on it, relating it to general patterns and synthesizing (Alinsky, 1972).

There are similarly a variety of approaches to strategic change. Strategy is often a term that is applied to top down and rational and formal approaches to change. Implied is deliberate and planned control in a search for optimal solutions based on sound information and planned targets. A contrasting view of strategic change is that it is a product of a series of actions that over time converge into pattern that receive legitimacy when they are recognized (Mintzberg, 1990). They are therefore the product of individual and collective sense making (Johnson, 1987).

Bringing about change for health in a society orientated towards disease and health care and where resources are perceived as limited or being reduced is a difficult task. The papers and workshops presented at the conference never the less demonstrated that effective action is possible and taking place widely and at a number of levels. Strategies for change are being implemented not only at the level of policy development but also at the local level through theme based or area based projects. A key theme that emerges is that the boldest strategies acknowledge and address the interconnectedness between these levels. As Pettigrew (et al. 1992) have stated, in order to achieve a high rate of change, policy development by itself is insufficient. Top down strategies cannot succeed unless bottom up action takes place and short term small scale projects cannot have an impact without a strategic framework that moves the resources to support the change. However there is a need to move from what Levy and Merry call first order change (1986) i.e. those minor improvements and adjustments that do not change the system's core and occur as the system naturally grows and develops to second order change or transformation which is multi-dimensional, multi-level, qualitative, discontinuous, radical change involving a paradigmatic shift.

Strategies for change at the policy level

Achieving a paradigmatic shift is dependent on there being a receptive context. The original raison d'etre of the WHO Healthy Cities Project was to take Health for All off the shelf on to the streets of Europe (Kickbusch, 1989). While some urban authorities are beginning to address strategies for health, there is little evidence at the national level of action on those factors that influence health despite the research evidence concerning their impact. Examples of the institutional constraints to change at the policy level is well illustrated by Peter Smith in the context of housing and health. Adrian Davis, however, in the context of transport policy and health, was able to demonstrate that change is possible if long in coming. Nevertheless, Mayer Hillman still feels there is long way still to go in the development and implementation of cycling policy at the urban level.

Even if the national context is not wholly supportive of change, three papers demonstrate how strategies for change might be developed at the urban level. The crucial role of a healthy economy, in the truest sense of the word, is well illustrated by the action taken in Sandwell. This important paper by John Middleton documents an innovative approach that could be easily replicated elsewhere, demonstrating how the public sector can work with the market to bring about change. A comprehensive approach to change is demonstrated by Lee Adams and Valerie Cotter in the case of Sheffield's Healthy City Plan, while Felicity Green and Donald Cameron describe how in Stockport, the Department of Health's national strategy for England, "The Health of the Nation", can be used as a catalyst for developing a local health strategy.

Marleen Goumans completes the papers on change at the urban level with a review of the impact of the Healthy Cities idea on policy development in The Netherlands. In it she demonstrates the problems of engaging the policy makers and politicians with the ideas of healthy public policy as encapsulated in the Healthy Cities agenda. This is despite the more receptive context of the national policy environment of the Netherlands.

Strategies for change at the local level

Feminists have drawn to our attention how the personal is also political. The interrelationship between personal change and change for health was well illustrated in a verbal presentation by M. Lakhdawala in one of the workshop sessions. The focus was on the participation of women in a health programme in the urban slums of Ahmadabad, India. Initially shy in discussing the issues important to them, the women gradually built up their confidence to go on and develop women's organizations and in the process reclaim some of their power from men. The groups started to address health problems across the slums and across the religious divide between Muslim and Hindu. As a result, over ten years, significant improvements were made in standards of water and sanitation.

Starting where people are at, lies at the centre of community development as a strategy for change. Ultimately, the future which such strategies are working for, are those of our children. In a workshop on Citizens of the 21st century the children of Speke Comprehensive in Liverpool talked about the activities that they were taking part in which were geared towards health and change. The workshop highlighted the importance of starting with children's own concerns too. This theme is mirrored in the report presented here by Clare Mahoney of the Children's Council in West Everton, also in Liverpool. A different approach to community change, geared to the American culture, is illustrated in the church based smoking cessation programme Heart, Body and Soul by Frances Stillman. Other examples of community development for health were reported throughout the conference and are referred to elsewhere.

It is clear that if change is to take place no amount of community development will be successful if it meets the impermeable barrier of existing organizations and the status quo. Organizational change is required too. In the final paper in this section Paul Thomas explains the basis of such a project geared towards the reorientation of primary health care, one of the key elements of the Health for All approach. There are only a few projects that currently pay attention to organizational issues. Yet organizational development for health requires greater attention in the future by those working in public health and health promotion if the benefits of community based projects are to lead to sustainable change.

Research as a strategy for change

Other writers elsewhere in this volume have pointed to the role research can play as a catalyst for change. Three papers are presented here which demonstrate examples where research has been deliberately chosen as a tool for change. The first is a report by Paulo Contu and colleagues of a project in Sardinia, itself an example of how innovation diffusion can lead to change. The second is by Margaret Jones and Shirley Judd highlighting the impact that a transnational action research project involving community participation had on the working practice of the local dietetic services. In this example the organization was permeable and open to change with positive results in terms of learning and action. In the final example, Rascha Thomas describes a cross sectoral collaborative project directly involving the researcher in the policy development team in a local neighbourhood in Amsterdam. Here the organizational constraints on change, as well as the potential available, are clear.

Evaluation as a strategy for change

If evaluation is treated as a process by which people learn through reflection and is best achieved if all those involved participate in the process then evaluation can also be a strategy for change (Springett et al. 1995).

A key feature of the organizational change which action to improve urban health requires, is collaboration between sectors. The final paper in this section reports on a Health Education Authority funded project which sought to develop indicators for evaluating what have come to be known as Healthy Alliances working with Health for All and public health practitioners. At the time of the conference the work was still in development and formed the basis of a workshop. The paper presented here by Viv Speller and colleagues records the completed project which ended in March 1995.

Conclusion

A key to transformation lies in the quality of direct relations among people, their capability to alter formative contexts of power and the skill to encourage and consolidate opportunities for substantive grass roots action. There was much reported at the conference that suggests that the seeds of such a transformation for health are already in place.

References

Alinsky, (1972), *Pedagogy for the Oppressed*.
Johnson, G. (1987), *Strategic Change and the Management Process*, Basil Blackwell, Oxford.
Kickbusch, I. (1989), "Healthy Cities: A Working Project and a Growing Movement", *Health Promotion International*, vol. 4, pp. 77-82.

Levy, A. and Merry, U. (1986), *Organisational Transformation*, Praeger, New York.

Mintzberg, H. (1990), *Mintzberg on Management*, Free Press, London.

Pettigrew, A., Ferlie, E. and McKee, L., *Shaping Strategic Change Making Change in Large Organisations, the Case of the NHS*, Sage, London.

Springett, J., Costongs, C. and Dugdill, L. (19??) "Towards a Framework for Evaluation in Health Promotion: The Importance of Process" in Ungar, R.M., "False Necessity", *Journal of Contemporary Health*, vol. 2, CUP, Cambridge.

20 Institutional impediments to improved housing in the UK

Peter F. Smith

According to Sheila McKechnie, former Director of Shelter, in the mid 1970s we had one of the best housing stocks in Europe, now we have dropped almost to the bottom of the league as measure by housing expenditure as a proportion of GDP. Fuel poverty is estimated to affect eight million households in the UK and that is before VAT on domestic fuel. Thirty per cent of all households are receiving benefit. In the opinion of Dr Brenda Boardman of Oxford University, the poor thermal efficiency of housing leads to condensation problems which in turn cause illness. She estimates that the cost to the Health Service due to condensation alone is £800 million per year. This does not take into account moisture penetration through the deteriorating fabric of the building. If you add to this the problems directly due to cold from inadequate heating, the total health bill comes to over £1 billion. The final macabre prediction is that the addition of the VAT on fuel will lead to an extra 5,000 deaths per year among the elderly and infirm, even after account is taken of additional benefits which the government may offer.

The impact of fuel cost on income is, of course, very unevenly distributed. The lowest fifth of the population in terms of income spend 13 per cent of their earnings on fuel; for the top 20 per cent the proportion is four per cent. A study by the National Childrens Home found that in low income families, mothers frequently had to choose between food and warmth. This position is exacerbated by the fact that it is the low income families that live in houses that are thermally the least efficient. The recent national housing condition survey shows that one in five homes in England and one in three in Scotland are seriously affected by damp and condensation. In Glasgow, half of all families with children were living in such conditions.

Ironically, low income groups tend to have to pay more for their fuel perhaps because they do not have gas central heating and have to rely on electricity or bottled gas, or the extra cost of prepayment meters and so called easy payment schemes etc. The dice is heavily loaded against them.

In an article in the British Medical Journal last month ("Health Implications of Putting Value Added Tax on Fuel", BMJ 22 October 1994) Professor Graham Watt of Glasgow University pointed out that workplaces can be closed down if they do not maintain a temperature of 16 degrees celsius, yet 37 per cent of households containing elderly people have winter temperatures below this level. He goes on to say that the crux of this problem lies, not in the relatively small numbers who are at high risk, but in the very large numbers for whom the effects are less extreme but slow and insidious and sometimes terminal.

At the same time, the way we do our accounting completely discounts the misery and suffering that are implied by these statistics. One day a monetary value might be applied to these "social externalities".

Housing, poverty and health are therefore inextricably bound together and a major cause of illness is the poor thermal efficiency of so many UK houses combined with inefficient heating appliances.

Changing focal length for a moment to the consider the health of the planet, in the UK buildings account for nearly 50 per cent of all carbon emissions and over half that total is attributable to housing - nearly 30 per cent of total UK carbon emissions. Targeting poor housing for radical upgrading would produce a fourfold benefit: reduction in the Health Service costs; reduction in the benefits burden especially through the alleviation of fuel poverty; a substantial contribution to enabling the UK meet its carbon dioxide reduction obligations under the UN Framework Convention agreed at Rio and a substantial boost to the construction industry.

So, when there is such an obvious case for treatment, why is so little happening? Most who are involved in housing know that the answer is to mount a national campaign to upgrade the thermal efficiency of existing housing beginning with the elderly and low income families. The target should be an average reduction of at least 40 per cent in the energy used for space heating across the whole UK housing stock.

A ten year programme of retro fitting was recommended by the House of Lords European Committee investigating the EC energy policy. It estimated that the cost of the work would be squarely matched by the price of the energy saved in the process. And this is where we crash headlong into the buffers of entrenched Treasury principles which will not allow such mathematical logic to affect policy.

When Michael Howard was Secretary of State for the Environment, he came to lunch at the RIBA. At that lunch I was able to ask him why the receipts from council house sales could not be used for retro fitting existing council houses. His answer was brief "because it would add to the PSBR" (Public Sector Borrowing Requirement). He was not prepared to explain why, but the reason is that the Treasury calculates PSBR in a way that would not have surprised Alice when she was in Wonderland. They operate under rules that can only be described as fiscal tunnel vision. Those involved in local government will know exactly what I mean.

Let me use the case of upgrading the thermal efficiency of a council property. The local council comes along and spends, say, £3,000 on upgrading the property which results in an energy saving of 50 per cent. Because the property has been substantially improved both in terms of its comfort standard and space heating costs, the council puts up the rent. However, the householder makes a net gain due to the reduction in energy bills as well as having a more comfortable house. At the same time, the householder now comes off in benefit because overall energy costs have been reduced. The family's chronic bronchitis is cleared up making them much less of a burden on the Health Service.

If the costs and benefits of this operation were considered in a unitary way, obviously it would make commercial as well as social sense. But the Treasury is not able to do this. It cannot weigh the cost of saved energy and of saved health and social security benefit costs against the capital cost of the retro fitting work. Such work is deemed to be an absolute addition to the PSBR.

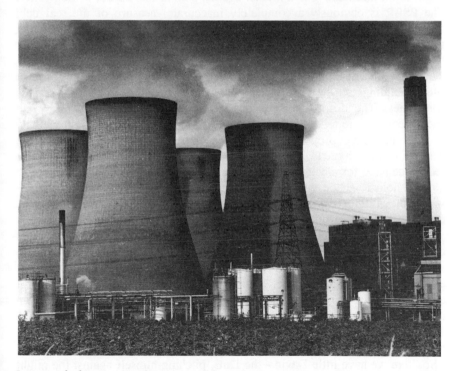

Improved house insulation could reduce energy requirements, carbon emissions and ill health

In effect that council house may well have caused injury to the PSBR at least three times; first when it was built, second, when it had routine maintenance work carried out and thirdly when the retro fit operation was executed. No account is taken of the fact that the local authority does not actually have money; it has to borrow and repay the loan at commercial rates set by the government.

The PSBR doesn't acknowledge repayments. A council house which generates income is treated in the same way as a school or a hospital which are pure cost because they are a social service.

Returning to Michael Howards's rebuttal, the fact that local authorities may have repaid most of the loan on a property then received capital on its sale does not affect the fact that any expenditure from such capital accumulation is deemed to be a cost to the PSBR. The result is millions of pounds lying idle whilst the housing stock deteriorates and consumes masses of energy and people die.

On the face of it this way of calculating the PSBR is a nonsense. However, there may be some arcane logic to it. Someone more cynical than myself might think that there was a hidden agenda behind this apparent illogicality. The PSBR is obviously a completely inaccurate measure of the real debt incurred by the government. But an artificially inflated borrowing requirement can be used by a government to justify to the electorate higher taxes and reductions in public spending.

In other countries, things are done differently. A common strategy for retro fitting buildings on the continent is through the operation of energy service companies. The idea is that an energy service company sells both energy and energy conservation. In the USA the utilities have found that it is frequently a better economic proposition to reduce consumption rather that increase generating capacity. In the UK for example it would be much cheaper to reduce demand for electricity than to build Sizewell C. But this requires the kind of holistic vision which is alien to our leaders. So, as the regulations stand, the utilities can supply electricity to homes but they cannot act as energy service companies.

Is this, I wonder, another example of schizoid government. The Department of the Environment wants to reduce the demand for energy; the DTI wants to sell as much energy as possible to push up GDP and to improve the sale prospects for Nuclear Electric. This is just one example of the adversarial ethos that pervades government from the Cabinet, through Parliament down to the ministries. Fighting your corner is the name of the game - the antithesis of the holistic approach to government. It seems the dynamics of confrontation form an essential part of our Britishness.

So, here we have little David - the DoE, pitching himself against the might of Goliath - the Treasury, Trade and Industry and Transport, sometimes called "the three terrible Ts". Whilst the financial muscle resides with the 3Ts we should nevertheless remember the outcome of that Biblical confrontation.

This compartmentalized approach goes even further. Not only is there discontinuity between energy supply and demand, energy itself is subject to being split into its discrete packages, so we have a coal revue which concludes effectively that coal is obsolete. We are currently having a nuclear revue, and this is despite the pleas of the experts to revue energy as a whole and devise policy accordingly. Of course there I've used the forbidden "p" word - policy. "Let the market decide" is the key phrase. As far as the market is concerned the elderly and infirm would greatly assist the PSBR if they died off. And as far as the planet is concerned, saving it by reducing carbon dioxide emissions to the level recommended by the IPCC is certainly not cost effective.

A national retro fit programme for housing would not only have an impact on health and benefits, it would also go a long way to resurrecting the construction industry from the dead. It is reckoned that one new job is created for every £20,000 spent on upgrading work. So here is another benefit which our methods of accounting will not allow to be included in the equation - thousands more jobs and the concomitant shift from an unemployment burden to substantial tax revenue.

I should say a little about new housing, focusing still on thermal efficiency. The government is keen to point out that our building regulations are sufficiently rigorous given our climate. They discount comparisons with, say, Denmark and southern Sweden on two counts. First, we are, it seems, habituated to lower comfort temperatures than others in northern Europe. Second, climate differences are such as to make direct comparisons of insulation standards invalid. Recently these assumption were examined.

First, as regards comfort temperature, it has been established that where homes have been built to much higher thermal standards than required under the regulations, the first benefit the householders take is in higher comfort temperatures. This was proved in the demonstration schemes in Salford and Manchester. Only after a higher comfort level was achieved did the householders decide to realize the benefit of reduced energy costs. Built in the 1970s these demonstration schemes made no impact whatever on the industry.

Second, a recent research project we undertook at Sheffield University in association with colleagues in Denmark, took a standard three bedroomed semi detached house and applied to it the thermal regulations of The Netherlands, Denmark and Sweden, using Sheffield climate data as the norm. The aim was to see how energy consumption differed in each case, bearing in mind they were all placed in the same climate. The result was that the England and Wales regulations were the least energy efficient. Danish regulations resulted in a 50 per cent reduction in energy compared with England and Wales. Swedish regulations were six times more energy efficient. Remember, this was after climate differences had been excluded.

If we look at climate data for the four countries the differences are comparatively small. For example, Malmo and Copenhagen are on about the same latitude as Berwick on Tweed but their longer summer days mean they receive more overall solar radiation. So, on all counts, our alibis in the UK have been blown.

Nevertheless, we have recently changed the Building Regulations after an agonizing period of consultation. What has transpired is that insulation standards for housing have barely changed except for windows which generally will have to be double glazed to fairly minimal standards. As over 90 per cent of all speculative houses have double glazing as a matter of market necessity, the real effect on thermal efficiency will be almost unnoticeable.

There is no doubt in my mind that the changes have been kept to a minimum due to pressure from the housebuilders who argue that higher insulation levels involve greater complexity which will cause great distress to the small builder. Also they argue thermal efficiency has a disproportionate impact on building costs. Not true. At most we are talking of between one and five per cent increase to produce a house that is at least 50 per cent more energy efficient than required by present regulations. Even at present day energy prices, the pay back time for these energy saving measures is extremely short.

There is, of course, another dimension to this situation. As I said earlier, housing accounts for almost one-third of all UK carbon dioxide emissions into the atmosphere. One of the outcomes of the Rio conference was the UN IPCC Scientific Report. This stated firmly that carbon emissions had to be cut by 60 per cent of the 1990 level worldwide to be reasonably sure of halting global warming. The Framework Convention agreed at Rio merely obliged us to return to 1990 levels of emission by 2000, and even this we seem to be unable to do. The UN Report goes into detail as to what is likely to happen if we continue with "business as usual" and its predictions make alarming reading. The fact that we are overloading the carbon cycle is due almost entirely to the industrialized countries. With 20 per cent of world population we account for 80 per cent of carbon emissions so we shoulder an urgent responsibility to change our habits in a radical way.

Reducing the energy used by buildings would offer the largest and most rapid returns in terms of reducing carbon dioxide emissions. Housing is the most profligate energy sector of the whole built environment. Targeting housing, especially that of the poor, would, therefore, make eminent sense for a government genuinely concerned to reduce carbon dioxide emissions.

Alas there are those in the construction industry who don't see it this way. Here is a quote from Roger Humber, Director of the Housebuilders Federation (published in Housebuilder, October 1993):

Sustainability is the ultimate fantasy of the green lobby ... sustainability means, in practice, no growth, deindustrialization, the reversal out of high tech into low tech, mending things not making them and a rather miserable life for us all, devoted to knitting blankets whilst sanctimoniously saving the planet.

Builders also point to the fact that energy saving features come low on the list of priorities of prospective purchasers. Unfortunately because of relatively cheap energy this is true. Location, style, etc. come top of the list; running costs are rarely a deciding factor. Perceptions will change as energy costs rise.

Two members of my RIBA Committee Robert and Brenda Vale have just completed a house in Southwell which is about 95 per cent more energy efficient than current houses and the cost was within the range for a normal detached house. When their photovoltaic cells and wind generator are installed, they reckon they will show an electricity surplus. This is a house, not in the countryside, but in a town centre on a constricted site and in the shadow of a famous Minster. It shows what can be done by an ordinary builder on an urban site within normal cost boundaries.

What I hope I have demonstrated is that our way of doing things within current Treasury rules and the market ethos has, in the housing sector, produced severe constipation. There are indeed small demonstration schemes taking place to show what can be done, but there is no hope whatever of an appropriate national programme of upgrading houses taking place unless their is a "Damascene" experience on the part of the Treasury. As a nation we are in the grip of tunnel economics; costs are never counterbalanced by benefits and until they are, the sums will continue to show that radical action over almost anything useful is prejudicial to the PSBR.

Perhaps we should balance the Roger Humber quote by a climate scientist which appeared in The Independent at about the same time. He predicted that the verdict on people today by future generations will be this "Why didn't those morons do something about it!"

We've explored one or two answers to that question.

21   Getting there: New policies and new alliances

Adrian Davis

To date the links between the health and transport have focused on the tangible and clinically identifiable impacts of road traffic casualties and air pollution. "Secondary" impacts, often the result of behaviour modifications, such as loss of independent mobility resulting in reductions in physical activity, and reduced social support networks, remain marginal.   Yet the combined effect on many people's quality of life has led some to believe that transport is now damaging health and well being more than promoting it (Hunt, 1989; IEHO, 1993).   This view has been vocalized by organizations and individuals as the effects of current transport are played out in society: witness concerns about asthma and air pollution, and opposition to new road schemes.   Transport policy is not meeting people's needs for access to the goods, services, and other people which facilitates and promotes health and well being.

This paper briefly reviews past and present transport policy developments in highlighting some of the health outcomes.   It then charts important changes in transport policy which may signal a move towards environmentally sustainable and health promoting transport policy.   Such changes bring with them new opportunities for intersectoral action and alliances between public health and environmental transport advocates in realising the vision of healthy cities.

The post war transport policy cul-de-sac

By the 1950s the car was becoming rooted in culture and society.   This was aided and abetted by the 1951 Conservative Government which shifted the emphasis away from the socialist ideology of collective good to that of individual values and consumerism.   The end of petrol rationing in 1950 followed by the cutting of purchase tax on cars, in 1953 both boosted the

277

process. The 1950s and 1960s saw the most rapid growth in ownership which more than doubled. By the 1970s the private motor car had become an apt symbol of the new affluence which stood in stark contrast to the austerity of the war years (Hamilton and Jenkins, 1989). Transport policy had clearly been decided. The forecasts for car ownership saturation, together with the largest roads programme since Roman times, were ample evidence of this. The car was implicitly assumed by government to be the desirable and normal form of travel. Yet there had been no public debate and virtually no policy for other modes of travel.

The Department of Transport's (DoT) revision of the road traffic forecasts in 1989 threw this policy into doubt, even within Whitehall. Adams (1989) illustrated the logistical and land take problems arising from attempts to meet a forecast of up to 142 per cent increase in road traffic by 2025, accommodating an additional 27.5 million motor vehicles. The new traffic, if stationary, could be placed on a motorway from London to Edinburgh, if it were 257 lanes wide. For movement, and the need for parking spaces at each end of the journey the space requirements are staggering. By the early 1990s the dichotomy between the tacit recognition of the unacceptable damage to the environment that this would require and the government's commitment to increasing the inter urban road network was widely apparent.

The forecast also raised major questions about access and equity of access. The enormous increase in car trips in recent years has not necessarily increased the number of activities undertaken. As May (1993) notes, a 60 per cent of all the increase in travel resulting from people making longer journeys simply to do the same things as at best of doubtful benefit to society. Moreover, at minimum a car based approach results in vastly increasing inequities in transport provision. It ignores the fact that 20 million people will be too young, old, infirm, banned, or poor. Adams (1993) has suggested what this might mean for this third of the population:

> ... a prototype of the programme envisaged by the government has already been tested in the health service, where they have an established system for looking after those who are mentally ill or otherwise incapable of caring for themselves. It is called "Care in the Community". One idea that is being developed for the transport version of this programme is the provision of large bus shelters in which the carless can congregate, and shout at passing cars, while waiting for the bus that will never come.

Primary health impacts: road traffic casualties and lung damage

While there are over 4,000 road traffic fatalities each year and a "guestimatible" number of casualties, current transport and "road safety" policies have, and continue to attack symptoms and not address the danger at source. As a result, what is meant by the term "road safety" has been questioned (Plowden and Hillman, 1984; Adams, 1985). Road safety, as guided by the dictionary, means freedom from the liability of exposure to harm or injury on the road (Davis, 1992). In contrast, Silcock (et al. 1991) have noted that "when writing or talking of road safety most people are referring to the lack of safety, usually expressed in terms of accident frequencies or accident rates ... road safety usually means the unsafety of the road transport system."

Such concerns have been heightened by the report "One False Move" (Hillman et al. 1991) which looked at children's independent mobility. Through a 19 year follow up study it found that parental perceptions of road accident risk had led them to restrict their junior school aged children's independent mobility. Walking and cycling had been reduced dramatically. For example, in 1971 80 per cent of seven to eight olds were allowed to go to school on their own, in 1990 this had dropped to nine per cent. More recently some road safety officers have also questioned traditional approaches, establishing a danger reduction charter for local authorities as a mechanism for shifting the agenda from treating symptoms to tackling danger at source. Wolinski (1994) has stressed that:

> ... this means looking afresh at what is measured and how. ... we need to recognise that there is a relationship between vehicle volume and speed and danger, not just accidents. Furthermore, we need to develop our appreciation of the full harmful effects of road traffic - pollution, community severance and health - as well as casualties, and of the inequitable way in which all of these operate. ... Most crashes are not "accidents"; many "safety" measures actually create more danger.

In general the focus of "road safety" on behaviourial modifications of the most vulnerable may be all to familiar to public health researchers (Tesh, 1988; Baum, 1994; Roberts and Coggan, 1994). Challenges to the behaviour modification lobby echoes The Black Report (1980) in stressing the need for a refocusing up stream to public policy and environmental modifications.

In the 1990s air pollution is also an increasingly central health concern (Ayres, 1994). There is a growing consensus that the alarming rise in child asthma is related to the ability of emissions to lower tolerance thresholds (Davies, 1994). Most recently PM10s (particles of less than 10 microns in diameter) associated with diesel have heightened concerns that such pollution may cause cancers (Savitz and Feingold, 1989; Phillips, 1994). A correlation between neighbourhood traffic volumes and child respiratory symptoms has also been reported by researchers (Wjst et al. 1993; Walters, 1994). The Department of the Environment (DoE) has recently suggested that local authorities may be given powers to control traffic when weather conditions are conducive to poor air quality (DoE, 1994).

"Secondary" health impact of transport

A focus on road accidents and air pollution follows a predominantly traditional bio-medical model of health and disease. Health and well being are, however, affected by a much broader range of transport impacts. Encouragingly, public health is increasingly adopting such a broad based model which incorporates environmental and social factors as well as bio-medical influences. The impacts include cumulative effects and lifestyle changes of which some are, arguably, largely responses determined by traffic. Additional impacts identified in the literature include:

1. Noise pollution.

2. Physical activity (sedentary car orientated lifestyles).

3. Community severance.

4. Access to healthy diets (and cost).

5. Land take (loss of green space).

6. Stress (to travellers and non travellers).

7. Personal safety (streets without pedestrians), including danger and fear.

8. Mental health and well being including longer term effects of noise.

9. Reductions in exercise (Biddle, 1993).

An example, community severance, how roads and traffic divide communities is one of the more subjective but no less important impacts of transport on health. Appleyard's studies (1981) show how environmental quality is inversely related to traffic density. The most vulnerable can be marginalized by a transport policy which undermines their ability to access facilities independently and to participate in community activities so reducing the ability to make and continue contacts with friends and acquaintances (Berg and Medrich, 1980). This may be an important "secondary" health impact because social support networks have been shown to be life supportive (Berkman and Syme, 1979; Fox, 1988). A further example may be seen in declining levels of physical activity in adults and children (HEA/Sports Council, 1992; Cale and Almond, 1992; Armstrong and McManus, 1994). While children have less freedom to walk and cycle many adults' mobility is expressed through habitual car use. In both cases this may itself significantly contribute to increase risks of coronary heart disease.

All change! - implementing the "new realism"

Increasingly because of transport impacts the dynamics of transport policy are changing. This has been termed the "new realism", the recognition of the impossibility (and undesirability) of meeting "demand" for road space with supply. An important confirmation came in June 1994 from the roads lobby's own central body, the British Roads Federation (BRF, 1994). In arguing the case for more road building their report admitted that even a 50 per cent increase from the £2 billion annual spend would not reduce the growing levels of congestion on the trunk road network. Later last year the highly influential Royal Commission on Environmental Pollution listed 110 recommendations for transport policy changes, many of which were aimed at reducing car dependency (RCEP, 1994). Two weeks later the DoT's own advisers report on Trunk Roads was published clearly showing that road building itself generates additional traffic over and above that calculated by the standard cost benefit formula. The DoT accepted most of SACTRA's findings. This puts into question much of the roads programme.

Such reports have also followed two favourable DoT and Department of Environment policy changes. In 1993 changes to the annual Transport Policies and Programmes (TPP) bids made by the 108 highway authorities in England for funds from the DoT introduced the concept of package funding. The "package approach" allows authorities to bid for funds for a variety of measures together, being assessed as an integrated "package". Importantly, a survey of the local authority responses to the criteria changes revealed that the most frequently quoted measure included in bids, by a significant extent, was bus priority (Cook and Davis, 1993). Traffic calming, cycle schemes and park and ride were also particularly popular. The most popular underlying objective of the package approach bids was improving the urban environment. By Christmas 1994 37 bids had been accepted. Another important policy change was Planning Policy Guidance Note 13 (DoT/DoE, 1994). A commitment from the 1990 White Paper, This Common Inheritance, the government has sought to introduce measures to help reduce the transport sector's carbon dioxide emissions. The guidance has consequently revived the connection between land use planning and transport. Locational policies favouring compact urban development make public transport, walking, and cycling viable alternatives to the car.

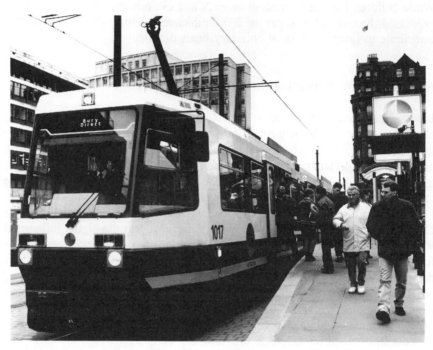

The new Metrolink in Manchester, one a of number of examples of a growing move to improve the urban transport environment

Conclusion: a proposal for intersectoral collaboration

Such changes exemplify the "new realism" in transport planning. Transport policy itself is currently undergoing change as the pressure for policies to address the environmental and health threats become transparent. The opportunities now exist to exert co-ordinated pressure to realize changes in transport policy, targeted at both central and local government. Pressure is needed to ensure that health is no longer a side issue in transport policy discussions. This can be most effectively achieved through intersectoral collaboration and action and alliances between health, and environmental transport advocates to generate, co-ordinate and exert such pressure.

The theoretical base is in place: health can be achieved through healthy public policy (Milio, 1981; Hancock, 1982; Draper, 1991). Specifically, transport has been identified (Transport and Health Study Group, 1990; Godlee, 1992). The test is whether public health advocates will accept such a proposal, challenging as it does the "great car economy".

Acknowledgement

This is a revised version of the paper presented by the author while working in the Sustainable Development Research Unit at Friends of the Earth.

References

Adams, J. (1985), *Risk and Freedom*, Transport Publishing Projects, Cardiff.
Adams, J. (1989), "Car Ownership Forecasting: Pull up the Ladder, or Climb Back Down", *Traffic Engineering and Control*, March, pp. 136-41.
Adams, J. (1993), "No Need for Discussion - the Policy is now in Place!" in Stonham, P. (ed.), *Local Transport Today and Tomorrow*, LTT, London, pp. 73-7.
Allied Dunbar National Fitness Survey, (1992), *Health Education Authority/Sports Council*, London.
Appleyard, D. (1981), *Livable Streets*, University of California Press, Los Angeles.
Armstrong, N. and McManus, A. (1994), "Children's Fitness and Physical Activity - a Challenge for Physical Education", *The British Journal of Physical Education*, Spring, pp. 20-6.
Ayres, J. (1994), "Asthma and the Atmosphere", *British Medical Journal*, vol. 309, pp. 619-20.
Baum, F. (1994), *Research and Policy to Promote Health: What's the Relationship?, Paper to Research and Change in Urban Community Health Conference*, Liverpool.
Berg, M. and Medrich, E. (1980), "Children in Four Neighbourhoods: The Physical Environment and its Effect on Play and Play Patterns", *Environment and Behaviour*, vol. 12, no. 3, pp. 320-48.
Berkman, L. and Syme, L. (1979), "Social Networks, Host Resistance and Mortality: A Nine Year Follow-Up Study of Alameda County Residents", *American Journal of Epidemiology*, vol. 109, pp. 186-204.
Biddle, S. (1993), "Children, Exercise and Mental Health", *International Journal of Sports Psychology*, vol. 24, pp. 200-16.
British Roads Federation, (1994), *The McWilliams Report*, London.
Cale, L. and Almond, L. (1992), "Physical Activity Levels in Young Children: A Review of the Evidence", *Health Education Journal*, vol. 51,

no. 2, pp. 94-9.

Cook, A. and Davis, A. (1993), *Package Approach Funding: A Survey of Highway Authorities,* Friends of the Earth/University of Westminster, London.

Davies, R. (1994), "What Exactly Does Vehicle Pollution do to the Lungs" in Read, C. (ed.), *How Vehicle Pollution Affects our Health,* Ashden Trust, London, pp. 12-24.

Davis, A. (1992), "Livable Streets and Perceived Accident Risk: Quality of Life Issues for Residents and Vulnerable Road Users", *Traffic Engineering and Control,* vol. 33, no. 6, pp. 374-9.

Department of the Environment, (1994), *Improving Air Quality,* HMSO, London.

Department of Health and Social Security (1980), *Inequalities in Health* (The Black Report), HMSO, London.

Department of Transport/Department of the Environment (1994), *Planning Policy Guidance Note 13: Transport, HMSO,* London.

Draper, P. (ed.) (1991), *Health Through Public Policy: The Greening of Public Health,* Green Print, London.

Fox, J. (1988), "Social Network Interaction: New Jargon in Health Inequalities", *British Medical Journal,* vol. 297, pp. 373-4.

Godlee, F. (1992), "Transport: A Public Health Issue in Health and the Environment", *British Medical Journal,* London, pp. 71-89.

Hancock, T, (1982), "Beyond Health Care", *The Futurist,* August, pp. 9-11.

Hamilton, K. and Jenkins, L. (1989), "Why Women and Travel?" in Grieco, M., Pickup, L. and Whipp, R. (eds.), *Gender, Transport and Employment,* Avebury Press, Aldershot, pp. 20-36.

Hillman, M., Adams, J. and Whitelegg, J. (1991), *One False Move ... a Study of Children's Independent Mobility,* Policy Studies Institute.

Hunt, S. (1989), "The Public Health Implications of Private Cars" in Martin, C. and McQueen, D. (eds.), *Readings for a New Public Health,* Edinburgh University Press, pp. 100-15.

Institution of Environmental Health Officers, (1993), *Transportation: The Route to Health,* London.

May, A. (1993), *Lifestyles: Transport,* Institute for Transport Studies, Leeds.

Milio, N. (1981), *Promoting Health Through Public Policy,* FA Davis, Philadelphia.

Phillips, D. (1994), "Can Vehicle Pollution Cause Cancer?" in Read, C. (ed.), *How Vehicle Pollution Affects our Health,* Ashden Trust, London, pp. 17-9.

Plowden, S. and Hillman, M. (1984), *Danger on the Road: The Needless Scourge,* Policy Studies Institute, London.

Roberts, I. and Coggan, C. (1994), "Blaming Children for Child Pedestrian

Accidents", *Social Science and Medicine*, vol. 38, no. 5, pp. 749-53.

Royal Commission on Environmental Pollution: 18th Report Transport and the Environment, HMSO, London.

Savitz, D. and Feingold, L. (1989), "Association of Childhood Cancer with Residential Traffic Density", *Scandinavian Journal of Work, Environment and Health*, vol. 15, pp. 360-3.

Silcock, D., Barrell, J. and Ghee, C. (1991), "The Measurement of Change in Road Safety", *Traffic Engineering and Control*, vol. 32, no. 3, pp. 120-9.

Tesh, S. (1988), *Hidden Arguments: Political Ideology and the Disease Prevention Policy*, Rutgers University Press, New Brunswick.

Transport & Health Study Group, (1990), *Health on the Move*, Public Health Alliance, Birmingham.

Walters, S. (1994), "What are the Respiratory Health Effects of Vehicle Pollution?" in Read, C. (ed.), *How Vehicle Pollution Affects our Health*, Ashden Trust, London, pp. 9-11.

Wjst, M., Reitmeir, P., Dold, S., Wulff, A., Nicolai, T., von Loeffelholz-Colberg, E. and von Mutius, E., (1993), "Road Traffic and Adverse Effects on Respiratory Health in Children", *British Medical Journal*, vol. 307, pp. 596-600.

Wolinski, A. (1994), "Danger: Road Ahead", *Surveyor*, 13th January, p. 9.

22   Urban community health and cycling

Mayer Hillman

At the Liverpool Healthy Cities Conference in 1988, the author of this paper outlined the wide ranging direct and indirect impacts of transport on urban health (Hillman, 1990). Special attention was paid to the disincentives to keeping fit by walking and cycling as part of the routine of daily life. A later report by the author, commissioned by the British Medical Association and published in its name, explored in detail the health and safety issues surrounding the use of bicycles (British Medical Association, 1992). The study on which it was based cited much evidence that people who exercise regularly are much fitter and can perform everyday tasks with less stress and fatigue. Physical activity is now well recognized to reduce not only the incidence of heart and respiratory diseases but also the risk of strokes. Mental well being has also been shown to be improved as exercise is beneficial in relieving depressive and anxiety states.

The BMA report suggested that the bicycle is the only realistic means for the majority of the population to maintain its physical and, to some extent, mental fitness throughout the year, and from childhood to old age. Alternative routes through the medium of recreational activity can not conceivably match the scope for doing so owing to the much greater potential for regular use of the bicycle as compared with, for instance, participation in sports, not to mention the deterrent aspects of access, cost and life long motivation.

It argued that cycling represents perhaps the optimal way whereby central and local government can contribute to the process of helping achieve national targets on reducing diseases (Department of Health, 1992) and of combatting the decline in the physical condition of the population: one in three adults overweight, no doubt owing to the increasingly sedentary nature of our lifestyles; three-quarters of the age group 35-64 at risk of a heart attack; and seven in ten men and eight in ten women below the age appropriate activity level necessary to achieve a health benefit (Health Education Authority and

Sports Council, 1992). Wider adoption of cycling as a main travel method can also improve the physical condition of children which is at an all time low, and declining: their metabolic rate is lower than it used to be (Armstrong, 1993).

Recent transport and health related research

In the last few years, research carried out by the author and colleagues examined the impact of the rising volume and speed of road traffic on children's independent mobility (Hillman et al. 1991). By replicating in 1990 surveys carried out in 1971 in state schools in different parts of the country, ranging from an inner London suburb to a rural parish in Oxfordshire, the study revealed a dramatic decline in freedom to travel on their own to and from school and to and from their social and recreational destinations owing to parental restrictions imposed principally because of an understandable desire to minimize the risk of their children being injured in a road accident. The decline in children's fitness resulting from the restrictions is probably exacerbated by the increasing time they now spend watching television. The study also recorded high levels of ownership of bicycles among children but remarkably little use of them as means of transport. This is regrettable on two significant health grounds. First, cycling can be particularly advantageous for children for whom the world is opened up once a bicycle can be used as their form of travel. And second, early life experiences are highly influential in the incidence of heart disease in later life and, for its prevention, childhood is the ideal time for acquiring the habit of regular exercise (Coronary Prevention Group, 1992).

The report of a Policy Studies Institute Conference held to discuss the implications of these findings of growing restrictions on children's independent travel highlighted the disturbing effects that the restrictions have on their physical, social and emotional development - as well as imposing a time consuming burden on the lives of parents, usually mothers, who see the escorting of their children (albeit the great majority of them able bodied) as an unavoidable element of child rearing for many years (Hillman, 1993a). It was noted that children's lives are becoming increasingly conducted under adult surveillance and that this was undesirable from the viewpoint of them acquiring coping skills from direct experience, promoting their innate sense of adventure, taking initiatives and risks, and gaining self esteem and confidence in the process, all of which are all key elements of the process of maturation into adulthood.

However, it is not only in the context of the personal health of children and adults that the virtues of cycling need to be seen. In marked contrast to travel by motorized means, every journey made by cycle results in a marginal improvement in public health owing to the consequent reduction in the risk of injury, danger and anxiety among other road users, and reduction in the environmental burden caused by pollution. It is the aggregation of literally millions of daily decisions to use a car without regard to the consequences of doing so which explains much damage to individual and community health. Indeed, it is ironic that the use of cars puts at risk road users such as cyclists whose travel does not contribute in any way to these undesirable effects. In particular, cycling is a form of travel that keeps the risk of injury and damage to health of other road users to a minimum. The continuation of an approach to the formulation and implementation of transport policy which is not aimed at promoting the use of the bicycle for every day travel is clearly questionable, and an approach which continues to encourage car use directly or indirectly can be seen as indefensible.

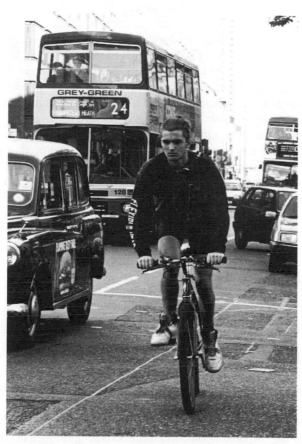

It is ironic that the cyclist, whose activity does not damage the environment, is put at risk by the car

Obstacles to society making more use of bicycles as a means of travel do not arise from difficulty in learning how to ride one: the great majority of both men and women can do so (Mintel, 1989). Nor does the ownership of a bicycle pose a major difficulty. Currently, there are 15-20 million bicycles in Britain, over three-quarters the number of cars, and cycle ownership has doubled in the last two decades (Department of Transport, 1993). But cycling accounts for only a paltry two per cent of journeys, and average mileage per bicycle has halved in the last 20 years (ibid.). Even on the most obvious journey for which it would be appropriate, namely children's school travel, cycle use accounts for only one per cent of journeys. For their journeys as a whole in the last five years, its use has fallen by one-third.

The relatively low ownership and use of bicycles in this country is largely explained by the adverse traffic conditions for cycling, in particular the fear of injury following collision with as motor vehicle. However, this concern needs to be seen in context. Analysis carried out during the preparation of the BMA report noted earlier showed that, even in the current traffic environment which constitutes such a threat to non-motorized road users, the number of life years gained by regular cyclists outweighs the life years lost in cycle fatalities by a ratio of about 20:1 (Hillman, 1993b). Moreover, there is considerable scope for increasing this ratio through two interrelated means: the environment for cyclists can be made more user friendly, as is being attempted in some UK cities following exemplary initiatives with the construction of safe and convenient cycle networks in Denmark, Germany and The Netherlands and the effect of that improvement is very likely to release the considerable latent demand for cycling among both current owners of bicycles and others who would like to cycle.

The analysis suggests that, far from it being irresponsible to encourage people to transfer from motorized transport to the bicycle, wherever this is feasible, owing to a concern about the risk of injury, it could be judged irresponsible not to encourage that transfer owing to the risk to health of not getting regular exercise by doing so.

Policies of successive governments in Britain

Oversight of the remarkable role that cycling can play in catering for personal travel is the predictable outcome of policies of the last 30 years. In determining how public resources for transport purposes are to be allocated, these policies have relied heavily on forecasts of traffic growth. These have been based on the extrapolation of past trends showing a strong link between affluence and car ownership to justify ambitious programmes of road building. Until recently, government has also made it clear that it does not see its task as promoting the use of the bicycle, hence, perhaps the omission of future levels of cycle ownership and cycle traffic from its forecasts!

Nevertheless, the Department of Transport in Britain is at long last acknowledging the role of the non-motorized modes, for instance in its recent guidance note on transport and planning (Department of the Environment and Department of Transport, 1994). It is clear that the cycle holds out far more scope than public transport for catering for the travel needs of the population when it is realized that three in five car journeys, and three in four bus journeys at present are no longer than five miles, a 25-35 minute cycle ride (Hillman, 1993c).

Local authorities are now encouraged to incorporate proposals to cater for cycling in their annual submissions for grants. In theory, far more expenditure could be ploughed into traffic calming on the 80 per cent of urban roads which are potentially eligible to be designated as 20 mph zones. and more cycle networks could be created and standards of road maintenance raised.

A rational transport policy

The government's policy approach may be compared with that in The Netherlands which decided 25 years ago to allocate a significant part of its transport budget to promote cycling. Indeed, anyone given the task of formulating a rational transport policy from the viewpoint of minimizing health as well as social, economic and environmental costs would have to conclude that cycling (and walking) should be not just catered for but should be given pride of place in the transport hierarchy, particularly in our towns and cities (Hillman and Cleary, 1992). Given its considerable virtues, it is no wonder that, in a recent book, a former Reith lecturer has expressed the view that "... the most important event in recent human evolution was the invention of the bicycle" (Jones, 1993).

The Dutch Government indicated its wish to encourage the use of bicycles in the coming decades (National Environmental Policy Plan, 1989). Its Master Plan Bicycle has the objective of both increasing cycle mileage by one-third above its 1986 level by 2010, and halving the number of cycle fatalities, by investing in more segregated routes for cyclists in recognition of the fact that about six in seven of their fatalities occur following collision with a motor vehicle (Welleman, 1992). Already, nearly all children, two in five men, and two in three women, own a bicycle (Centraal Bureau voor de Statistiek, 1990). About 30 per cent of journeys there are now made by cycle, including 60 per cent of school journeys and 25 per cent of the journeys of women pensioners, cycling is thus not just a mode largely for young people. Some may observe that it is generally easier to cycle in The Netherlands because of its relatively flat terrain. But it should be noted that the great majority of people in Britain also live in urban settlements where journeys do not entail riding up steep hills. Whilst not being able to establish cause and effect, it is salutary to compare the incidence of heart disease in the Dutch and British populations. There is of course a wide range of contributory factors to death from this cause and no one of them can be isolated to show that that is the explanation for any observed difference. Nevertheless, the fact that exercise plays a major part in terms of lowering this risk suggests that, as its incidence in The Netherlands is half of that in this country and 15 times as many journeys per person are made by cycle there, cycling may well deserve some credit.

Conclusions

Until recently, the Department of Health and the medical profession have largely ignored the considerable benefits to the health of the nation that would be likely to ensue from promoting regular cycling owing, first, to the conventional emphasis on curative medicine, and second, insofar as the exercise element of health promotion does feature in the advice provided for the general population, owing to an understandable concern about the risk of injury in the current traffic environment.

Nevertheless, a strategy on promoting the health of urban communities has greater prospects through the medium of transport policies aimed at improving the safety, convenience and attractions of cycling (the costs of which would represent only a small proportion of current transport expenditure), than through the medium of health policies. At the same time, the objectives of policy on environment, energy conservation, equity and economy, would also be furthered. The outcome of such a policy would not only directly improve the fitness of people responding to the wider opportunities to do so. It would also lead to improved community health by lowering the adverse impacts of motorized travel.

References

Armstrong, N. (1993), "Independent Mobility and Children's Physical Development" in Hillman M. (ed.) (1993a), *Children, Transport and the Quality of Life,* Policy Studies Institute.

Centraal Bureau voor de Statistiek (1990), *Mobility of the Dutch Population in 1989,* Voorburg/Heerlen.

Coronary Prevention Group (1992), *Prevention of Coronary Heart Diseases: Recommendations for National Governments.*

Departments of the Environment and Transport (1994), *Planning Policy*

Guidance Note 13. Transport, HMSO.

Department of Health (1992), *The Health of the Nation,* HMSO.

Department of Transport (1993), *Transport Statistics Report: National Travel Survey: 1989/91 Report,* HMSO.

Health Education Authority and Sports Council (1992), *National Fitness Survey.*

Hillman, M. (1990), "Transport and the Healthy City" in Ashton, J. and Knight, L. (eds.), *Proceedings of the First UK Healthy Cities Conference, Liverpool 1988,* University of Liverpool.

Hillman, M. (1992), *Cycling: Towards Health and Safety,* British Medical Association, Oxford University Press.

Hillman, M. (ed.) (1993a), *Children, Transport and the Quality of Life,* Policy Studies Institute.

Hillman, M. (1993b), "Cycling and the Promotion of Health", *Policy Studies,* vol. 14, no. 2, pp. 49-58.

Hillman, M. (1993c), *Public Transport: An Unrealistic Substitute for Most Car Trips, Proceedings of PTRC XXIst Summer Annual Meeting,* University of Manchester.

Hillman, M., Adams, J. and Whitelegg, J. (1991), *One False Move ... a Study of Children's Independent Mobility,* Policy Studies Institute.

Hillman M. and Cleary, J. (1992), "A Prominent Role for Walking and Cycling in Future Transport Policy" in Roberts, J. et al. (eds.), *Travel Sickness: The Need for a Sustainable Transport Policy for Britain,* Lawrence and Wishart.

Jones, S. (1993), "The Evolution of Utopia", *The Language of the Genes,* Harper Collins.

Mintel, (1989), *Bicycles,* Mintel International Group, September.

Netherlands Ministry of Housing, Physical Planning and Environment (1989), *National Environmental Policy Plan: To Choose or to Lose.*

Welleman, A.G. (1992), "The National Bicycle Policy and the Role of the Bicycle in the Urban Transport System" in Michels, T. (ed.), *Still More Bikes Behind the Dikes,* CROW, The Netherlands.

23 Sandwell's experiences researching a healthier local economy

John Middleton

Sandwell was formed in 1974 from the amalgamation of the county boroughs of Warley and West Bromwich. It has a population of about 300,000. It lies between Birmingham and Wolverhampton in the West Midlands.

Sandwell's Public Health Department includes the public health physicians and policy advisors, and health promotion services; prior to April 1994 it included occupational health and drug prevention and control services which have now been devolved to NHS trusts. We seek to operate to the Acheson definition of public health as "the science and art of the prevention of disease, the prolongation of life and the promotion of health, through the organized efforts of society" (Department of Health, 1988). Our working definition of health promotion is "any combination of social, political, economic or organizational activity which will improve the health status of individuals or of communities" similar to our definition of public health, but simply for practical, operational purposes, excluding treatment and care services (Middleton et al. 1989).

We have published six public health reports. The first four dealt with broad economic, environmental and social influences on health (Middleton et al. 1989; Middleton et al. 1990; Middleton, 1991; Middleton, 1992; Middleton, 1991; Middleton, 1990). "Life and Death in Sandwell" used a WHO, Health for All format with emphasis on major prerequisites for health including peace, education, food, clean water, housing, employment and income. The public health diagnosis it described was the same as the economic health diagnosis given by the urban policy unit of the local authority (Middleton et al. 1989; Middleton, 1990).

The first annual report suggested targets for "Healthy Sandwell 2000". "Ten Years to Health" the second public health annual report (Middleton et al. 1990) confirmed the locally agreed Healthy Sandwell 2000 targets following a year of consultation and discussion. Ten Years to Health also presented two years of research in the economics of health, its production and consumption in Sandwell with evidence presented under headings: "Conditions for Health?" including, environment and employment; "Producers of Health?" including local studies of tobacco retail and the food industry; and "Consumers of Health?" including the Sandwell lifestyle survey, the Sandwell AIDS and young people survey and the Sandwell shopping survey (Middleton et al. 1990).

Sandwell is heavily reliant on traditional manufacturing industries, the foundry industry, metal casting and moulding industries, and chemical industries. Much of the work is in dangerous and dirty conditions and is poorly paid. Five foundries have pollution control orders upon them.

An economic strategies for health group met between 1989-91. Its role was to: study the effects of health on work; study the effects of work on health (risks from work on health); study the effects of unemployment on health; local economic strategies on health, e.g. anti-poverty and local shopping; to research health and local economic vested interests, e.g. food, alcohol and tobacco. In all these cases, it was to advise on policies to improve the health of Sandwell residents through the influence of the health and local authorities on local economic forces (Middleton, 1990).

Within our health promotional activities in Sandwell we consider that the local economy is a powerful force for ill health, and potentially for good health. Public health practitioners cannot ignore economic and political influences on health (Draper, 1991) preferring to explore only comfortable lifestyle based health promotion programmes with well motivated individuals. This paper is mainly concerned with the "producers of health" surveys. It reports the findings of the first three studies we have undertaken in Sandwell:

1.   "Curing the Tobacco Economy" (Press and Field, 1991) - a study of tobacco retail and local economic dependence on tobacco sales.

2.   "Good Health: A Study of the Drinks Retailing Industry" (Research Partnership, 1993).

3.   "In search of the Low Fat Pork Scratching" (Maton and Jepson, 1990) - a study of the food industry, jobs, outlets and proposals for growth with the expansion into healthier food lines.

Curing the tobacco family

The Sandwell survey

Sandwell has no tobacco manufacturing industry, but has wholesale distribution and retail. In 1989 The Research Partnership was commissioned to undertake a review of extent of tobacco retail in Sandwell. The survey sought information about the number of people employed in tobacco sales, the income generated, the total turnover and profit levels. The study generated estimates of numbers of jobs dependant on tobacco sales and profits and ascertained views on alternative products and services which retailers felt they would offer if tobacco sales were to continue to decline. The study estimated that Sandwell's market for tobacco products was between £36.4 million and £41.6 million per year, in 1989. Around £4,500 was spent per hour on tobacco products in Sandwell. For each smoking related death in Sandwell, £70,000 was spent on tobacco in 1989. Sandwell retailers made between £1.27 million and £1.45 million in 1989, with an average overall profit margin of 3.5 per cent. About one-third of all tobacco sales were attributable to single outlet, locally owned retailers in 1989. Dependence upon tobacco sales differed according to outlet type. For newsagents, tobacco accounted for 32 per cent of sales, but less than ten per cent of profits. General stores were around 20 per cent reliant on tobacco sales for turnover and for supermarkets, the figure was only five per cent, with a profit margin of less then two per cent. Between 300-400 whole time equivalents in Sandwell's retailing sector were estimated to be dependent on tobacco sales in 1989. It was considered that the jobs identified would be unaffected by any further decline in tobacco demand, as expenditure would shift to other products with a higher profitability and mark up. The study showed that the efforts of multiples to control the availability of news supplies, the rationalization strategies of some chains and the uniform business rate were regarded as much greater threats to the viability of small local retail enterprises than any marginal reduction in tobacco sales.

National issues

The study supported other work which has suggested that the tobacco lobby has greatly over stated the industry's economic significance in supporting retail jobs at the local level.

The study showed that far fewer retail jobs were dependent on tobacco sales in Sandwell than national tobacco industry estimates would have suggested. The sales of cigarettes were shown to be important for cash flow, and for "traffic building" to encourage people into a shop. There is therefore a need to establish other entry points to small retail outlets for cash turnover, and also for other traffic building: examples might be returnable bottles and video hire which require customers to come into a shop twice, giving opportunities for other purchases. The study suggested that the tobacco lobby over states the retail jobs dependent on every job in cigarette production, they gave a figure of about 180,000 retail jobs dependent on tobacco sales, a ratio of seven retail to one manufacturing job. Godfrey and Hartley estimated 26,000 retail jobs were tobacco dependent (1 to 0.87 in 1988). Our study suggested that about 40,000 retail jobs were dependent on tobacco manufacture about 1.3:1. During the period 1982-86 tobacco product sales fell by 9.6 per cent, during the same period, jobs in manufacturing cigarettes fell by 34.1 per cent but in the same period, retail jobs rose by 5.6 per cent. This is further confirmation that as tobacco consumption falls, consumption switches to other goods which support greater profits and higher potential to sustain jobs.

Further work

The Sandwell tobacco retail study is seeking to recruit tobacco retailers to the "Sandwell Smoke Watch" project to monitor tobacco sales over time and in relation to public health campaigns. We are also seeking to continue the discussion of alternative products and services in retailing. However, in parallel to the dialogue, an aggressive campaign against cigarette sales to under 16 year olds is being mounted in 1995. The Health Authority supports at the borough planning level the enhancement of local shopping centres and community developments. Each time the budget day debate on tobacco taxation comes along we are able to refute local tobacconists arguments about job losses, because we have the locally obtained data.

Good health: the drinks retail industry

Sandwell findings

This study used industry data and a local survey of publicans to look at drinking patterns, trends and problems. It sought particularly to develop solutions to problems which were of concern to health and the industry.

The survey found that Sandwell people consumed 180,000 bulk barrels of beer per week in 1987, almost a million pints per week. An additional 20,000 bulk barrels were being consumed by non Sandwell residents in Sandwell pubs. The report suggested a higher consumption of traditional beers, mild and ales in Sandwell than elsewhere in the West Midlands and nationally. Alcohol consumed by Sandwell by men by units was slightly higher than national estimates, but women drank less and did not follow the national trend toward increased drinking. There appeared to be more home drinking by men and women. Official employment statistics showed 4,166 employed in the industry in 1989, but our survey suggested 5,501. This higher figure reflected a better estimation of part time workers, who were calculated to making up 80 per cent of the total workforce. Off sales employment has increased between 1981-89 (from 621 to 803 people). Average turnover for pubs was £3,530 per week in the highest quarter (the fourth) of the year (range £1,500-£6,500). Lower estimates for each of the other quarters were £2,660, £3,060 and £3,200. This gave an annual on sales estimate of £100,338,000. Publicans reported trends in consumption reflecting the trade surveys, a decline in ales, from the higher local base, and a rise in lagers, wines and soft drinks. Asked about new facilities, 36 per cent of publicans reported new family rooms in planning, 7 per cent reported plans to remove the distinction between lounge and public bar areas, 7 per cent planned special food areas and 10 per cent planned garden improvements. This was in addition to 19 per cent already with a family room, 64 per cent with gardens, 28 per cent with no bar separations and 38 per cent with food areas. Concerns were expressed by some about the loss of traditional drinking venues, but others anticipated more family oriented services. Concerns were expressed about more drunken behaviour, particularly by young people, and in the bar areas.

Conclusions and local policy implications

Overall, the study showed a major local economic influence, in a state of transition, presenting areas of common concern and scope for co-operation between the brewers and publicans and public health services. Actions to reduce public drunkenness and promote community safety would be welcomed. Trends towards family oriented pubs gave opportunities for the promotion of sensible drinking, in more controlled social environments and opportunities to promote healthy eating and smoke free areas. Trends towards increasing consumption of soft drinks suggested opportunities for publicans to profit whilst reducing drinking and driving, promoting the pub as a new and different social venue and attracting new custom. A parallel study by occupational health colleagues suggested publicans knowledge of safe drinking levels was poor and that their known occupational risks of alcohol were compounded by their lack of understanding about the problems of alcohol use. Since the study, sadly, there has been no progress in the dialogue with the industry and local retailers. Renewed efforts to involve the industry are being made through the newly reconstituted Sandwell Drugs and Alcohol Joint Planning group.

The food industry

The tobacco industry is one industry to "do battle with" accepting as it does, no common ground or shared aims with the public health lobby. The alcohol industry seems reluctant to find the common ground with public health. Everyone needs food, so the food industry seems to offer opportunities for co-operation to improve the public health.

The Black Country is the UK capital for pork meat products including sausages, faggots, pork scratchings and pork pies. "In search of the low fat pork scratching" (Maton and Jepson, 1990) became the title and the quest for the Sandwell food industry study, undertaken on behalf of Sandwell Public Health Department, by West Midlands Enterprise Board.

United Kingdom national trends in the food industry

The food system can be influenced at all levels for the promotion of health. At the national level, the consumption of food remains relatively static, but there are large shifts within the market.

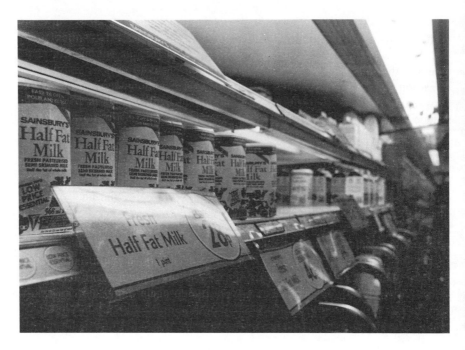

Food consumption patterns do change, and the food industry offers opportunities for co-operation to improve public health

Table 23.1 shows the relative decline in consumption of milk and cream,

300

butter and lamb and bread and the increase in consumption of poultry, vegetable products and fruit over 25 years; this indicates that patterns of food consumption are not static, but can be altered, for better, or worse, over time.

Table 23.1
Index of changes in consumption of food products

Product	1961	1971	1985
Milk and cream	114	113	90
Lamb	150	120	73
Poultry	36	73	102
Butter	153	137	70
Vegetable products	61	73	136
Fruit products	88	92	118
Bread	145	115	108

Source: Social Trends (100 = 1980 figures)

Table 23.2 indicates the dominance of large chains in food retail. There is also a growing trend within these chains towards increasing sales of "own brand" products and towards control by the retailer of all stages of production, processing, distribution and sale of food.

Table 23.2
Market shares 1987

Multiple	Outlets	Market Share
J Sainsbury	279	13%
Tesco	380	12%
Dee Corporation[1]	1,173	10%
Asda Group plc	111	9%
Argyll Group plc[2]	890	9%
Kwik-save plc	721	3%
Waitrose	84	3%
Co-op Societies	1,540	15%

Source: Keynotes

Table 23.3 shows the dominance of a small number of companies on sales of selected foods in 1989. Sales of bread and freezer foods have particularly dented independent manufacturing.

Table 23.3
Market share of leading firms in selected foods

Bread	45%	(2 firms)
Biscuits	76%	(3 firms)
Breakfast cereal	73%	(3 firms)
Confectionary	80%	(3 firms)
Sugar	100%	(2 firms)

Source: Keynotes 1987

Table 23.4 shows investment in food industries by regions in the U.K. The West Midlands had the lowest level of investment in the food industry in the UK in 1987.

Table 23.4
Level of food investment by region -
Capital inv/emp/£ sterling

UK	100	2,048
South East	79	2,001
East Anglia	187	2,398
South West	120	2,331
West Midlands	61	1,192
East Midlands	88	2,398
Yorkshire and Humberside	139	1,676
North West	77	2,077
Wales	77	3,251

Source: Regional Trends 1987

Sandwell survey findings

The major findings of the Sandwell survey were that the food industry employed around 5,000 people in 1989, four per cent of the Sandwell workforce compared to 12 per cent nationally. This indicated considerable under representation of the food industry in the district and suggested scope for new jobs to be created by the attraction inwards of new companies and also through the protection and enhancement jobs in the industry in Sandwell at that time. A need was suggested for existing companies to diversify their product ranges into healthier food products. There are some doubts about the estimates of the jobs in food retail from the study, but even with a much higher estimate of retail jobs, the under representation of the food industry in the Sandwell workforce would still be present.

The study report recommended increased local support for the food industry which should include technical support - food technology, microbiology and environmental hygiene and nutritional advice and economic and commercial support - marketing, packaging, product development, placement and distribution. To provide these, a Sandwell food team was proposed, and the concept of a "food park" was suggested where firms would come together in custom built clean accommodation; facilities which might reasonably be shared, like packaging and distribution, could be made available.

A series of seminars for the food industry were held in collaboration with the Black Country Development Corporation and Sandwell Economic and Environment departments. In 1990-91 these focused on healthy food, food safety and the 1990 Food Act; further seminars have been held subsequently, including ethnic minority foods and further sessions on food safety.

The survey suggested potential areas for local expansion of the food industry - healthy snack products, alcohol free cocktails and sugar free drinks, ethnic minority foods and low fat meat products (Sandwell has the UK champion low fat sausage maker in Bill Bowkett, a butcher from Oldbury). A mixed economy should be encouraged and proposals for food manufacturing, retailing and consumer co-operatives should be supported.

Sandwell Health Authority is now the major purchaser of the Sandwell food co-operatives initiative. This is bringing healthy fruit and vegetables to large numbers of poor, disadvantaged, disabled and elderly people at affordable prices. It is meeting health promotion, community care and economic development objectives after its first year of operation. Sandwell Health Authority, Black Country Development Corporation and the Council are seeking to develop a food industry support team; a food policy officer has been recruited to support this.

The study criticized proposals to development out of town mega retailing centres, fearful that these could damage job prospects in the many smaller shopping centres in Sandwell, increase reliance on motor vehicle transport and reduce access to good shopping facilities for the poor, the disabled and the elderly. The report recommended increased investment in local communities and their shopping facilities; this recommendation has again been made in the second and fourth annual public health reports (Middleton et al. 1990;

Middleton, 1992).

"Swords to ploughshares" - "swords to shopping centres"

This brings me nicely to my final theme. In 1991, Safeway built a new megastore on the site of the former Alvis armoured car factory in Coventry; this I have called a case of "swords to shopping centres" as a modern day variant of the biblical theme of "beating swords into ploughshares". If ever there was an industry which could be described as unhealthy it is military industry. By definition, the products of the industry are "unhealthy"; but the industry itself is a drain on natural resources, a major source of pollution, a poor employer for the sums invested and a massive contributor to poor economic performance, high inflation rates, high interest rates and world debt (Sidel, 1985; United Nations, 1981). It is the most florid example of an anti-health vested interest for which alternatives must be found in socially useful, peaceful, environmentally friendly products and services (United Nations, 1981; Renner, 1990).

The Lucas Aerospace combine shop stewards alternative plan (Wainright and Elliott, 1981) in the 1970s showed the way for what products could be made using the skills and resources of a high technology military manufacturer. The products fell into five broad areas: oceanics, (including marine agriculture and mineral extraction), telechirics (the application of remote handling techniques for tasks to be done in dirty and dangerous conditions), alternative energy systems and advanced batteries, public transport systems (including the road rail bus). Many of the products were "green" and all were socially useful. Subsequently many similar alternative plans have been produced in the UK, the United States, Italy and Germany (Renner, 1990); a consistent theme throughout these has been the search for environmentally friendly products: most of the alternative plans place considerable emphasis on alternative and renewable energy generation, energy conservation, recycling wastes and pollution control.

The conversion of military industries for peaceful purposes is therefore a major local, national and international public health issue, and one which requires urgent attention. It is the most obvious example of my overall theme: that economic diversification can be a powerful force for the public health; whether it is in the tobacco, alcohol, food, armaments, or other anti-health industries (Middleton, 1992). Paul Field and I call this the "health dividend"- in the same way that there logically a social dividend to be gained from redirecting the resources for warfare into welfare, so there is a health dividend to be gained from converting industry for disease into industry for health.

Conclusions

In some cases, the ultimate goal should be conversion of the industry out of "anti-health" production or services. Economic forces are powerful determinants of health and disease. The new public health movement needs to educate itself about the effects of economic vested interests and develop a cohesive force against those economic forces which endanger the public health. Our three local studies on food, alcohol and tobacco retail are small scale studies which might be regarded as pilots or as examples to be followed elsewhere. They have enabled us to gain an insight into the problems faced by these industries locally and enabled us to begin a dialogue with influential sections of the local economy who might otherwise have regarded us as working against their interests.

Where dialogue is possible we will seek it; diversification of the food industry towards healthier, safer products is one potential area for co-operation. Work with the tobacco industry is plainly more difficult; cigarettes are lethal, there is no such thing as a safe cigarette and we are asking the tobacco manufacturer to stop making and selling cigarettes and effectively to go out of business, unless he or she can find alternative business.

However, our survey of tobacco retailers demonstrated that there is scope for diversification and that dependence on tobacco sales is not as crucial to retailers as the tobacco companies would have us believe.

The work of the Sandwell Economic Strategies for Health Group has been subsumed into other working relationships between the health and local authorities, the Trade and Enterprise Council, the Black Country Development Corporation and Tipton City Challenge. This has culminated in the establishment of the Sandwell Regeneration Partnership. This body is seeking to set up an overall strategy for economic, educational and quality of life improvement for Sandwell. The partnership recognizes the inter-relationship between health, economic, social and educational problems. It seeks to tackle these in a multi-disciplinary and collaborative fashion, with the formulation of shared strategies.

There are signs that the new public health movement is gaining in the sophistication of its approaches to political and economic issues which are at the root of all public health problems; but there is still a very long way to go. We in Sandwell will be pleased to work with any other interested groups or individuals to develop these projects and ideas further.

Notes

1.   Now Gateway Corp. - included Fine Fare, Shoppers Paradise.

2.   Includes Presto, Lipton, Lo-Cost and (during 1987) Safeway.

References

Department of Health (1988), *The Acheson Report*, HMSO, London.

Draper, P. (1991), *Health Through Public Policy*, Merlin, London.

Maton, K. and Jepson, D. (1990), *In Search of the Low Fat Pork Scratching*, Birmingham: West Midlands Enterprise Board and West Bromwich, Sandwell Health Authority, (Public health technical reports series No. 7.)

Middleton, J. (1990), "Life and Death in Sandwell: Where Economic Health and Public Health Meet", *Journal of Local Government Policy Making*, vol. 16, pp. 3-9.

Middleton, J. (1992), "The Weapons of Public Health", *Medicine and War*, vol. 8, pp. 100-8.

Middleton, J., Rao, J. and Donovan, D. (1989), *Life and Death in Sandwell*, Sandwell Health Authority, West Bromwich.

Middleton, J., Rao, J. and Donovan, D. (1990), *Ten Years to Health*, Sandwell Health Authority, West Bromwich.

Middleton, J. (ed.) (1991), *Sandwell Health - The Album*, Sandwell Health Authority, West Bromwich.

Press, M. and Field, P. (1991), *"Curing the Tobacco Economy", Birmingham, National Association of Health Authorities and Trusts, and Sandwell Health Authority, Research paper no. 3*, NAHAT.

Renner, M. (1990), *Swords to Ploughshares, World Watch Institute, Washington, Paper no. 96*.

The Research Partnership (1993), *Good Health: A Study of the Drinks Retailing Industry*, Sandwell Health Authority, West Bromwich.

Sidel, V. (1985), "Destruction Before Detonation", *Lancet*, vol. ii, pp. 1287-9.

United Nations (1981), *Report of an Expert Committee on Disarmament and Development (Thorsson Report)*, United Nations Organisation, New York, pp. 1287-9.

Wainwright, H. and Elliott, D. (1981), *The Lucas Plan*, Allison Busby, London.

24 Developing Sheffield's city health plan – process, content and lessons to be learnt

Lee Adams and Valerie Cotter

"Healthy Alliances" has been a watch word of the government's health policy in the last few years. However, there are still comparatively few district wide examples of Healthy Alliances in the UK. Sheffield has been the setting for a Healthy City project since 1987 and is still a strong interagency initiative. A latest step forward has been the publication of the "Our City Our Health - Framework for Action" - a plan for health improvement subscribed to by all Healthy Sheffield partners. Healthy Sheffield has once more showed itself ahead of the field in this endeavour. This article describes the plan and the process of community participation leading to it; it also argues that for real health improvement, strategic alliances at local government level are essential, rather than just interagency co-operation for health promotion projects, which is how healthy alliances are often interpreted.

Developing Sheffield's health plan - "our city our health"

With the publication in January 1992 of "Our City Our Health (OCOH) - Ideas for improving Health in Sheffield" a booklet, summary and supporting materials, Healthy Sheffield embarked upon a process of consultation, debate, education, research, negotiation and planning in pursuit of the city's first interagency health plan. In January 1994, the OCOH initiative reached a major milestone with the launch of the City Health Plan - entitled "Our City Our Health - Framework for Action".

About Healthy Sheffield

Healthy Sheffield is an interagency Health for All initiative that was established in response to two local reports - Poverty and Health Report 1985

(Sheffield City Council) and a Health Care and Disease Profile 1986 (Sheffield Health Authority). Both documented the relationship between poor health and levels of deprivation in the city, and indicated levels of preventable illness, premature death and inequalities in health. Healthy Sheffield was also inspired by the World Health Organisation's Health For All 2000 initiative and the linked Healthy Cities project.

From its inception Healthy Sheffield has worked within a broad, social model of health, asserting that health is influenced by a range of factors - most importantly social, economic and environmental factors. Healthy Sheffield's aim is "to improve the health of Sheffield people and significantly reduce health inequality". Important areas of work have included interagency planning, project and service development, community and organizational development, information and research as well as national and international liaison and advocacy.

Notable successes have included:

1.   The development of a strong intersectoral partnership (Sheffield City Council, Sheffield and Rotherham Chamber of Commerce, Community Health Council, Sheffield Health Authority, Family Health Services Authority, Sheffield Hallam University, Sheffield University, Racial Equality Council and Voluntary Action Sheffield).

2.   The establishment of interagency health promotion programmes.

3.   Setting up effective demonstration projects such as community health neighbourhood schemes.

4.   Provision of training and information in both organizational and community settings.

5.   A positive influence over partner organization's agendas and plans which have an impact on health.

6.   The establishment of forums and networks for education, debate, planning and consultation on health issues.

7.   Work on strategic planning and policy development e.g. a Community Development and Health Strategy and the City Health Plan.

Why develop a city health plan?

In Sheffield, as in most cities, a diverse range of organizations influence health through their work and the services which they provide or commission. Although much was already being done to protect health and well being in Sheffield, there was also a clear need to develop a wider understanding of the health needs and problems in the city and to define how they might be more effectively addressed.

The development of an intersectoral public health strategy was perceived as having a number of benefits. A strong argument was made to ensure that it would arise out of effective public and organizational consultation to determine key factors affecting health in the city and to seek ideas about what could be done to improve it. It was expected to: create opportunities for community participation through consultation; provide a focus of debate in the city around health issues; provide a coherent framework to which all agencies could refer to support their planning on health; raise organizations' awareness of their role in the protection and promotion of health and identify commonly agreed objectives on health which would improve existing collaborative working and which would influence more effective collaboration on health in the future.

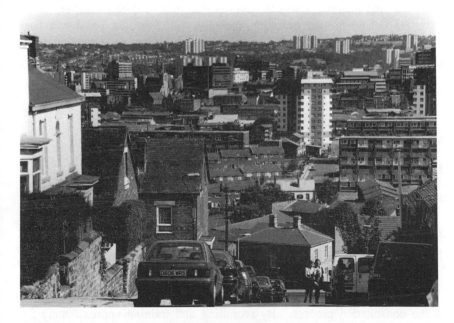

The key to developing Sheffield's city health plan was effective consultation with the public and the city's organizations

"Our city our health"

A number of clearly definable stages have marked the progress of the "Our City Our Health" initiative.

1.   Development of OCOH model and supporting materials.

2.   Consultation.

3.   Analysis of consultation responses.

4.   Synthesis and planning.

5.   Ratification and agreement.

6.   Launch.

7.   Implementation.

An interagency group, the Healthy Sheffield Public Health Strategy Working Group (PHSWG), was established to steer the development of a City Health Plan. Its first major task was to develop materials to raise awareness and to stimulate debate around health in the city, which would provide a basic resource to the consultation. The main document was very comprehensive and produced with an emphasis on accessibility. Materials developed included

1.   "Our City Our Health" - Ideas for improving Health in Sheffield - main document.

2.   Summary document of OCOH.

3.   Information leaflets.

4.   Briefing paper and newsletter.

5.   Translated documentation.

6.   Exhibition and tape/slide show.

The effective dissemination and use of these materials was an essential part of the consultation process. By recruiting and training approximately 250 individuals both within and outside Healthy Sheffield organizations from various walks of life, it was hoped that information about the process would quickly reach as many groups as possible. These trained facilitators worked in a number of ways, talking to people about health, holding discussion groups and focus groups, designing and distributing questionnaires and stimulating responses from within their organizations. Creative and imaginative approaches to collecting information were encouraged - from interviewing shoppers in the local covered market to involving community groups in graphically designing their vision of a healthy city.

Publicity was another important factor in ensuring that information about the "Our City Our Health" consultation reached as wide an audience as possible. A public launch was held to attract media coverage, and the local press were briefed in the process and themselves encouraged to participate. Publicity and consultation materials were sent directly to statutory organizations, voluntary and commercial organizations, academic institutions, professional and trade union bodies and industrial and commercial organizations throughout the city.

The time initially allowed for the training, dissemination and consultation process proved to be an under estimation. After the launch in January 1992, responses were still coming in to the Healthy Sheffield team in November 1992. The development of an analysis protocol to draw effective conclusions from the materials received also proved time consuming. The variety of formats in which responses were received, contributed in no small measure to this, as did the breadth and range of the topics covered by responses.

Consultation responses

Structured responses were received in six different questionnaire formats - primary questionnaires which had been distributed with the discussion and summary documents and questionnaires designed by the following participating organizations - Youth Service, Recreation Department, Community Health Council, Central Health Clinic. In addition to the 89 per cent of responses received on structured questionnaires, unstructured responses arrived in the following formats - letters, reports, memos, video and audio tape. Many of the questionnaires contained a considerable amount of unstructured text in the form of free comment.

Responses came from the following categories of respondent:

Individuals	1,421
Groups of individuals	56
Community groups	36
Professional groups	11
Intersectoral groups	6
Organizations	84

We know that many of the group responses involved large numbers of individuals, for example the Health Authority response counted as one response but involved the participation of over 100 individuals and we calculate that between 4,000 and 5,000 people took part in the response process.

A qualitative analysis was carried out of all unstructured text enabling a specialist programme (text based Alpha) and the structural data was also interrogated to provide detailed information about respondents contributions on the following:

Factors which affect health

Income	Environment
Products and activities	Education
Social support	Social rights
Care	Work place health

Health of population groups

Women	Men
Children	Older adults
Black and minority	Young people
ethnic communities	People with disabilities
Lesbians and gay men	

Methods to improve health

Organizational development	Community development
Education and training	Information and research
Planning	Advocacy

The key themes emerging from this qualitative analysis were published in Summer 1993 in a document called "Our City Our Health - What you Said". Publication of this document enabled feedback to be given to consultation respondents and others with an interest in "Our City Our Health" and provided an opportunity to keep people in touch with the process and to attract continuing support and publicity.

Drafting the plan

The next challenge was to use the findings from the consultation to inform the process of drafting a City Health Plan. In fact, this was a process which had started as the members of the Public Health Strategy Working Group worked together to produce summary versions of the consultation data. It was also crucial to ensure that other key sources of information were identified and considered, particularly around parallel and complementary strategic development which would influence the partner's priorities and ability to deliver on the emerging health plan: for instance, information about Health of the Nation, community care, and urban regeneration and economic development strategies for the city.

"What You Said"

a summary of the Responses to the Our City - Our Health Consultation

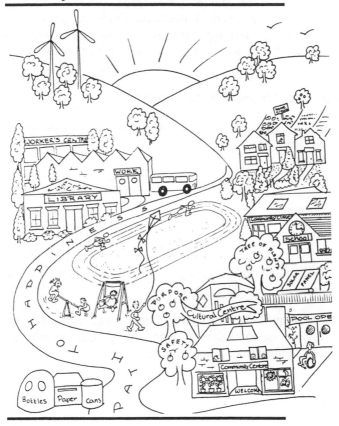

"What you said", the report summarizing the responses to the consultation process

The first draft of the framework was circulated for comment to all Healthy Sheffield partners in April/May 1993. Based upon the analysis structure, it proposed objectives and potential goals for factors which affect health, population groups and method areas. This, it must be admitted, while producing a very comprehensive proposal for future development, was seen to be overly long, sometimes repetitive and too prescriptive for the tastes of some of the partners.

It was clear that a radical rewrite was required, yet one which would not lose sight of the messages emerging from the consultation. The resulting draft "Framework for Action" was designed to focus on a number of distinct health themes and to present clear objectives and ideas for common action which were accessible to a wide range of interest groups. The needs of specific population groups were integrated into each theme area. Three themes were accorded greater prominence -poverty, discrimination and environment. These emerged overwhelmingly as priorities through the consultation process. It is hoped that they will inform the future development and implementation of each of the other theme areas within the framework.

Contents of the "framework for action"

Using the key themes of poverty, discrimination and the environment the action areas were as follows:

Accident prevention	Carers' health
Care services	Community safety
Education	Health promotion
Housing	Mental and emotional
Nutrition	well being
Physical activity and leisure	Sexual health and fertility
Smoking, alcohol and drugs	Violence and aggression
Work	

Within the framework, each of these areas for action are described in terms of their importance to health, problems for population groups, objectives; cross reference are made as appropriate.

Ratification

The next step in the process was to gain the ratification of each of the partners in Healthy Sheffield to the content and format of the document. In ratifying the framework they were expected to endorse the broad objectives outlined and to agree to collaborative and individual work to develop appropriate responses to implementation within their roles and resources.

The ratification process took place in October/November 1993. It entailed each partner considering the document at its most senior executive and member levels. It provided an opportunity for increasing awareness and ownership of Healthy Sheffield, and of establishing a greater political commitment to implementing the plan. For example, groups involved in ratification included the City Council's Policy Committee, members of the Health Authority and Family Health Services Authority, Community Health Council members, trustees of Voluntary Action Sheffield and similar groups within the other partner agencies.

Engaging chief executives of partner organizations

As well as securing political support, the ratification and subsequent launch process for the framework provided an opportunity to engage the active and public support of chief executives of each of the partners and to involve them in discussions about effective implementation of the framework. To this end a meeting, attended by all partners chief executives along with relevant chief officers from Sheffield City Council, was held in December 1993. This was the first of what is hoped will be many future opportunities for this group to meet with members of the Healthy Sheffield board to take forward issues related to the City Health Plan and other aspects of Health for All development in the city.

(The Healthy Sheffield board is a committee of representatives at a very senior level - but below chief executive - of the partner agencies, e.g. the Director of Public Health, Director of Health Promotion, Director of Strategy represent the HA's on the board).

Chief executives discussed and agreed a number of priority areas for collaborative effort within the framework for action for the first year of its implementation. While it is acknowledged that a great deal of activity was, and is, occurring and needs to continue to happen within each of the theme areas, it was felt that by identifying three special areas at the launch of the framework, a boost could be given to some focused work in areas which would derive particular benefit from collaborative activity. Specific partner agencies were identified as project champions to lead interagency task groups in these priority areas:

1.   Work - led by Chamber of Commerce.

2.   Mental and emotional well being - led by Voluntary Action Sheffield.

315

3. Carers' health - led by the City Council's Social Services Department

These groups have been convened and are working on detailed implementation plans for each of their areas, and will make recommendations on resource allocation, target setting, timescales, lead agency responsibility, and project priorities within the next few months.

It must be said that much work is also going on to implement the framework across all of the other activity areas as well, e.g. accident prevention, smoking, sexual health.

The launch of the city health plan

The launch of the "Framework for Action" provided an ideal opportunity to bring together local community groups and individuals to celebrate the best of the existing joint working in the city to improve health and well being, along with the organizations who are expected to deliver on many aspects of implementing the plan. Over 600 people (including representatives of 68 individual organizations) took part in the launch event, which included healthy activities, a range of information stands, displays and exhibitions as well as the more formal launch. Through a series of workshops, participants were involved in a close examination of the framework, and explored their role and their expectations of the implementation process.

The launch event attracted positive media coverage and extended awareness of the "Our City Our Health" process. Most importantly, it was an event to celebrate for all those who had contributed to the development of the framework - facilitators, respondents and workers within each of the partner organizations - and it provided an opportunity to acknowledge the considerable commitment and effort invested in the process. It also ensured that, through a signing ceremony by political representatives of each of the partners, a visible public commitment to implementation. We were fortunate that Dr Graham Winyard from NHSME was able to attend the launch.

Future of the city health plan - implementation

The process of implementing the framework for action, and of reviewing and refining the structures which will assist the process, has already begun. Key elements of current and future work are:

1. A review of Healthy Sheffield infrastructure with the aim of ensuring that existing and new intersectoral working groups have a clear and effective role in implementation.

2.   The development of Healthy Sheffield partners' action plans and work programmes to integrate the objectives of the Framework for Action.

3.   The development of further overall targets for health in the city, and within the partner organizations, against which progress can be measured. Specific target setting will be piloted within the three task group areas.

4.   Establishing effective mechanisms for monitoring and evaluating progress.

5.   Reporting progress and collaboratively reviewing priorities.

6.   The provision of appropriate training - training sessions have been undertaken or are planned for example for link officers from departments within the City Council, for Health Authority planners and for workers who will disseminate information to black and minority ethnic communities in the city.

To conclude, there are a number of important factors which can be identified which both helped and hindered the conception, planning and production of the "Our City Our Health" process which are summarized below.

What helped?

Public health progress has often been characterized by charismatic personalities and it was certainly the case for OCOH attracted visionary individuals who were prepared to take risks.

The Healthy Sheffield Development Unit, a small team of staff who facilitate Healthy Sheffield work, and trained consultation facilitators to work throughout the city in an educative way, was vital.

An interagency committee structure which provided the necessary mechanisms for decision making helped.

Support was given by senior managers and politicians. This was vital as OCOH was a major undertaking at a time of upheaval in many partner organizations, coupled with severe financial constraints.

Time for team building with the Healthy Sheffield board, the staff and networks was prioritized.

Adequate resources were important. Obviously very little finance was available for this initiative and most of the work was undertaken within the small Healthy Sheffield Development Unit budget. However, a definite

317

budget is required for such work and again it is to the partners' credit that with all Sheffield's financial troubles this work was supported.

Effective promotions and communications were crucial.

Accountability to partners and engagement of partners in every step of the process was a must.

A climate of openness and trust which has been developed through Healthy Sheffield over the last few years.

Key individuals showed an understanding of a process of change - which can be slow and frustrating. Strong members of the Healthy Sheffield board were invaluable to steer this process.

Co-terminosity of boundaries (between FHSA, Health Authority and Local Authority) was an asset.

Shared commitment to principles and agreement on aims and a common agenda provided a strong foundation.

Time was taken for conceptual development as well as practical projects.

Healthy Sheffield prioritized community development and the processes of involving people in the city.

A balance was struck between developing a long term plan, but at the same time engaging in a wealth of short term actions (which we have not the space to specify here).

A national lobbying role in the objectives of the Healthy Sheffield initiative was included, recognizing that only so much can be done to improve health within Sheffield itself.

Finally, we have gained agreement for a commitment to action by all partners.

What hindered?

This was a time of enormous organizational and policy change within key agencies and this affected progress - e.g. Community Care legislation, NHS reforms, LEA and educational institution changes.

The economic climate was a major factor. Finance was, and is, very tight in our city, and with the ending of Urban Programme funding, new and innovative work for health improvement is difficult to resource.

Obviously not everyone was enthusiastic and there were negative personalities who felt threatened and were difficult to engage.

Distrust - there was some sense that individual organizational authority was/is being usurped by the process of collective planning.

Early theoretical development was not always valued or its importance was not understood.

There was a limited understanding of health (medical model accepted rather than a social model) even within the Health Service sector, so much educational work was and is vital.

For some it has been difficult to see "Healthy Sheffield" as not a separate project but a new approach which partners are part of and which should inform all their other activity.

We would have liked a national framework to which Healthy City initiatives like Healthy Sheffield could and can relate. The Health of the Nation helped in putting healthy alliances on the agenda but also took a rather narrower perspective than the ethos informing many Healthy Cities particularly around the social, environmental and economic basis of ill health. In this respect it has been less than inspirational.

Understanding locally of realistic timescales is often a problem with different partners wishing for progress at different rates.

Consultations create expectations and people can feel let down if organizations don't deliver; this was a constant fear for partners, particularly in our economic climate.

The process has taken time and we lost committed people along the way, through reorganizations, redundancies and people moving on. This hindered continuity.

Support for target setting is a problem, as many of the objectives in the framework relate to well being, for which there is little base line data. Some partners are more enthusiastic than others about target setting and who can be released to undertake this very time consuming work is an issue.

Was it too ambitious? Probably! Could it have been simplified? - probably!

Conclusion

If cities or districts are to plan for the health of their populations then this must include economic and environmental and unitary planning as well as health service and community care planning. This can only be achieved by joint structures and joint commitment of a variety of agencies at local level. This kind of planning structure deserves much more attention by policy makers if we are really to improve health and reduce inequality. We hope this paper has given an overview of the "Our City Our Health" process and some of the lessons we have learnt. There is much practical activity as well as the strategic planning process going on which has been inspired as developed by the Healthy Sheffield initiative that we have not had space to describe here but publications on our activities are available from:

Healthy Sheffield Development Unit, Town Hall Chambers, 1 Barkers Pool, Sheffield, S1 1EN

25 The development of a boroughwide health strategy in response to the health of the nation

Felicity Green and Donald Cameron

The purpose of this paper is to describe how one borough with a population of 300,000 has developed a health strategy in response to the government health strategy The Health of the Nation (HMSO, 1992) with a view that the process of developing the strategy and the lessons learned may be of use to other towns, boroughs and cities. The paper will begin by outlining the context and frameworks in which the strategy was developed, then to describe the development highlighting the advantages and disadvantages of this approach and the lessons learned.

Stockport is a borough in Greater Manchester with a population of 300,000. Overall Stockport could be seen as an affluent borough with many wards at the top of the affluence/deprivation rankings (Townsend, 1989). However this statistical tool of averaging belies the real truth about the borough, which is that it is one of contrasts and that those wards neighbouring the city of Manchester are as deprived as some of the most inner city areas of their close neighbour. In order to improve the health of the borough as a whole it is imperative that we address the inequalities and target our health promotion initiatives to areas experiencing the highest levels of ill health.

The strategy was developed as a response to the Health of the Nation and is owned by all those agencies in the borough which have a health promoting role. At its launch on 3 June 1994 it was publicly endorsed at a signing ceremony by Secretary for State for Health, Chair of Stockport Health Authority, Chair of Stockport Family Health Services Authority, Chair of Stockport Healthcare NHS Community Trust, Chair of Stockport Acute Services NHS Trust, Mayor of Stockport Metropolitan Borough Council, Chair Community Health Council, Chair of Council for Voluntary Service and President of the Chamber of Commerce and Industry.

Although The Health of the Nation highlights the statutory responsibility of purchasing Health Authorities to improve the population's health this has been accepted ideologically and in practice as a narrow view and not the way we will achieve good health in Stockport. It is however worth pointing out that all the key agencies mentioned above are co-terminus and therefore have the interests of the same population at heart and we have not been involved in the merging of purchasing Health Authorities. The significance of these two factors cannot be underestimated.

In addition Stockport undertook a major review of its joint collaboration machinery in 1991, by a process of several public meetings, resulting in the structure shown in Figure 25.1. The development of the health strategy has been the responsibility of the JHPG and facilitated through the JHPTs. The membership of the JHPG is shown in Table 25.1. These are all senior officers within the key agencies.

Table 25.1
Composition of the joint health planning group

Agency	No. of Representatives
Stockport Health Commission	4
Stockport Healthcare Trust	3
Stockport Acute Services Trust	2
Chief Executives Dept., SMBC	1
Leisure Services Division, SMBC	1
Social Services Division, SMBC	1
Education Division, SMBC	1
Technical Services Division, SMBC	1
Environmental Health Division, SMBC	1
Voluntary Sector	2

Over the past ten years there has been a history of joint projects between the health authority and the local authority within the borough. There are too many to give the detail of, but some are listed below:

> School and Youth Service Health Education project
> Hand of Hearts
> Fun in the Sun.
> Exercise on Prescription
> Swimbus
> Corporate Challenge
> INTO HEALTH town centre Health and Information shop
> Central Youth
> Healthy School Award

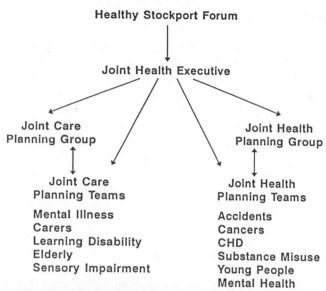

Figure 25.1 Stockport joint collaboration machinery

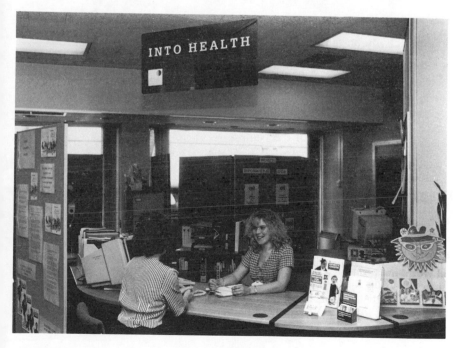

INTO HEALTH is an information centre which is one of a number of joint health and local authority projects in Stockport

Development of the strategy

After the publication of the government green paper The Health of the Nation, the Pump Handle group (public health workers within the Commission and Trusts) decided that a local health strategy would be an appropriate response. The starting point for development was an identification of the major preventable disease problems in the area together with their major risk factors. It became apparent that there were many common risk factors for the problems and it was agreed that the focus of the strategy would be to develop targets to reduce these risk factors in those groups within the population at greatest risk. It was recognized that this was a very "top down" approach to improving the health of the population seated within an epidemiological base but with the imminent publication of outcome, reduction of disease targets by the government it was felt to be an entirely appropriate approach. Consultation with and ownership by lead agencies was seen to be the backbone of the strategy alongside dissemination to the public but not direct consultation.

The aim of the strategy is to improve the health of Stockport people and the objectives:

1.   To provide a focus for NHS, local authority and voluntary sector activity on the Health of the Nation.

2.   To act as a local management tool for making progress on the Health of the Nation objectives.

3.   To facilitate the monitoring and accountability role of the NHS regarding Health of the Nation.

4.   To encourage partnership working.

Progress targets to improve health were set for each of the identified risk factors and a process of consultation began with the other agencies. This process was underway when the White Paper on Health of the Nation was published in July 1992 and it was then agreed to focus our attention on the five key areas proposed by the government with the addition of another key area covering social conditions and population groups. We did not feel in a position to betray our fundamental beliefs about the influence of poverty, housing and environment on the population's health.

Examples of targets set in the strategy are:

1.   From 1994 to run a yearly campaign on safe cycling.

2. By 1994 all pharmacists to have been approached to disseminate educational materials on preventing cancers.

3. By December 1994 all schools to have been encouraged to gain the Healthy School Award.

4. By 1998 50 per cent of first parents to have access to a child development programme.

5. By 1996 50 per cent of primary health care workers to have undergone welfare rights training with an 80 per cent uptake by 1998.

It was recognized that the targets being set needed to be:

1. Relevant to Stockport and to the groups in the population which they apply.

2. Developed within a framework which allows for reassessment and revision so that they retained their relevance.

3. Related to the primary targets in the Health of the Nation.

4. Monitorable with clear indicators of progress identified.

Coincidently the revised joint planning machinery was in place by July 1992 and the targets were categorized under their key area and discussed fully in the JHPTs. All agencies were represented on the JHPTs and it was the responsibility of each member to ensure that the targets pertaining to their agency were discussed and agreed at the highest executive level of their organization. This process of revising and agreeing the targets too just over a year and in some instances the new targets bore little resemblance to those originally written by the Pump Handle group. The targets were now altogether more realistic and relevant to Stockport than they had ever been. An extremely encouraging part of this whole process was that contrary to deleting targets many agencies were actually prepared to do more than was originally suggested. For example, targets for Leisure Services Division of SMBC were primarily around increasing uptake of exercise but senior Leisure Services Officers also wished to include targets referring to the Library Service and the Arts and Entertainment Section in the promotion of mental health.

By October 1993 a draft strategy was ready to go to the health authority, the trust boards and to the committees of the local authority. Members of these bodies warmly welcomed the strategy and made minimum changes to it so at last we were nearly ready to print the document and disseminated it to Stockport people. In March 1994 the Stockport Health Promise was finally ratified by the Commission (with whom the statutory responsibility lies) and was launched at a signing ceremony on 3 June 1994. A popularist newspaper version of the strategy has been posted to every household in the borough and 100 volunteer speakers will be trained up to talk to staff groups, voluntary groups, etc. about the strategy. Any comments received during this public consultation period will be recorded and the document will be revised in June 1995. It is hoped that by then some of the targets will have been achieved and that new ones will be added. It is intended that this will be a dynamic and evolving health strategy.

What we learned during this process

It was useful having potential targets as a starting point for negotiation even if they were completely rewritten. The development of the strategy within the joint planning framework lent importance to the whole procedure. Spending over a year negotiating with all agencies through the JHPTs was well worth the relationships that were built up during that time. More time needed to have been spent negotiating with the Acute Services about their role as they were preoccupied with getting their house in order pending trust status. Similarly the GPs were in the midst of negotiating fundholding relationships with the Health Commission which blocked a high level of involvement from them. Listing the targets under the responsible agency has clarified the interpretation of the document. An unrealistic shopping list of wants was not presented to the council, who in the present economic climate, would have felt under siege. More work could probably have been done with Social Services who play a smaller role in the strategy than other local authority departments. It was important to stress from the beginning that the document would be under constant revision so that all the health gain measurers for the next millennium did not have to be included.

References

HMSO (1992), "Health of the Nation - A Strategy for England and Wales", *Secretary of State for Health.*
Townsend, P. (1989), "A Study of Deprivation in Greater Manchester", *Tameside Borough Council.*

26 Putting concepts into the (health) policy practice ...

Marleen Goumans

The Healthy Cities project offers a conceptual framework for the development and implementation of local health policy. Indeed, two of the main goals of the WHO Healthy Cities project in Europe are to put health high on the political agenda and to develop a new health policy in cities. To achieve this means influencing many of the key actors involved in the process of policy development. A key focus for research is how politically responsible people and policy makers who are already working in a this way perceive "Healthy Cities" and what impact its ideas and activities have actually had on health policy development. This is fundamental because the implicit reasoning behind the Healthy Cities initiative is that through concrete community activity, change would be achieved in local policy making, which would in turn support and influence national implementation of Health for All 2000. This bottom up approach would compensate for the lack of action achieved following the production of national health policy statements such as the Dutch "Nota 2000" (de leeuw, 1989).

The research reported here is a pilot study undertaken in The Netherlands. It is part of a research project on the development of health policy by local governments in ten cities selected from cities that are either part of the WHO/Euro Healthy Cities project or the National Networks of Healthy Cities in The Netherlands and the United Kingdom.

The purpose of the substantive research is to explore development and implementation of health policy by local governments, looking in particular - at the influence innovative ideas such as the Healthy Cities concepts has on policy makers, the use of those concepts and their influence on health policy development. This paper takes some of the key concepts and activities seen as relevant to policy development contained within the Healthy Cities project and examines the extent to which they are used in practice by those involved in policy development. Finally it makes some suggestions based on the preliminary research on how those professionals and others involved in the

Healthy Cities movement can gain political support for health policy at the urban level.

The underlying assumption of the research is that policy development can be regarded as iterative and dynamic. In an iterative or dynamic view of policy the activities and the involvement of actors, including their motivation, are under consideration. Policy is not a decision (Allison, 1971), policy is produced in, with, and through negotiations between participants in their environments. The strength of this type of analysis is that it is possible to investigate all the movements, either intended or not, that were stimulated because of the intended policy.

Background to the study

In May, June and July 1993 a pilot study took place in five cities in The Netherlands. In these cities, key people who are professionally involved in policy making in the health sector, were interviewed. These included policy makers working with municipal health services, directors of the municipal health services, a director of the municipal welfare service, and the responsible aldermen for health. The interviews were guided by a checklist. Checklist items included their vision of health policy in general and, more specifically, their vision on the implementation of Healthy Cities concepts and health policy in their city.

In The Netherlands there is an obligation under the Collective Prevention Act for local government to develop health policy. Of particular interest, therefore, is the extent to which healthy cities projects influence policy development. The data from this pilot study provided impressions of, and some key words within, innovative policy processes (Leeuw de, 1989; WHO/Health, 1986; WHO/Euro, 1992; Worldbank, 1993). Like for example individuals, institutions, concepts, communication, politics, decision rules, healthy cities as a political instrument, healthy cities as content for policy, structure (finances and organization), unpredictable, projects, roles, working procedures, uncertainty, enthusiasm, personal commitment, multi-actors, competition, no uniform policy domain, mobilization. In addition it gave some insights into the following which forms the basis of this paper; the main reasons for starting or not starting a Healthy Cities project and the perceptions held of four of the basic health policy concepts underpinning Healthy Cities ideology (data, community participation, political commitment and intersectoral collaboration).

328

Main reasons for starting or not starting a healthy cities project

The main reasons for starting a Healthy Cities project were: curiosity; the ambition of a city; to use it as a framework for existing activities and policy; to promote the city and to give policy a nice "flag" (e.g. "War on drugs").

On the other hand there were general complaints that it is too theoretical, it looks nice, however, it has no hands and no feet, and health policy is too much concentrated on resources and not on content.

At the operational level the main arguments were concerned with the content of the project. At the political level the arguments were formulated in terms of political gain or loss, for example, the promotion of the city or the responsible individual politician. Participation at the managerial level was determined both by the need to promote the service they represented as well as the content of the programme. It is clear that if only the operational level has an active role, the activities they undertake tend to be separate projects that are not integrated in a shared political vision. Whereas if only the political level supports the Healthy Cities idea, it may result in the operational level is not able to make this "flag" a lively one with content. This leaves the managerial level with an important role in interacting with the other two levels. This is because the managerial level can provide the support needed for political relevance as well as provide a proper translation of ideas into concrete activities. In time the arguments may reinforce one another.

It is not surprising therefore that those interviewed at the political level needed other arguments to convince them, and these were different from the arguments at the operational level:

> My position as Alderman for health was an "empty role", had no body, I wanted something more.

> If Healthy Cities had not been available we would have searched for something else.

> I don't know if Healthy Cities is the reason that things happen in this city. The title Healthy Cities as such does not mean anything to me. However you can use it as a label to get people enthusiastic about certain ideas.

This raises the issue as to whether Healthy Cities be considered as a result of present activities and policy or whether the ideas are meant to stimulate activities and policy? Some informants said that they regarded Healthy Cities to be the recognition of their policy and activities. This recognition can be used on the one hand by the managerial level to remind the political level to remain supportive. On the other hand the political level uses it as a stimulus for the local health services and other municipal services.

All the interviewees questioned whether their policy and activities would have been very different if they had not have been part of the Healthy Cities movement. A key issue was whether Healthy Cities should mean new activities, or whether it should mean continuing old activities and adding a new dimension to them. The key question was whether one should stay within the regular budget or whether Healthy Cities should go hand in hand with new financial resources and a separate project office.

In The Netherlands, the four year programme (1990-94) of the national government included the notion of realizing governmental and social innovation. Extra financial resources were available to support this. Both the city of Rotterdam and Eindhoven achieved a lot of what they have done so far because they used, both in their own way, the idea of social innovation to raise awareness for Healthy Cities. This alone, however, does not provide a guarantee that this strategy will work as well for other policy issues. Municipal health services that proposed integrated policy and action for the implementation of the "Physically Disabled Supplies Act" received a negative response from their local government. Apparently the idea of using Healthy Cities as a conceptual framework is not (yet) a rule of the policy game. Indeed, there are only few municipalities that consider the main reason for being involved with Healthy Cities is to use it as the conceptual framework to implement their legal task to develop health policy in their city. In the end the reasons for politicians and policy makers to get involved with Healthy Cities therefore are as expected political, personal and pragmatic.

Suggested health policy components

According to the WHO, Healthy Cities should have six characteristics in common (WHO, 1992): the generation of intersectoral action; to emphasize community participation; to work through processes of innovation; to work towards a healthy public policy; based upon a commitment to health and to require political decision making for public health.

Within Healthy Cities the health policy concept has four basic components. Those components are the use of information for decision making, intersectoral collaboration, community involvement and political support. The perception by policy makers and politicians of each of these concepts are as follows:

Supportive information for decision making

It was felt that both qualitative and quantitative information on the determinants of health should be used in the development of policy and political decision making. The role of epidemiology in relation to policy decisions received more attention. Policy makers and decision makers needed this information on the one hand to justify their decisions and on the other hand as information that can point at a direction for action. However, there was not always a balance between qualitative and quantitative information on a certain subject. The power of figures and facts was seen as very strong. In reality, however, policy is not a science that can be driven by facts and figures alone. There are many more factors that influence the policy development, especially when you consider this to be dynamic and iterative. There is often as mismatch between perceptions as to the use of hard facts and the actual use in informing decision making.

The problems many people have with regard to Healthy Cities is the difficulty in "measuring the health of a city." However, efforts are being made to develop indicators for this purpose. Some cities are developing a geographical information system in order to map out the location, the severity and content of problems. This can result in an indication and direction for policy decisions. Other ways of gathering information are through organizations and health professionals in the city or by means of a community health inquiry.

Based on the information politicians and policy makers receive about their city, the following subjects are mentioned as major health problems and target areas in The Netherlands:

1.   Addiction - gambling and drugs.

2.   Elderly - prevention, isolation, care, housing, facilities, integral policy and accidents.

3.   Unemployment.

4.   Youth - gambling, drugs, future perspectives, second generation problems, food and prevention of accidents.

5.   Public mental health - homeless people and drifters, ex-mental health patients and problems in the neighbourhood.

Intersectoral collaboration

There were several examples of activities that were organized and implemented by so called "intersectoral groups". However this was mostly at the operational level and occasionally at a managerial level. At the political level intersectoral collaboration is not common.

An example of intersectoral collaboration is the policy on gambling addiction. Key participants were local government, the police, the local health service and the bureau for alcohol and drugs consultation. Those groups do not only work together on concrete activities, they formulate together plans and they do this at all levels. Moreover every actor is responsible for the implementation of the policy.

The several local public health services do make some efforts to put health on the agenda of other organizations and municipal services in their city. Their advice is appreciated, however, never asked for. In other words the local health authority has to show the initiative. A form of collaboration between welfare and health is regarded as "normal." Within other departments, however, question marks are raised when the health authority asks them for co-operation and/or provides them with advice concerning their policy decisions on possible consequences for the health of the city inhabitants:

> Other services are not likely to pay attention to the health aspect, however it is the prime task of the health service to do so ...

> I do not agree with the idea that health is an issue within all the municipal departments and services. At some stages we can speak of some increase in cooperation. Why should we integrate with services that we do not consider to be relevant for the tasks we have to perform?

It was recognized that it was necessary initially to discuss what a department can win or loose by investing in this specific activity. A Housing Department is not judged and budgeted for their contribution to health matters. Health policy development should go hand in hand with reallocation of resources and identification of new indicators for monitoring the activities of the departments. The traditional organizational structure and financing system does not stimulate collaboration and facilitate policy, everybody has his or her own "store." Integration within the departments of one municipal service was thought to cause already enough difficulties.

In only one city of the pilot was the municipal health service represented in the key management group of the city. This means in concrete terms that the municipal health service was regarded as one of the key actors that should be involved in every city policy that is developed. This was the only example of integrated policy development.

It is rare that a city plan was judged on its consequences for health. Some cities were trying to achieve this in the near future and some are already very close to it but there were difficulties: "at a certain stage there are so many aspects against which your decision should be judged, that it is no longer possible to make your decision. Let's be honest, who is able to work with this concept of policy?"

It would seem therefore that one of the key aims of Healthy Cities which is to cross the boundaries of the departments, is at present more theory than practice. And if it happens, it is more for practical reasons i.e. projects than for policy development.

Participation of the community

In "traditional policy" in The Netherlands, the community can give its comments on certain policy proposals by means of hearings. However, there is a chance that the comments as made by the community are filtered by the department before they reach the agenda of the municipal council. City inhabitants can also raise questions in government committees on health affairs. Their questions reach the city council through those committees. When plans are made on specific issues, the planning group will always consult the target groups. The question is, however, is this community participation?

> I question if services and organizations in general are truly willing to collaborate with the community.

> People want to be healthy, however they will not organize themselves and demonstrate in front of the city hall for the promotion of their health. They will demonstrate when something threatens their health.

> For a health service we consider it important to have good contact with organizations within the community. If they are excited about our plans it can sometimes be more effective than any kind of decision within the local government.

Community self administration is considered to have potential for the near future. This means in concrete terms that a neighbourhood has its own steering committee that discusses problems and tries to solve them. This can be in collaboration with public and private services and organizations. In theory, they can even develop their own neighbourhood plans with regard to daily activities and social affairs which they can discuss directly with the city government.

As shown above, in practice the community has more involvement at the operational level (implementing concrete activities) than at the managerial or political level.

> How can we speak about community participation in health affairs if they do not yet participate in greening or city planning?

333

Indeed, some activities do not even ask for community participation and the community does not always want to participate.

> I pay my taxes in order that the government can sweep the streets etc., so do not bother me with questions that I have to give them a hand.

In reality there is a need to find the balance between the possible and the preferable.

Health on the political agenda

The WHO considers this as one the major goals in the Healthy Cities project. As indicated earlier the managerial level can play an important role in integrating operational and political commitment. It was clear from the interviews that political interest in an issue can increase by the growing visibility of a project, through providing information, use of media, organization of events, presenting plans in terms of political gain and positive financial consequences, inviting politicians to meetings and gatherings, attending (informal) meetings.

Political interest for a subject can be measured in terms of finances, policy papers, health related items on the agenda of the city council. If a local government truly accepts a broad definition of health it would provide the opportunity to force other services than the health services to judge their plans on certain health indicators.

Prevention and protection has always been considered to be a task of the municipalities. In The Netherlands, however, the interest of the local government in health care is growing, partly due to the economic recession and decentralization. If a government is able to create health care facilities in its city, it creates employment as well.

Decision makers lack of information, thus a health professional has the task of filling in the gaps. This can be done by means of presentations or small seminars where a municipal service provides the members of the city council, or a part of the city council, with information on their activities and their progress and their ideas of addressing a certain problem. The problem can be highlighted from several points of view, several possible solutions can be discussed and the problem can be visualized. By means of providing them with information and knowledge, the support required to address a certain problem can be increased. One must not forget that the scope of a municipal council influences their decisions, so it is important that their scope is "correct".

The political colour of the responsible person may influence the position of health on the political agenda. "Political commitment is influenced both by personal characteristics and party politics."

Thus in essence, it is due to the efforts of professionals that health increases in visibility, however health is still not really an issue for the politicians. As can be seen from Table 26.1 health is following the same pattern of policy development and political decision making as other issues and still is in an early phase. The content of policy is always the first decision point if policy is going to be made. If it comes to political decision making, costs and benefits in political, financial and governmental terms are the most important decision points. Effects, feasibility and local political pressure are the second group of influencing factors at that stage.

Table 26.1
Decision points in (health) policy development

No decision point	Decision point of the first order (pre-phase)	Decision point of the second order (phase of political negotiations)
Statute or law	Content (almost in 100% of the cases)	Costs/benefits: -financial -governmental -political
	National developments	
	Expected effects	Local political pressure
	City workplan	
	Questions from the community	Feasibility of the plan
		Position/charisma
	Political pressure	
		Law
	Attitude of people/ charisma	
		National developments
	Idea of the management	
		Expectations
	Local politics/political parties	
		Party programme
	Law	

Conclusion: what does healthy cities offer policy makers and politicians?

It is clear that if a professional is to receive political support for a project, he/she should know how his/her key decision maker perceives the concepts and ideas that are behind it. This would increase understanding and enable policy decisions to be more effectively guided. It must be recognized, however, that in the end politicians are opportunists. Thus instead of putting health on their agenda, it is probably more productive to focus on looking for the health dimension in the issues that are already on it.

Politicians are not very likely to change the way they approach policy. If they perceive the project as innovative they mostly see only the consequences at service and the operational level. By showing the relationship between different kinds of public policies and health, politicians may be convinced of the potential Healthy Cities has to offer. Emphasizing the health aspects in other policy fields can bring political gain. Gaining political support probably can best be achieved by providing information on what they can win through developing health policy, what concrete outcomes it can offer and how it can fit with their regular and legal tasks.

Policy development is dynamic and context related. It is clear from this preliminary study that the ideals of Health Policy development as encapsulated in the ideology of Healthy Cities are not currently part of mainstream health policy.

There are far more examples of intersectoral collaboration at the operational level than at the political level. Health policy as opposed to health care policy at the urban level is still considered to be innovative and generally has not yet had an impact on the decision making process. If health or a health issue gains a place on the agenda, it is because "the right person was there at the right place at the right time" and because they were "ready for this subject". Whilst the health sector is not different from any other policy sector in this regard it would appear to be more difficult to get it to receive any attention at all. A focus on disease is more attractive because the short term cost and benefits seem more concrete.

What is clear is that more policy research is needed so that we can increase our insight and understanding of how politicians and decision makers reach their decisions, what they do, and why they choose these actions, i.e. how they put health policy concepts into practice. A major task remaining, for both research and practice, is how to find the balance between the health policy goals of the Healthy Cities project on the one hand, and what is practical and possible on the other.

References

Allison, G.T. (1971), *Essence of Decions: Explaining the Cuban Missile Crisis,* Little, Brown and Company, Boston.

de Leeuw, E. (1989), *Health Policy,* Savannah, Maastricht.

Rogers, E.M. (1983), *Diffusion of Innovations,* (third edition), The Free Press, New York.

WHO/Health and Welfare Canada, Canadian Public Health Association (1986), *Ottawa Charter for Health Promotion.* An International Conference on Health Promotion - The Move Towards A New Public Health, Nov. pp. 17-21, Ottawa.

World Health Organisation/Euro (1992), *When a Project Becomes a Movement,* FADL, Copenhagen, pp. 7-8.

Worldbank (1993), *Investments in Health.*

27 The West Everton Child Health project

Clare Mahoney and Ann Roach

The Liverpool Child Health project takes as its framework a broad definition of health which includes environmental, social and political influences. Its action is based on the principle that poverty is the single biggest cause of ill health. It is run from two community bases, West Everton Community Council (WECC) and Rotunda Community College for Adults. It does so founded on principles that reflect the aims and ethics of the organizations where the project is based, as well as the broad aims of Save the Children Fund.

The main aim of the project is to influence the provision of services which can contribute to good health. It does this by supporting young people and children in their efforts to participate in the design and delivery of services. The services which promote good health are many and varied. Some are more accessible than others. Some service providers, although willing to work with community groups find it a daunting prospect. The project therefore helps this process both by developing the community in various ways so that it can contribute effectively and by acting as a bridge between service providers and the community. By making links with providers of services, it is investing in relationships which promote partnership and multi-agency working, so called "Healthy Alliances". The aim of these alliances is to encourage communication between communities and service providers so that all parties concerned look at the ways in which they can each get the best out of each other. Experience suggests that although health authorities in particular are currently expressing a great willingness to listen to community defined needs, they are unclear how to go about it and how to make use of the information gained.

For that dialogue to take place community involvement needs to be nurtured. A key element is education and access to information, both of which are central to empowerment and a person's feeling of control over their life. It enables people to believe in their ability to change things that they are unhappy about. Self confidence and self belief are known to be central to achieving a sense of well being. Using the structures of the Rotunda Community College, the Child Health project is working on the development of projects which combine these elements. It supports the overall work of the Health Strategy Group, and is closely involved in the setting up of a Lay Health course and Patient Rights group. It is establishing two networks of local people, one of adults and one of children, both made up of people who are interested in health.

Participation is not just about adults. Children and young people have the right to put their views forward and be taken seriously. They should be included in the planning of services which affect them. They too have the potential to participate in community action. Children and young people should be encouraged and supported in the development of their own agendas. This means that they identify issues which are of importance to them in their own language and their own way. It is not the sole responsibility of the children to adjust to the ways of an adult run world; adults must meet them half way.

The children's council

An example of a community initiative which embodies these principles is the Children's Council in West Everton. The Children's Council is a group of local children who meet regularly to discuss and make decisions on points of concern. The role of the Child Health project has been to give support at weekly meetings, provide training and skills development workshops and to build up a network of local adults, paid and unpaid, who will help develop this work.

The idea of the Children's Council first arose at the annual weekend away review of the West Everton Community Council, held at the Ozanam Centre, North Wales in October 1990. Concern was expressed about the lack of facilities for children in the West Everton area, particularly in the Langsdale and Islington section of the patch, and of the temptations which surrounded them. The Mansfield Youth Club had closed down; the Salisbury Club had been demolished earlier to make way for new build housing. Drugs presented a major problem and stolen cars were often driven at speed throughout the area. Concerned residents felt that it was simply not safe for the children to be out on the streets.

The problems, and the possible solutions, was referred to the wider network of neighbourhood groups in West Everton for discussion and feed back, and it was included on the agenda of the WECC steering group. It was discovered that there were pockets of children from each of the eight areas who were reluctant to "cross each others boundaries". So it was decided that some attempt should be made to break through these individual barriers and at the same time provide them with adequate play facilities. Two workers from the WECC, together with the Community Development Unit from Liverpool City Council, consulted closely with parents and others for solutions. The idea of a Childrens' Council, run on similar lines to the WECC steering group, began to emerge at this stage. The basic idea was to create a system through which children would be able to express themselves and to have some sort of input into decisions that affected their lives.

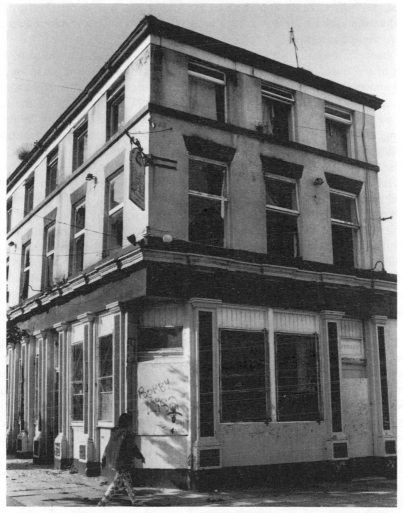

The formation of the West Everton Children's Council was stimulated by the poor social and environmental conditions in the area and the lack of facilities for the children

A special meeting for all children across the area was called on in February 1992. It was attended by over 100 children. Their enthusiasm was apparent. The organizers broke them up into area groups to get them to say what was "good" and "bad" in their particular district, and also what they would like to see happening in the whole community. Using a flip chart, they were then asked to prioritize the ideas they had suggested. Building on this event, and to show community involvement was not all about meetings, the children were encouraged to organize and run their own disco. All the arrangements, bookings, buffet, disco and cleaning up afterwards was undertaken by the children themselves. It was a huge success. They sent out thank you letters to everyone concerned and asked for more activities.

A feedback meeting was arranged a week later to look into the pros and cons of the event. Other issues came up such as road safety, green issues, their concern for the elderly and the lack of facilities for children right across the area. Difficulties had arisen in organizing the event, some of the kids dropped out, and the remainder realized that it was not as easy to make arrangements for activities involving large numbers of their peers. Smaller meetings were arranged by and for them, with the children rotating as chair and secretary.

At this point in the development of the idea, the UK Based charity Save the Children Fund became involved and suggested that a Children's Community Worker be funded by them who would provide support for the initiative. At the same time one of the local community worker's job description was amended to include outreach work with children. Save the Children backed up their interest with a donation of £1,500 and a children's account was opened at the local bank. Significantly when the Children's worker was appointed in early 1993, parents were actively involved in the interviews.

The "Kids Council" (as they prefer it to be called) started monthly meetings that have continued ever since. Every "kid" in the area is considered a member, and even if they're only two years old. Most of the activity has taken place in Langsdale and Islington, the southern part of West Everton where the facilities have been particularly bad. The area and its housing had been in very bad condition with half the houses and maisonettes either vacated or vandalized. It was an area that was being looked at for redevelopment by city planning officials. The children decided to approach the local neighbourhood group, the Islington Action Group, which was in consultation with Liverpool City Council over the development of the area through new build and some demolition. On the children's suggestion sleeping policemen were included in the plans. Other action included starting a Bingo sessions in Friary House each Sunday afternoon for the adult population, particularly the elderly, following expressions of concern by the children. The attendance is between 30 and 40 people each week.

Training for empowerment took many forms. A leader from the Yellow

House Drama Group in Bootle was invited to work with the children. This enabled the quieter children to express themselves in a positive way, have fun, and experience the self discipline required in that profession, something they found difficult. Another three day course for 20 children was held in West Derby. The focus there was getting children to discuss issues that affected them including: working together; listening to each other; setting their own rules; organizing events; writing up and reporting back; each members playing an active part; planning discos; and learning from mistakes.

As a result the children came up with a number of suggestions such as the use of the former housing office in William Henry Street, now empty and unused as a play area. They wrote letters to the local Councillor and Council Officers seeking action.

Conclusion

The Children's Council received widespread publicity in the national press as being the first of its kind in the UK. While its continued existence is evidence of its potential, setting up the Children's council was not easy and not without difficulties. Like any other organization, revamping was needed from time to time, targets needed to be set and analysis needed to take place. Indeed there was a lot of hard work that needed to be done. There have been a number of conflicts, not least between the adults and the children. In part this has been the result of the natural process of growing up. But there have also been some concrete outcomes. The "Jenky Way" play area that has long been a dream of locals has now become a reality, opened naturally, by a six year old child. Over the years, children have been involved in all sorts of activities on all sorts of occasions, for example the fight to save good four bedroom houses from demolition, street clean ups, the local Gala, etc. More recently there has been another well attend disco and a relaunch of the council in the form of a gigantic "fun day".

28 Health behaviour research in minority communities: A brief summary of experiences from heart, body and soul and project BLESS

Frances A. Stillman

Purpose

This paper summarizes a health behaviour research project that is a partnership between an academic institution, the Johns Hopkins University School of Medicine, and the African American community of east Baltimore. The first phase of the project, "Heart, Body and Soul", focused on developing and evaluating culturally specific smoking cessation programmes implemented through the African American churches. The first initiative of Heart, Body, and Soul was a randomized clinical trial of an intensive smoking cessation intervention compared with minimal self help intervention (Stillman et al. 1993). The second phase of the project, project BLESS, continued the smoking cessation activities in the churches and developed, implemented, and evaluated other culturally relevant smoking cessation activities in housing developments, food distribution programmes, literacy programmes, and senior citizen centres in conjunction with other community organizations. In addition, a targeted media campaign and an advocacy campaign focused on the macro level issues related to tobacco control policy and legislation. This paper highlights the activities with the churches and our successful effort to ban outdoor tobacco advertising in Baltimore, Maryland.

Background

African Americans remain at high risk for tobacco use, and continue to suffer disproportionately from smoking related diseases and death (Center for Disease Control, 1987; State of Maryland Department of Health and Mental Hygiene, 1986-89).

While the most recent Maryland Behavioral Risk Factor Survey indicates that current smoking rates are similar among whites (26 per cent) and blacks

(28.4 per cent), there are far fewer former smokers among African Americans (18 per cent) than among whites (26 per cent). Furthermore, the Risk Factor data do not reflect the higher smoking prevalence and smoking mortality rates present in our inner city regions (Novotny et al. 1988). Our 1991 random digit dialling survey of approximately 1,000 urban African Americans found a current overall smoking prevalence of 35.5 per cent; 42.9 per cent in males and 32.9 per cent in females. Urban African Americans have the highest smoking related mortality and morbidity of any race or ethnic subgroup in Maryland.

Maryland leads the nation in cancer deaths and is among the states with the highest cardiovascular morbidity and mortality. Lung cancer rates among African American males are approximately 505/100,000 (compared to 79/100,000 in white males). Asthma is consistently among the three most common reasons for absence from school in Baltimore City as well as in the rest of Maryland (Novotny et al. 1988).

Targeting of African Americans by the tobacco industry

It is well documented that the tobacco industry in the United States has targeted African Americans at the individual level with culturally specific marketing campaigns and strategies. The industry has also targeted the African American community with well planned and executed strategies to influence the political, educational, and social sectors. In addition, the outdoor advertising companies (billboards) have lucrative contracts with both alcohol and tobacco companies. The inner city areas have the highest prevalence of advertisements and billboards promoting tobacco and alcohol consumption (U.S. Department of Health and Human Services, 1994). A recent survey of all outdoor advertising in a four square mile area surrounding the Johns Hopkins Medical Institutions in Baltimore, Maryland, found almost 1000 outdoor billboards, signs and advertisements for cigarettes and alcohol. On one street alone we counted 151 cigarette advertisements alone we found 30.

Involving African Americans in smoking cessation and tobacco control

Unfortunately, there has been a lack of interest in and almost no research on smoking cessation in and tobacco policy research focused on urban African Americans. Little attention has been paid to understanding how the tobacco industry influences community organizations. Furthermore, no research has been done on how the various sectors of the community can develop a working coalition to reduce smoking prevalence and affect tobacco control legislation. These initiatives should include implementation of clean indoor air legislation to reduce exposure to environmental tobacco smoke, reducing access of youth to cigarettes, and eliminating outdoor cigarette advertisements, as well as providing easy access to culturally specific cessation programmes or self help materials.

Since the health of individuals is interrelated to the health of their communities, smoking cessation and tobacco policy research that works in partnership with the African American community (i.e. pastors, city council members, housing developments, community organizations), incorporating culturally relevant and specific interventions identified and implemented by the community, are a highly effective means for behavioral and societal change.

Establishing a working relationship with CURE

Churches are an important institution in the African American community (Lincoln, 1984; Frazier, 1963). In East Baltimore there are often two churches per block and 65 per cent of the population attends church regularly. Even among those who do not attend church, a strong spiritual ethic remains. Over 80 per cent of African Americans cite prayer as a major coping mechanism and place religion as the highest priority in their lives.

One of the goals of our project was to establish and maintain a relationship with Clergy United for the Renewal of East Baltimore (CURE), an organization of approximately 200 churches. CURE is an established lead agency that had previously mobilized to work on other community issues, such as housing. We thought CURE would be an effective means of gaining access to a large number of churches, community leaders, and community members. To build trust among the community, we found it necessary to share control of important project decisions and to incorporate identified community objectives as project objectives. This meant that the project expanded its focus into areas that were not part of our original plan.

The clergy group wanted to be part of the planning, hiring, implementation and evaluation phases of the project. We also realized that the research team and the church group had unrealistic perceptions of each other. We viewed the community as a homogeneous group of impoverished people, and they viewed us as a monolithic organization with unlimited resources. Both groups had to come to the realization that inaccurate perceptions of each other were a problem.

Gaining access to churches

Once we decided to work with the churches and CURE, we had to schedule

347

individual meeting with pastors and church leaders, a very important but time consuming process. Some churches had gatekeepers that protected the pastors. The church calendar also was an important factor, since many churches had activities booked well in advance. Major holidays and other important church events also had to be taken into consideration when planning project events. Furthermore, church calendars may not be accurate, or unplanned events, such as funerals, can alter the calendar.

Because scheduling meetings with clergy members took much longer than originally planned, and clergy were often available only in the evenings, project staff had to be flexible and dedicated (since a regular work schedule is not consistent with how churches operate). Staff attended church services and events, in order to meet church members and pastors. These efforts facilitated our acceptance.

One of our first tasks was to help CURE obtain an up to date listing of all their member churches, since their list was not accurate and did not reflect the changes that were occurring in the community. They did not have the resources to conduct a survey of all their churches and to establish a computerized data base to assist in mailings. In the process of compiling a more accurate list we learned more about the churches and the community than we would have by just working from a pre-existing list. This work demonstrated to CURE that we were interested in assisting them in accomplishing their goals and not just interested in using them to accomplish our research agenda.

Project BLESS

Project BLESS (Baltimore Leading Everyone to be Safe and Smoke-free) is a city wide smoking cessation and tobacco control initiative that will ultimately benefit the health of the entire community. By mobilizing an inner city community to bring the force of its efforts to change tobacco policy, the project has formed a local coalition. The project also encompasses a clinical trial of an intensive smoking cessation and tobacco control intervention versus a minimal intervention, which is being conducted in Prince George's County, Maryland, an urban centre with high concentrations of African Americans. Prince George's County is serving as our reference community. In project BLESS, process data, including minutes from all meetings, attendance records at all events, time utilization logs from staff and volunteers, types of services, and numbers of materials provided, are collected to evaluate the project components. Cross sectional community wide surveys and tracking of a cohort of smokers are also being conducted annually to determine outcomes associated with change in smoking prevalence.

Advocacy to ban outdoor tobacco advertisements

Baltimore has just recently become the first city in the United States to ban all outdoor tobacco advertising. The legislation was just signed into law a few weeks ago. This landmark endeavour was the result of a coalition that brought together community organizers, academics, city council persons, lawyers, community members, and religious leaders. This required a great deal of planning and preparation since previous attempts to ban advertising resulted in legal action based on constitutional issues related to freedom of speech. The academic institution provided an invaluable service, but the actual change could not have occurred without local, grassroots involvement.

Pastors and other community leaders were provided with training on how to be effective advocates, how to work with the media, how to interact with local politicians, and how to activate their churches or community organizations to take some action. Pastors were asked to give sermons in favour of this legislation, to encourage their congregations to write letters to their city council representatives, and to make telephone calls to the Mayor in support of this legislation. Scientific literature related to advertising and consumption of cigarettes by children was provided along with specific data on how tobacco affects African American youth and their communities, in order to assist pastors and other community members in their support of this legislation. The process of enacting this legislation was carefully monitored for our evaluation.

Reconciling the multiple scientific and community needs

The relationship between the community and an academic institution needs to be a partnership. The partnership must be a true partnership, with each partner having equal input into the process. This is easier said than done. The community and an academic institution have different operational styles and cultures that affect how tasks are approached and conflict is resolved. Developing a working relationship requires time, tolerance, and the ability to adapt and change (Mittelmark, 1991).

The research team should clearly define and articulate the research aims and communicate them accurately to the community. The project staff needs to listen to the community and adapt or develop programme components based on this interaction. The community needs to understand the time limits of the research funding, while the researchers need to make every effort to develop programmes that are sustainable. Researchers have time lines to follow and stated research objectives to achieve. They must also work with the community to accomplish goals deemed important to the community. This requires a commitment of time and energy on the part of the research team and their staff to accomplish additional tasks. For example, pastors and other community leaders sought out project investigators to assist them in securing funding for grants for literacy programmes, a drug abuse centre, a youth programmes, etc. Community leaders were given the opportunity to present these additional goals to the senior administrators of the Johns Hopkins University, the School of Medicine and the Hospital, who then helped them get funding. These relationships facilitated donations to CURE, the establishment of a joint effort to train community members to serve on a volunteer security network, and the obtaining of additional resources, such as buildings in the community and a van. In all endeavours the community fully expected to be an equal partner. They did not want to be viewed as just being research subjects or the beneficiaries of the researchers' largesse. They wanted to be heard and to participate in all discussions. As stated by one of our pastors, "The community is not being empowered, it is in power".

The researchers also had to educate the funding sources as to the true nature of community based research. Pastors were involved in the grant writing process and participated in the scientific review process of our grant application by going with the research team to the National Institutes of Health and made presentations to assist us in securing funding. In return we became committed to assisting the community in securing separate funding.

What we learned from our initial efforts

Over all, we have learned that flexibility is necessary and rigid protocols are unrealistic. We had to stop being the "experts" since the pastor's role in the community necessitated that they be viewed as the leaders. The research team needed to stay in the background and become consultants and advisors. At every opportunity, the community leaders wanted to be viewed as being in charge of the project. In some instances, the designated spokesmen were articulate, well informed, participatory, and fulfilled the responsibility of this role. They devoted their time to prepare letters, testimony, and meeting agendas, to assist with grant applications, and to make media appearances. Unfortunately, in other instances the designated spokesperson failed to appear, did not make use of briefing materials, and made statements that were inaccurate. Part of the explanation for this is that the pastors are often in competition with each other for church members and demand that their members be given preferential access to job opportunities or other project resources. These incidents needed to be resolved with sensitivity.

Communities represent more than a local, they are constituted of people who share cultural and social relationships. Understanding that culture influences perceptions, behaviours, and operational styles is important since culturally mediated differences often lead to irritation and frustration between "partners". Thus, how things happen is as important as what actually happens (Thompson and Kinne, 1990).

Hiring staff that either went to church in the community or lived in the community was a key factor in facilitating access to the community. Providing jobs and training opportunities was essential. This also necessitated that the researchers facilitate changes in hiring policy at the institution, which had formerly made it difficult for community people to be hired except in the lowest levels of the institutional structure. Community leaders are now included on University review committees and are invited to teach classes, and three pastors have been given faculty appointments at the School of Medicine. To bring about behaviour change in an entire community, it is useful to view the community as a system in which relatively stable structures co-operate to achieve common goals and establish norms. To bring about effective tobacco policy controls, community systems theory would posit that the most influential sectors of a community need to be mobilized simultaneously. The sub-systems identified in our efforts include the political, educational, health, religious, communications, and housing systems, along with grassroots community organizations (Green and Raeburn, 1990). Most important, we learned that the community is very diverse and the members of the community are a great resource.

To change social norms and to change the socio-cultural environment as it relates to promoting smoking cessation, implementing and enforcing clean air legislation, banning tobacco sales to youth, and banning tobacco advertisements, we need to continue fostering culturally relevant cessation programmes and skill development among the community members and their sub-system leaders. Our research with the community is seeking to accomplish these goals as well as to document the process.

Acknowledgements

This project was funded by the National Institutes of health, National, Heart, Lung, and Blood Institute Grant RO1HL4360, "Church-based Smoking Cessation Strategies in an urban Black Community".

References

Center for Disease Control (1987), "Cigarette Smoking Among Blacks and Other Minority Populations", *Morbidity and Mortality Weekly*, vol. 36. p. 403.

Frazier, E.F. (1963), *The Negro Church in America*, Schocken, New York.

Green, L.W. and Raeburn, J. (1990), "Contemporary Developments in Health

Promotion: Definitions and Challenges" in Bracht, N.B. (ed.), *Health Promotion at the Community Level*, Newbury Park, California, pp. 29-42.

Lincoln, C.E. (1984), *Race, Religion and Continuing American Dilemma*, Hill and Wang, New York.

Maryland Behavioral Risk Factor Survey (1986-89), *State of Maryland Department of Health and Mental Hygiene, Baltimore, Maryland*.

Mittelmark, M.B. (1991), "Balancing the Requirements and the Needs of Communities" in Bracht, N.B. (ed.), *Health Promotion at the Community Level*, Newbury Park, California, pp. 125-37.

Novotny, T.E., Warner, K.E., Kendrick, J.S. and Remmington, P.L. (1988), "Smoking by Blacks and Whites: Socio-Economic and Demographic Differences", *AJPH*, vol. 78, no. 9, pp. 1187-9.

Stillman, F.A., Bone, L.R., Rand, C., Levine, D.M. and Becker, D.M. (1993), "Heart, Body and Soul: A Church-Based Smoking Cessation Program for Urban African Americans", *Preventive Medicine*, vol. 22, pp. 335-49.

Thompson, B. and Kinne, S. (1990), "Social Change Theory: Applications to Community Health", in Bracht, N.B. (ed.), *Health Promotion at the Community Level*, Newbury Park, California, pp. 45-61.

U.S. Department of Health and Human Services (1994), *Preventing Tobacco Use Among Young People: A Report of the Surgeon General*, UDHHS, PHS, CDC, NCCDPHP, OSH, Atlanta, Georgia, pp. 179-84.

29 Re-orienting primary medical care towards primary health care

Paul Thomas

This paper looks at the lessons to be learned from the attempts in Liverpool between 1989 and 1994 to facilitate the transformation of primary medical care (especially the GP services) towards primary health care - a holistic and integrated approach to addressing the health of people in localities. In 1989 as in most deprived cities, most Family Practioner Services in Liverpool were isolated, crisis driven and disease focused. Despite some pockets of excellence, for the most part there was little team work and little in the way of co-ordinated relevant on going educational support. The 110 practices (240 GPs) between them employed only eight practice nurses and very few had attached health visitors or district nurses. In addition the health involved organizations worked in relative isolation from each other - there was little history or experience of co-ordinated collaborative work anywhere.

By contrast, Liverpool general practice in 1994 can claim to be team work conscious with an appreciation of non-medical approaches to health care: all practices include in their team a health visitor, a district nurse and a practice nurse; almost all practices have a practice manager; and all have had some experience of multi-disciplinary learning; all practices have had some contact with a wider perspective on health including some understanding of mental and social health needs. The health involved organizations which were once so far apart are conscious of the need to operate together and are committed to allowing localities to develop in their own unique way, inside a co-ordinated framework: the locality purchasing process involves people from public health and general practice, but also has input from people from a non-medical background. It is widely understood that interventions must promote and support team work and intersectoral collaboration as well as addressing topics and there is a growing understanding of the importance of the facilitation role in the change process.

This change does not mean that Liverpool has arrived at Utopia, but it does mean that significant change has taken place in the way people think about their work and how they relate to others. The health service reforms provided opportunities for local people to bring about this change and it was the result of the work of many people. The focus here is on the Liverpool Primary Health Care Facilitation project in order to tease out some principles of how to facilitate such a change in culture.

The primary health care facilitation project as a tool for change

The Liverpool Primary Health Care Facilitation project developed the idea of a multi-disciplinary facilitation team: people from different disciplines (health visiting, district nursing, practice nursing, practice management, general practice) became a team to facilitate development in a defined geographic area. They drew on established theory and practice from management of change, team building and organizational development, using educational methods which involve the principles of adult learning and participatory research. They were aware of policy implementation theory which shows that effective cultural change is best helped by "creating coalitions and allowing street level discretion" (Elmore, 1979/80).

The project recognized that sustainable change requires simultaneous and complimentary change, at all levels, in three separate dimensions that we have called quality, quantity and consensus:

1. The dimension of quality - personal skills, personal confidence and sense of self value.

2. The dimension of quantity - rules and roles, protocols and targets.

3. The dimension of consensus - the organization of general practice (and other groups), the sense of common purpose and the level of teamwork.

So, for example, improving immunization uptake (quantity) requires improved skills of individuals (quality) and improved systems in the practice (consensus). Neglect of any of the areas results in a slower change process. These three dimensions are named after the evaluation methods used to detect change - qualitative and quantitative methods and shared statements. This notion of three separate but interdependent dimensions of change finds echoes in the writing of the so called "hermeneutic" continental philosophers such as Habermas and Gadamer (Wulff, 1990).

The importance of identifying these three dimensions is to appreciate that change in each of them, and at different levels, needs to be linked so that they are compatible with each other. If this does not occur, change is resisted because people have difficulty in appreciating the reason for change. This understanding prompted the project to work closely with senior managers of health involved organizations as well as at the "grassroots" and to ensure that the three dimensions were linked in all interventions initiated by the project itself.

The approach to change

Conscious of the need to consider primary health care as a complex system requiring an intervention that involved everyone, the project adopted a bottom up approach - listening, involving and problem solving - asking health care workers and others what future they would like to see and they perceive to be the immediate priorities for action. This information was amalgamated and fed back to people to arrive at a consensus for action inside practices, across localities and inside the health involved organizations. So, for example, practices and individuals with similar interests were put in touch with each other and commonly perceived problems in practices were communicated to health service managers.

In addition the facilitation team operated a number of discrete interventions including:

1. Interactive bulletins sent regularly to everyone in the target group in order to maximize participation.

2. Repeated personal contact with individuals and the target groups and consciously building networks inside and outside of the city to develop relationships.

3. Multi-disciplinary forums where local health care workers learn the skills of participatory group work while exploring health issues and new ideas of the moment.

4. Multi-disciplinary workshops where local health care workers learn the skills of participatory group work while examining a specific problem and developing relevant action.

5. Models of local collaborative activity were used to exemplify quality practice and encourage adoption of such models.

6. Importing ideas, models, people and skills from other places for local use.

7. Road shows, in practice multi-disciplinary workshops where one aspect of the work of the practice is subjected to a team audit and action for change initiated.

8. Residential team building workshops where practice teams explored their shared ˙vision of the future, shared understanding of their problems and develop shared objectives as a team.

9. Consensus statements and coalitions which can be effective at articulating a vision for the future.

10. Examples of collaboration between different sectors, e.g. health and education sectors, to demonstrate that even groups that are far from understanding each other or regularly working together can produce "win win" outcomes. These are used as a legitimising role model and a force for policy change.

The impact of the project

The tangible outcomes which resulted from this activity are many and together they have the effect of changing people's perceptions about their role in the whole health care system. It offered people an alternative model of primary care away from a hierarchical disease preoccupied approach, towards a more holistic and participative approach that is also concerned with mental health and social health - an Alma Ata vision of Primary Health Care.

The specific outcomes of the project are of less significance than the change in culture but mentioning a few of these may give some idea of the kind of things that happened:

Women's health conference

A gathering of 50 plus people, half of whom were from the medical sector and half from local groups, to explore issues related to women's health in a geographical area. The amalgamated report was then distributed widely and influenced the local debate about local health needs. This then effected the locality purchasing process.

The health promotion clinic attendance project

An anthropology trained PhD student interviewed staff in four health centres about the reasons why they perceived that women did or did not attend for cervical cytology. Their views were then amalgamated and fed back to the practice team in the multi-disciplinary workshop where they devised action plans to address the issues that they found. At the next stage the same interviewer visited a number of women who had not attended (and those who had attended) to find out their views on the same question. These views were similarly amalgamated and fed back to all of the practices in multi-disciplinary team workshops to demonstrate that there is a mis-match between the understanding of practice staff and patients. The realization of this plus the fact that there were things that could be practically done to address them resulted in a galvanizing of the practices to address the issues.

Heart disease discussion document

Forty people from over 20 different disciplines over a number of meetings discussed the issues related to heart disease prevention. Working from a common data set which was not solely medical, they arrived at a form of words that was acceptable to all sectors about the way forward. This resulted in a public acknowledgement by the health authorities, trade unions, private employers, the local authority, church and voluntary groups. This consensus statement still many years later has been the authoritative document from which further activity can take place.

Occupational health project

Lay health workers interview patients about their perceptions of their own occupational hazards from the waiting rooms of health centres and practices in the city. Up to one-quarter of all the practices of the city have been involved at some stage. In addition to giving individual advice both to patients and to health care workers, the project team would develop suspicions about trends or common themes in the hazards they are hearing, and would commission extra research into these. This research was then used to cause policy changes. So, for example, they identified and highlighted the problems that caretakers in high rise blocks have in respect of violence. The subsequent research and report related to this was influential in forming housing policies for the Housing Action Trusts. In a similar way they were able to highlight and arrange action around war pensions for Somalis, asbestosis and smoking related cancers, and noise induced deafness.

Describing projects and models of activity does little to understand the power of cultural change. When moods and attitudes change, when it becomes common for people to talk about their work in a collaborative and enthusiastic way that understands and respects people that they did not know before; when people chose to align their efforts with others, the force for change is very great. Some of the comments from key informants contained in the report of the project (Thomas, 1989-94) bear witness to this.

Conclusion

The recurring theme in all of these projects is the involvement of all people relevant to health care (managers, workers, allied groups, patients) as informants and focusing and packaging their collective insights in a way that is useful to them and can influence policy. This non-expert participatory approach has been as effective in Liverpool Primary Health Care Facilitation project as it has been in other "Large Group Interventions" which apply whole system methodology (Journal of Applied Behaviourial Science, 1992).

Perhaps the most telling piece of evidence of the change of culture has been the development of the LMFTs - four part time Local Multi-disciplinary Facilitation Teams have operated since September 1993 in four of the seven planning areas of the city. Most of these are made up of a general practitioner, a health visitor, a district nurse, a practice nurse and a practice manager (each employed for five hours a week) although two community psychiatric nurses and a school nurse are involved in the total project. This network of 20 people operates in a similar way to the previous facilitation project and is held together by multi-disciplinary learning tied to a university course (the Certificate of Facilitation of Primary Health Care). This initiative marks the end of Primary Health Care Facilitation as a project - recognizing that an infrastructure of facilitation and communication is an essential part of Primary Health Care in a complex world, easing the interfaces, among others, between the "bottom up and top down" processes, different disciplines and different world views, involving many organizations and influencing the policy making machinery.

References

Elmore, R.F. (1979/80), "Backward Mapping: Implementation Research and Policy Decisions", *Political Science Quarterly*, vol. 94, no. 4, pp. 601-16.

Thomas, Dr. P., *Liverpool Primary Health Care Facilitation Project 1989-1994*, Liverpool FHSA, Liverpool.

Special Issue: Large Group Interventions, (1992), *The Journal of Applied Behaviourial Science*, vol. 28, no. 4, December.

Wulff, H.R., Pederson, S.A. and Rosenberg, R. (1990), *Philosophy of Medicine*, Blackwell Scientific Publications, Oxford.

30 Health promotion through the community participation: Project for Sardinia, Italy

P. Contu and C. Congiu

Sardinia is the second largest island of the Mediterranean, it covers an area of about 24,000 square kilometres and has about 1,600,000 inhabitants.

Through personal contact with two participating cities in the Healthy Cities Network (Liverpool and Valencia), a small group of researchers, working in the Department of Hygiene and Public Health of the University of Cagliari, started to develop the Health Promotion ideas in our region.

In this paper we will describe the initial step of our health promotion project whose aim is to develop some small healthy community initiatives that can represent models of good practice and, in a second stage, develop a network (Ashton, 1992; Ashton and Seymour, 1988; WHO, 1985). So far the project has been implemented in two communities.

The project: health promotion through community participation

The main goals of the project were: to start a process of active participation in the community; to improve the intersectoral co-operation among agencies, services, institutions and voluntary associations and to improve health conditions of the population.

Six criteria of success were considered: increase of the community activities (meetings, groups); increase of intersectoral activities (public services, volunteers); increase of the overall number of health and social activities; reduction of the prevalence of risk behaviours; reduction of the number of risk conditions and reduction of the incidence of disease. Appendices 30.1 and 30.2 summarize the framework of the project resources, constraints, opportunities and the anticipated project milestones (Eurispes, 1993).

The project in practice

Realization

Our project involves a small town and a low income district of the city of Cagliari. The town is Paulilatino (2700 inhabitants), which is located in a rural area of central Sardinia, and characterized by an old population, a low levels of crowding, and a high migration rate (Contu, 1992). The second area is the district of Sant'Elia, that originated in the 1950s and developed through the activity of the Institute for Working Classes Houses. The population is young; infectious diseases (particularly hepatitis A), mortality rates and juvenile delinquency are high and public services inadequate (Congiu et al. 1994; Contu et al. 1996). The choice of these two zones is related to the fact that the researchers were deeply involved in these areas.

In both cases the project started with a formal meeting between the local political leaders and the University. So far, we have worked to fulfill the first six project targets differently in the two communities. In both cases we took particular care to contact the community leaders and to include the researchers in this process, in order to be able to establish a formal relationship with them and to constitute an intersectoral committee. Meanwhile, we started the analysis of the community.

Paulilatino From the very first, the contact with the community leader took place through formal meetings. So far the City Council has stated formally its support to the health promotion project and some bilateral agreements between University and Municipality, University and Comunità Montana, University and School, University and Local Health District were signed in order to provide a legal framework. We also involved the general practitioners, the parish, some voluntary workers. An informal Intersectoral Committee, co-ordinated by the University Health Promotion Team, was established early on in the process.

The two main activities we have started so far are further community diagnosis, and school health education.

The community diagnosis aims not only to inform needs and resources, but also to improve community participation and to generate a public debate, and therefore we try to involve the community leaders in all the steps of the analysis. A questionnaire, administered by means of interview to a representative sample of citizens, will play a central role in our assessment.

In order to promote better integration among the different service workers, and between them and the researchers, we have started health education activities in the schools.

S.Elia The second area of our project is an urban neighbourhood where

360

several different services and institutions operate without proceedures for co-ordination. It may happen for instance, that the service workers responsible for a given group have to deal with different politicians at the same time or that the original group may change unexpectedly, thus causing confusion about overlapping responsibilities and competencies.

Here the contact with the community leader took place in a different way, and confirmed the importance of the difficulties stressed in the project including political confusion, lack of collaboration, interpersonal conflicts, a sense of hopelessness, and a bureaucratic attitude.

One of the main problems was the political crisis that occurred in December 1994. The City Council of Cagliari was dissolved and a government representative took care of the city council, waiting for the new elections which due in June 1995. So it was very difficult to establish any infrastructure for the work.

A second difficulty was the lack of intersectoral cooperation. Both public services and voluntary associations are used to working alone and are very defensive about their work. This has resulted in a history of personal and political conflicts.

A third problem was the passive habit of the population and of some professionals who after such a long history of disillusionment preferred to sit down and wait for a miraculous intervention from above.

The burden of all these difficulties was so great that it jeopardized the development of the whole project. The risk of failure was overcome however, by trying to carry out the projects through different means. The local neighbourhood leader suggested that we should act as a transitional government project dedicated to adolescents as a mechanism to break through the impasse. This was achieved through the creation of an informal intersectoral committee. This project provided experience of intersectoral working and co-operation in the community, making it possible for people who had been used only to conflicts to share some common interests and activity. Gaining small achievements in short periods strengthened their confidence in the community as such and in the service workers, thus overcoming the hindrance of the present political crisis.

Discussion

We described the initial mobilization process of the two communities that were involved in the project. The process started recently, so that it is still not possible to provide a complete and rigorous analysis.

Nevertheless this experience can offer some themes for our reflection:

1. A detailed protocol for planning and implementation is very useful. A

clear presentation of the project assures a common vision, and provides some time pressure to carry out specific activities to deadlines.

2. At the same time, considerable flexibility, diversity and local creativity are also necessary. Every community is unique and so all constraints, opportunities and solutions vary from one community to another.

3. A major step is the building of a formal infrastructure that assures the continuity of the project, independently of who started the project and what political forces were dominant at the time.

4. The acceptance and completion of some temporary projects with limited scope can strengthen co-operation and establish self reliance in the community, making possible, in this way, the start of the global project.

5. A very important problem is the relationship between the project group and the political authority. A firm commitment to the project requires a personal relationship between researchers and politicians, but sometimes this can create an identification between the health promotion project and one political party and cause strong opposition among the other parties.

References

Ashton, J. (1992), *Healthy Cities*, Open University Press, Buckingham, United Kingdom.

Ashton, J. and Seymour, H. (1988), *The New Public Health*, Open University, Buckingham, United Kingdom.

Congiu, C., Contu, P., Argiolas, F., Cintura, R. and Scarpa, B. (1994), "Community diagnosis: The City of Cagliari", Paper given at Health in Cities: A Global Conference - Liverpool.

Contu, P. (1992), *Analisi fattoriale e analisi di cluster per un modello di programmazione basato sui problemi sanitari e ambientali*, Doctorate thesis.

Contu, P., Cintura, R., Congiu, C. and Scarpa, B. (1996), *Diagnosi di comunità: la città di Cagliari*

EURISPES 1° (1993), *Rapporto sulla qualità della vita in Sardegna - La Nuovissima Edizioni*.

WHO (1985), *Targets for health for all*, WHO, Copenhagen.

Appendix 30.1
Project framework

Sponsor - Institutions   Municipality, Administrative District, City Association, Region
University
Educational services
Health and social services
Professionals and Volunteers associations

Team   Intersectoral Committee and Technical Staff
Academics
Politicians
Health Service Responsible
Social Service Responsible
Educational Service Responsible
Informal leaders of the Community
Health promoters
Citizens and Volunteers

The promoters team and the technical staff can work together, occasionally overlapping or even totally coinciding, according to the community's own aims and characteristics

Constraints and difficulties   Passive attitude: the community waits for an intervention from the outside
Diseases are often caused by some of the community rooted habits and culture (alcohol, uncooked seafood)
Lack of intersectoral co-operation with possible personal conflicts
Political instability
Bureaucratic attitude (limits imposed by the law)

Opportunities   The Department of Hygiene plays a traditional role in the prevention of infectious diseases as does the School for Social Workers in social interventions in the territory
Interaction between Department of Hygiene and School for Social Workers
Voluntar workers: they represent an important and qualifying point of reference, which will bring, after the introduction of

363

	the new regulations, a stronger co-operation with the institutions Political renovation Personal involvement of the researchers with voluntary workers and in the studied community
Financing	Funds from local corporations (plan of social assistance) National Health Service: epidemiological activity and health education of the service staff and general practitioners Funds for health education programmes in the schools University research funds
Resources	Staff and students of Department of Hygiene and School for Social Workers Staff from the local institutions, schools, social and health services General practitioners, Pediatricians Voluntary workers

Appendix 30.2
Project milestones
The protocol for planning and implementation

Milestone	Who	How
Community analysis: needs, resources, behaviours, culture	Researchers	Routine statistics, surveys
Contact with the community (politicians, renown personalities), and service responsible	Researchers meetings	Personal contact, informal leaders
Engagement of the researchers inside the community	Researchers	Sharing the community life and activities
Definition of a formal vagreement	Researchers, services responsible, community leaders, voluntar workers	Meetings, consensus
Constitution of the Intersectoral Committee and Technical Staff	Researchers, services responsible, community leaders, voluntary workers	Meetings, consensus

Opening of an office chair in the area	Intersectoral committee	
Creation of a monitoring system	Intersectoral committee, technical staff	Routine statistics, surveys
Community analysis carried out by the community itself: needs, resources, behaviours, culture ...	Intersectoral committee	Routine statistics, surveys questionnaires, interviews
Project reassessment, presentation of specific aim projects, definite approval [1]	Intersectoral committee, technical staff	Consensus
Project campaign through the mass media	Intersectoral committee, technical staff	Press conferences, interviews articles
Constitution of a Health Promoters Team [2]	Intersectoral committee, technical staff	Consensus
Health promoters training: knowledge, behaviour, co-operation and communication ability. [2]	Intersectoral committee, technical staff, experts	Regular training activity, lessons, work groups, conferences, practical training

Health promotion in the community. Providing information, and improving behaviour	Technical staff, promoters team, experts, services responsible and workers	Advertising, health education in schools, churches ..., involvement of GP and social workers
Health promotion in the community: environmental cares	Technical staff, promoters team, experts, services responsible and workers	Political doing and services co-operation
Project evaluation. Results diffusion and planning	Intersectoral committee, technical staff	Consensus

Notes

1. Prevention of infectious diseases, promotion of healthy life styles, environmental education, Healthy Nutrition Promotion, Raising people's awareness of their health rights.

2. Can become more or less relevant according to the community specific aims and characteristics, but whenever the team and staff coincide they are no longer needed.

All aims can be differently structured according to the community's own aims and situations. Later on, the process may lead to projects with new aims.

31 Healthy eating in West Everton, Liverpool, England: An inner city community nutrition project

Margaret Jones and Shirley Judd

Abstract

Community participation is reviewed and evaluated for the West Everton phase of SUPER-project, healthy eating initiative. The SUPER-project is a collaborative venture in which countries exchange ideas, information and experiences concerning dietary promotional activities.

The Department of Community Nutrition and Dietetics (North Mersey) Community (NHS) Trust, were particularly interested in using the process of community participation to raise the profile of nutrition and develop new communication and working networks in the city. This paper discusses the outcomes of the project and examines the effect of the project on future working practices of the dietetic service.

Background

The relationship between diet and the development of coronary heart disease, strokes, some cancers, obesity and bowel disorders is well documented in Britain and an estimated 50 per cent of all premature deaths in European adults under 65 result from diet related disorders (James, 1988). In Liverpool heart disease accounted for 27 per cent of all deaths during 1989. But this rate varied greatly across the city wards, and the rate for Everton, an inner city area with high unemployment, was 1:245. This compares very unfavourably with the national average of 1:550 for England and Wales (Liverpool Healthy Cities, 1991).

Eating habits are influenced by social, economic and cultural factors (Ashton, 1987). Eating habits were found to be strikingly similar in Liverpool and Valencia, Spain (Vaandrager and Ashton, 1989; Vaandrager, 1990; Vaandrager et al. 1992). In these cities people living in affluent areas had both a greater access to healthy food and were more informed about their nutritional requirements than those living in poorer areas. These studies led to the development of the European SUPER-project. This is a collaborative venture in which countries exchange ideas, information and experience concerning dietary promotional activities (Vaandrager et al. 1991).

Vaandrager (et al. 1993) outlined a four step health promotion approach for changing dietary patterns in Europe. The four steps are:

1.   Intersectoral organization and collaboration.

2.   Environmental interventions i.e. interventions to remove barrier to healthy eating.

3.   Community action to facilitate health promoting behaviour.

4.   Efforts to encourage individuals to adopt and maintain health promoting behaviour.

This paper concentrates on the mechanism of community participation (action). Previous health promotion projects have been criticized for using the rhetoric of participation and empowerment whilst failing to lead to any action by the community (Stern, 1986; Brownlea, 1987; Hancock and Draper, 1989). In West Everton efforts were made to develop a "bottom up" approach. Researchers aimed to provide advice, without imposing solutions on nutritional choice. In all community participation projects, care must be taken to ensure the community and not the researchers or sponsors are the primary beneficiaries (Swantz and Vainio-Mattila, 1990). Ultimately the community were to feel empowered to make choices, and in so doing, take control of their own community health issues

SUPER-project aims and objectives

The above theoretical considerations underpin the aims of the project, which were to: reduce nutrition related diseases by improving the availability of healthy foods; improve public awareness of healthy foods and to develop nutritional self help resource packs for the use of local communities throughout Europe.

Methods

The method or process used in action research is doubly important as it is itself a mechanism to promote participation. For this reason the method is discussed in some detail.

The initial SUPER-project research in West Everton was carried out by Röling and Smit (1992). They began by "rapidly appraising" the health status of the area. This involved reviewing existing health and social data, interviewing "key informants" i.e. people within the community, either professional or informal community leaders, and finally compiling a qualitative diary describing their observations and experiences of working in West Everton. Detailed guidelines for using this technique are described by Annett and Rifkin (1988). The pooling of both the quantitative health information and the qualitative personal accounts created a wider picture of health issues. This view is also supported by Baum (1988) who favours an eclectic approach to researching health issues. The benefits of this method are that it can be carried out quickly, with little professional input, and is consequently less expensive (Röling and Smit, 1993).

Following the rapid appraisal locally employed interviewers carried out 160 face to face interviews. It was felt that local people would be better received when visiting people at home. The questionnaire consisted of 67, mostly closed questions relating to three main topics, life in West Everton, eating behaviour and factors which influence eating behaviour. Every fourth household was selected from the local electoral register. Subjects interviewed were aged 18 and over.

Inventories of two local shops, KwikSave supermarket and a small corner shop, were also carried out. Availability, price and situation of food in the shops were recorded.

With this information Röling and Smit hoped to evaluate the feasibility of using community networks to promote healthy nutritional practices. Also it would provide an insight into factors which influence eating patterns, identify communication networks and develop relevant nutrition promotional activities.

Findings and subsequent health promotion activities

The rapid appraisal and questionnaire identified the following key points:

1.   West Everton is a deprived area with high levels of unemployment.

2.   At the time of the study shopping facilities were poor.

3.   Low levels of car ownership and poor public transport limited access to better shopping areas.

4.   Nutritional knowledge was poorer than other areas of Liverpool.

371

5.   Healthy food was perceived to be expensive.

6.   Food was not a salient subject. Health was not considered when choosing food.

7.   The diet was high in fat, sugar and salt and low in fibre.

8.   A strong social cohesion existed within West Everton.

The nutrition promotion activities were planned by Röling and Smit in collaboration with West Everton Health Forum, local tenants groups, schools, community health workers and the Department of Community Nutrition and Dietetics (North Mersey) Community (NHS) Trust. Full details of the activities are listed in Röling and Smit (1993) and Bergman (1993).

As interest in healthy eating was low, it was decided to work with established local groups to raise the profile of nutrition. Activities were spread over a four month period. Each month a stand with information, food to taste and competitions was set up for one or two days in the KwikSave store. This was manned by the community dietitians and a local resident.

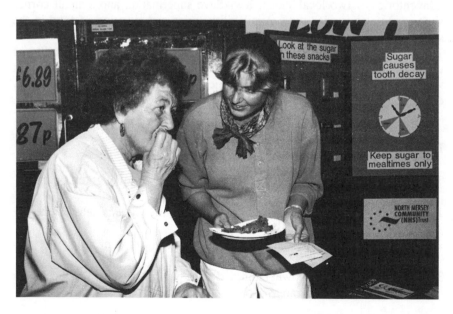

A healthier food tasting session at the KwikSave supermarket in Everton

The days were promoted by posters placed in the local health centres, library, community centres and the KwikSave itself. Poster displays on specific nutrition themes, for example, how to use less fat were also placed in public buildings, community centres, church halls, schools and health centres each month.

The local schools became involved in a number of ways. The first year of the local secondary school took part in a competition to design the cover of, and suggest a slogan, for a leaflet encouraging people to eat more fruit and vegetables. The finished leaflet with the title "Super Fruit" was launched in March 1994. Two primary schools also took part in a series of four sessions on healthy eating. The community dietitians worked closely with the class teachers to ensure the sessions complemented work around nutrition already covered in class.

One of the primary schools had an active Parent School Partnership programme. Between 10-15 parents attend the school on a daily basis to take part in vocational, recreational and social activities. During the four months a series of cooking sessions were organized, looking specifically at cooking with less fat, less sugar and more fibre.

These activities were co-ordinated by the project workers and the Department of Community Nutrition and Dietetics, with most of the resources and information coming from the latter. However, various individuals and groups also participated, namely, student dietitians, dental health promotion, parent school partnership key workers and one local resident.

Evaluation and future of community participation in nutrition health promotion in Liverpool

Bergman (1993) evaluated the effectiveness of this collaborative approach. She identified the popularity of group cooking sessions and school based activities. There was also considerable media interest in all the competitions, in researchers and in the project itself. The authors believe the "neutrality" of the researchers, i.e. the fact that they were independent of local health and government authorities, made them a non-threatening external influence in the community.

Despite initial interest, the response for local activists was poor and only one local community helper was committed to assist at planned events. There was, however, no shortage of key actors who were keen to act as "sign posts" for the SUPER-project work. That is they identified others, mostly professionals e.g. teachers, health workers who could participate. For example, school children and parents were identified by members of West Everton Health Forum as groups who would appreciate and enjoy working with community dietitians. Although this was useful information for researchers, it did not lead to community ownership at the operational level of the project.

The above would seem to indicate the existence of a heavy dependence on health professionals. This is understandable as previous agendas for health promotion issues have been set by medically dominant health professionals (Farrant, 1991). This professional dominance undermines the growth of community participation (Stern, 1986). As well as disempowering local communities to take ownership, it can lead to high expectations of project workers to achieve changes in a short time scale. Lack of community ownership also leads to a vacuum when the health workers leave. Activities in West Everton were temporarily suspended when the student researchers and a key community dietitian left.

The process involved in the SUPER-project work in West Everton has been a learning experience for dietetics in Liverpool. Networking, although invaluable, is difficult, time consuming and can lead to disappointments. Communities are often suspicious of projects, wondering "what's in it for them?" This may explain why there was a low response to the call for community participants for activities.

It was a worthwhile process though. As well as raising the profile of nutrition and its importance to health, the project has widened the net of influence accessible to dietitians. The Dietetic Department has been able to network with key community leaders and workers not previously identified, e.g. school teachers, health forum etc.

Dietitians have gained the confidence to "let go" of the lead and work with groups rather than "on" them to facilitate and not drive projects. They have also had to accept that people cannot be hurried. Community members who wish to join in will come forward when they can take the lead.

The rapid appraisal technique has been built into the City's Nutrition Strategy and incorporated into the City Health Plan. This has formalized the intersectoral collaboration and secured funding for on going nutrition research in Liverpool. This is vital to develop a nutrition needs assessment that guarantees long term commitment to the community. Such is the value of this process in identifying community nutrition needs and opening communication and working networks for dietitians to operate, it has become a key first task for any new dietetic post in Liverpool.

There is also recognition that examples of good practice should be shared. This should not be for the benefit of researchers or professionals alone. The profile of initiatives should be raised through all working networks to sustain momentum and pride in all participants achievements.

The emphasis on community participation has also strengthened Liverpool's dietetic role within the field of public health and underlined the need for nutrition facilitation as opposed to exclusive therapeutic services.

The work of the SUPER-project has now moved to the Picton area of

Liverpool. This information gathering process has been refined to give a clearer picture of lifestyle influences on food choice and a more accurate dietary analysis. The contacts made in West Everton have been maintained and both clinical and health promotional services have increased.

References

Annett, H. and Rifkin, S. (1988), "Guidelines for Rapid Appraisal to Assess Community Health Needs", *Geneva: Division of Strengthening of Health Services*, WHO.

Ashton, J. R. (1987), "Making the Healthy Choices the Easy Choices", *Nutrition and Food Science*, July/August, pp. 2-5.

Baum, F. (1988), "Community Based Research for the New Public Health", *Health Promotion*, vol. 3, no. 3, pp. 259-68.

Bergman, G. (1993), *Healthy Eating in West-Everton; the Evaluation of Nutrition Promotion Project as Part of the SUPER-project*, Department of Public Health, Liverpool University, Liverpool.

Brownlea, A. (1987), "Participation: Myths, Realities and Prognosis", *Soc.Sci.Med*, vol. 25, no. 6.

Farrant, W. (1991), "Addressing the Contradictions: Health Promotion and Community Health Action in the United Kingdom", *International Journal of Health Services*, vol. 21, no. 3.

Hancock, T. and Draper, R. (1989), *Participatory Research: A Key Strategy for Health Promotion, A Report from Conference on Community Participation and Empowerment Strategies in Health Promotion, Centre for Inter-Disciplinary Research*, University of Bielefeld, June.

James, W.P.T. (1988), *Preventing Nutrition-Related Diseases in Europe*, WHO Regional Publications, Europe series, no.24.

Liverpool Healthy City (1991), *Heart Disease ... A Discussion Document*.

Röling, S. and Smit, M. (1993), *Communication Networks and the Promotion of a Healthy Diet: A Baseline Research for the SUPER-project in Liverpool*, Nijmegen University, Nijmegen.

Stern, R. (1986), *Debate and Dialogue: Enlarging Public Participation, Reducing Professional Dominance in Proceedings of the first International Conference on Health Promotion; Ottawa 1986*, WHO.

Swantz, M. and Vainio-Mattila, A. (1990), "Participatory Inquiry as an Instrument of Grass-Roots Development" in Reason, P. (ed.), *Human Inquiry in Action: Developments in New Paradigm Research*, Sage Publications, London.

Vaandrager, H.W. (1990), *The Nutrition and Supermarket Research in Two Different Social Class areas of Valencia*, IVESP, Valencia.

Vaandrager, H.W. and Ashton, J.R. (1989), *Healthy Eating in Liverpool in*

1984 and 1989: Knowledge, Attitudes and Choice, Department of Public Health, Liverpool University, Liverpool.

Vaandrager, H.W., Ashton, J., Colomèr, C. and Koelen, M. (1991), *SUPER - The European Food and Shopping Research Wageningen*, Department of Extension Science, Wageningen Agricultural University.

Vaandrager, H.W., Koelen, M.A., Ashton, J.R. and Colomèr Revuelta, C. (1993), "A Four Step Healthy Promotion Approach for Changing Dietary Patterns in Europe", *European Journal of Public Health*, vol. 3, pp. 193-8.

32 Differences in health promoting activities

Rascha Thomas

Background

Studies dating as far back as 1977 have shown a substantial and persistent pattern of health differences between the various boroughs of Amsterdam. In these studies health was measured by standardized hospitalization and mortality ratios. The pattern of health differences coincided almost exactly with the pattern of social economic differences. The social economic status of a borough was measured by number of unemployed, percentage of housing stock built before 1906 etc. Boroughs with a relatively high social economic status were relatively health and boroughs with a low social economic status were relatively unhealthy.

Although these studies did not prove a causal relationship between the variables health and social economic status, in 1989 the city government was eventually convinced that something had to be done about this disturbing relationship. The Municipal Health Authority was asked to investigate this relationship and to come up with possible policy measures to improve the health of residents with a low social economic background. In 1990 the government system in Amsterdam was decentralized and borough councils were installed. This provided a new opportunity for co-operation between a borough rather than a city council and the municipal health authority. The first borough where this collaboration actually took place was Westerpark. Westerpark is a relatively small borough of roughly 32,000 inhabitants, located just west of the centre of Amsterdam. It is an area where extensive urban renewal has taken place. About 28 per cent of all residents are immigrants mainly of Turkish and Moroccan origin, 20 per cent unemployed, 60 per cent single person households, 40 per cent of all households with children are single parent families.

The health authority began with a great deal of research: existing statistics were gathered for a health profile at borough level, many local key figures in the fields of health, welfare and education were interviewed about the health and social problems in the borough and thirdly a large health survey was carried out among 1,000 adult residents of the borough. As expected on the basis of earlier research, the health indicators used showed a health situation in Westerpark that was far worse than the results of the same indicators measured in other areas in the Netherlands.

Production team

The borough council, when presented with the results of this research, were not exactly pleased to be confronted with this situation because they felt obliged to do something about it but really didn't have a clue where to begin. Several discussions with resident platforms and with the borough council took place about the possible action that could be taken. However it soon became clear that this was not the way to make a selection from the large number of problems shown by the research and it certainly was not an effective method to find practical solutions to these problems. In April 1992, the chairman of the borough decided he did not want to ignore the results of this study, he used his influence to proclaim a year of health promotion in Westerpark. The Municipal Health Authority was prepared to join with the borough council in the formation of a project team that would initiate, co-ordinate and if necessary carry out activities that could improve the health situation of the residents.

The borough and the Health Authority both saw this year of health promotion in Westerpark as an experiment in translating research into actual local activities. For the Health Authority working at neighbourhood level rather than city wide was new and a ready made protocol was of course not available.

Problems

The project team was formed by a researcher and a health promotion worker from the Health Authority and a policy worker from the Borough Council. Luckily the three members of the project team were soon able to agree on methods and goals. We interviewed a large number of local experts about their experience of the health (related) problems in the borough and more importantly about their ideas for possible solutions. The results of these interviews combined with the results of the survey gave us a long list of problems to be tackled. In retrospect, these problems could be grouped according to three of the determinants of the Lalonde model of health:

1. Social and physical environment

   - too much rubbish on the streets
   - not enough greenery
   - too much traffic
   - too many drug addicts
   - not enough contact between neighbours
   - not enough suitable play areas for children

2. Behaviour/life style

   - not enough women's health education for immigrant groups
   - not enough aids education for immigrant groups
   - alcohol problems in community centre and home for the aged
   - not enough information about available services for the elderly
   - too many people smoking

3. (Health) services

   - 50 per cent of the immigrant population do not visit the dentist regularly
   - many parents have problems concerning the upbringing of their children
   - relatively large number of residents with chronic respiratory diseases
   - lack of support for family and neighbours caring for the chronically ill
   - pharmacy assistants are not able to give the necessary information about the prescribed medication to immigrants who hardly speak dutch
   - no prenatal courses for immigrant mothers to be

It also became clear that each of these groups of problems entailed a different way of tackling the problems.

Social and physical environment

The installation of the borough council has meant that problems of this nature are tackled more effectively and with less delay than when the city council was responsible. The departments of the borough council involved such as refuse collection, planning department etc. were meeting the challenge of improving the borough with enthusiasm and inventiveness. When these departments were approached by the production team there was a little irritation as the problems and complaints presented were already familiar to the departments, they were working hard at solving these problems and the perspective of health improvement did not offer an extra incentive or means to solve these problems. Solutions to problems in the physical and social environment:

1. Neighbourhood attendants.

2. House meetings.

3. Refuse inspectors.

4. Playground action plan.

5. Adventure playground.

6. Renovation and expansion of existing park.

7. City guards to control traffic and general order.

8. A complaints centre where residents can report nuisance caused by neighbours.

The project team agreed with the various departments that many of the problems were being tackled effectively and except for keeping an eye on the progress of these initiatives there was no further involvement of the project team.

Behaviour/life style

Most of the activities falling under this category were a result of the interviews with local experts. Leaders of local immigrant organizations and workers in the community centres requested health education programmes in the language of the respective target groups. In most cases existing forms of health education in Dutch, Turkish or Moroccan could be offered such as:

1. Women's health education programme for Turkish women.

2. Women's health education programme for Moroccan women.

3. Health education on aids, gambling and diet for Surinam residents

380

organizations.

4.   Special health information meetings and brochures for the elderly still living independently on: taking medication, visiting your GP, safety in the home and safety on the street.

One of the community centres experienced problems with the drinking habits of visits and voluntary staff. Once the Amsterdam Office for Prevention of Alcohol and Drug abuse was called in to help the centre, it became clear that the local old people's home experienced similar problems. The GPs in the area also complained that they felt unequipped to deal with alcohol addiction among their patients. The Amsterdam office for prevention of drug and alcohol abuse developed an integrated approach in which: the staff, visitors and volunteers of the community centre and home for the elderly were involved in finding a way to bring the alcohol consumption back to a reasonable level; the GPs were offered a training course; a borough wide information campaign about alcohol was organized in local media and residents were able to visit an alcohol counsellor free of charge in the local health centre.

In this case the project team borough in a professional organization, normally working on a city level, which met the challenge of working on a neighbourhood scale. This office is now prepared to offer similar services to other boroughs i.e. developing a suitable approach for and with local residents and workers.

In this category, as in the category mentioned before there was really very little work for the project team other than making sure that activities were being carried out. Work in this category mainly consisted of bringing local parties into contact with professional organizations working at city level. Knowledge of the (free) services of these professional city wide organizations was often lacking. Although most of these activities are one off events and therefore not likely to have a structural effect on the health of the residents, many and local institutions now know what services are available from city wide professional health promoting organizations and know how to contact them.

(Health) services

Under this category a number of activities were developed involving more structural change. The most common denominator of these activities was that local demand was not met by the present supply of services offered.

Dental project for immigrants

Under this category a programme was carried out in which immigrants were informed about the Dutch system of dental care in which half yearly check ups and treatments are free once a dentist has cleared that their teeth are in a good condition. The costs of getting teeth into this condition have to paid by the patients themselves. This system was not clear to most immigrants and during the interviews with local immigrant experts this was posed as the main reason why immigrants did not visit the dentist regularly. The dentists in Westerpark, when interviewed, all stated that there practices were full and that there were not enough dentists in the borough. The project team was able to convince the health insurance company to reserve a contract for a new dentist in the area. Furthermore, at the information meetings all those interested were offered the opportunity to visit the dentist for a dental inspection and an estimation of the costs of the necessary treatment before a declaration of healthy teeth could be given. To assist participants of the project Turkish and Moroccan volunteers from the neighbourhood made appointments with the dentist and accompanied patients during their visits to translate between dentist and patent and to repeat information given during the meetings if necessary. This project worked reasonably well and resulted in a booklet about the development and the practice of the project so that it can be carried out in other areas.

Chronic respiratory diseases

During our interviews one GP from the neighbourhood indicated that care for the many patients with respiratory diseases was inadequate as GPs did not have time to regularly check on correct intake of medication, social counselling, help with stopping with smoking etc. He suggested that a practice nurse, trained especially for this category of patients would be a good idea. At the same time we were informed about the plans of the district nursing organization to station a district nurse especially for chronic respiratory disease patients in the area. This district nurse felt that early diagnosis of respiratory disease in children could be improved at the Health Authority's children's clinics. In discussions about the results of the health survey residents had complained about air pollution from traffic and industry in the area and felt that this was the cause of many respiratory diseases. The medical environment specialist from the Health Authority stated that the level of air pollution in the area was not excessive, but he did draw attention to the enormous amount of urban renewal that had taken place in the area and the possibility that this often lead to lack of natural ventilation in houses (through cracks and faulty windows). He advised a campaign to instruct residents of new housing about good ventilation practices and offered to look over renovation or new building plans to give advice on simple construction details that could improve the quality of air inside the home. The project team interviewed all the GPs in the area about their experiences with this group of patients and about the possible ways in which they felt that treatment and guidance of this group could be improved. Most of the doctors stated that they would like to see their respiratory patients with the district nurse during special consultation hours, in order to discuss, with the patient, the medication programme and whatever other needs the patient might have so that the nurse would have all the necessary information for further guidance of the patient. The Asthma Fund (a charity for chronic respiratory diseases) was approached and was interested in organizing an exhibition about coping with respiratory disease in the local library and in funding a full colour brochure that distributed door to door informing all residents about various aspects of chronic respiratory disease and local services available such as special sport facilities for these patients and the open consultation hours of the district nurse.

All of these suggestions were brought together by the project team and most of them were carried out, except for the joint consultation of GPs and the district nurse. Despite early enthusiasm from the nurse herself, her superiors decided that she was to stick to the new protocol of a number of open consultation hours to which GPs could direct their patients. The housing corporations were also not yet prepared to offer their plans to Health Authority experts for advice, they did however include information about good ventilation practice in the general information they give to residents of new housing.

There were other activities but these two examples demonstrate, clearly enough, that the project team's main role was to negotiate between various local and city wide professionals so that they would actually organize and carry out the changes suggested by the local experts (residents and professionals).

Conclusions

Usually a researcher delivers her/his report with some policy recommendations that are generally far removed from daily reality in the neighbourhood and he or she has very little to say about what happens with the results of this research.

Participation in this project team was a rare opportunity to actually do something with the results of one's own research. A big challenge, out of the office and away from the improvement of the health situation in an area. At best it serves to get the subject onto the local political agenda. It creates unrest which hopefully leads to action. Once this (political) choice for action is made the research becomes background information, and the local demands, ideas, possible solutions to problems etc have to be gathered.

In order to do this well extensive knowledge of the local situation is necessary, not only formal knowledge about who is officially responsible for which tasks, but also which people are most likely to want to take an active role in improving the health situation. This information was provided by the participation of a very enthusiastic and well connected borough policy worker. Of course extensive knowledge of the health care and health promotion fields was also essential.

For the parties participating in the project team, this year of local health improvement in Westerpark was an experiment that has revealed certain productive mechanisms and also some barriers which now pose a new challenge for the Amsterdam Health Authority and for the councils of local boroughs.

Working in a multi-disciplinary team consisting of experts on the local situation and experts in the field of public health (promotion) is a good way to initiate activities that are aimed at influencing the behaviours or life style of residents. We found that many local organizations were not aware of the health promotion facilities in the city. This problem was easily solved when this became clear during the interviews. In some cases new health promotion products were developed to meet the specific requirements of the residents in the borough.

Improving the physical and social environment towards a more health environment was a task that was already being tackled effectively without it being labelled as a "health issue". The goals of the national policy programme of "social economic renewal" which is carried out on neighbourhood scale are practically equivalent to the goals aimed for when improving health conditions by changing the social and physical environment i.e. less people unemployed, cleaner and safer streets, more people participating in all aspects of society, good education and facilities for children, especially in deprived areas. The project team's very minor role in these activities consisted of following them closely and in a few cases offering advice on certain details.

The third determinant that the project team tried to influence in order to improve health was the health care system. This was by far the most difficult category of activities, usually involving many different parties, each with their own specific work styles and protocols. It soon became clear that the local health practitioners like GPs and dentists were overloaded with work, most practices were full and could not accept new patients. When we approached them about the health problems and possible solutions practically everybody indicated that although the work pressure was enormous, they were prepared to try new ways of working if we were prepared to organize this taking their wishes and needs into account. As the example about the activities concerning respiratory disease shows, this often entailed encouraging city institutions like the district nursing agency, to change and adapt their services to the requirements of the local situation. For this type of organization working on a made to measure basis, rather than with one standard package of services is new, probably more expensive, difficult to organize because of the inflexibility of the organization, and risky (e.g. will this new method achieve better results than the standard service offered and secondly, better results for whom?). The project team usually managed to convince the people who worked for these organizations in the neighbourhood, they often came up with good ideas for improving work methods. The problems arose when the management of these organizations had to give permission and funding for these new activities. The combined strength of a local borough council and the Amsterdam Health Authority participating in the project team at least gained access to the managers of city wide health organizations and individual health professionals, but it did not give the members of the project team any real power to force these organizations to adapt and change their services or working methods. Encouragement and enthusiasm from our side did not always result in the necessary changes.

The future

If the city of Amsterdam and its health authority wish to continue this type of health improvement in socially and economically deprived areas it will have to create better tools. At this moment the city council and the health insurance institutions finance and therefore control, most of the health services in the city. The borough councils have no control over these organizations. If borough councils decide to actively pursue better health (care) for their residents they will have to be given some negotiating power. Whether this done directly by decentralizing funds and responsibilities for health from the city to the boroughs or indirectly by allowing the local boroughs to make their demands during the negotiations between the city council and/or the health insurance institutions on the buyers side and the health services on the seller's side.

A second dilemma is that the borough councils are, at present, not equipped to investigate and determine their own health needs. They need help and the Health Authority has to decide whether she is going to provide this help as a public health institution. If so the Health Authority would have to begin by breaking open its own standard package of services such as the baby clinics, school health, school dentists, drug addiction programmes, pest control, etc and adapting the services to the specific wishes and needs in the various boroughs. For an organization used to working in a top down manner this is quite a challenge. However, the fact that the health authority has so many workers stationed in the clinics in the neighbourhoods, gives them an advantage in developing a bottom up approach.

33 Multisectoral collaboration for health: Evaluative project

Viv Speller, Rachel Funnell and Lynne Friedli

The English national strategy for health, Health of the Nation (DoH, 1992) gave support to the concept of multisectoral working and acknowledged its debt to Health for All by the Year 2000 (WHO, 1981). The term "healthy alliances" was coined for joint working between health services and other agencies, and purchasing health authorities continue to be encouraged to establish healthy alliances to develop joint health strategies and investment programmes. However the central attention paid to the development of healthy alliances has brought with it a preoccupation with NHS performance management. The focus on the measurement of activity and progress towards objectives has been sharpened to assess the effectiveness of investment in particular alliance interventions.

In 1993 the HEA commissioned the Wessex Institute of Public Health Medicine to research into evaluation in healthy alliances. The Multisectoral Collaboration for Health - Evaluative project aimed to develop evaluation processes and suggest indicators that could be used by alliances. Criteria for indicators of intersectoral work had been proposed, however many were conflicting and untested. Indicators were required to cover health status and health promotion, and yet should be simple, sensitive to short term change, and capable of application at target group, small area and population levels (Kar et al. 1988; WHO, 1988a; WHO, 1992). Analytic methods should include quantitative and qualitative methods and subjective and objective assessments, whilst capturing a dynamic process (Hayes and Manson Willms, 1990). There was also a need to look at the processes of intersectoral decision making as well as their outcomes (Ziglio, 1991). Ashton (1988) proposed five sources of data: NHS, organizational, special survey, analytically derived and "soft" data. "One size fits all" indicators were thought to be unlikely owing to the different physical, social and cultural contexts of healthy cities (Hayes and Manson Willms, 1990; WHO, 1988b). This range of requirements exposed a number of underlying conceptual confusions about health and health promotion that were not being addressed by a purely technical consideration of indicators (Noack and McQueen, 1988; McQueen and Noack, 1988).

In the Canadian Healthy Communities Project (Hayes and Manson Willms, 1990), participating·communities were concerned about lack of guidance, expertize and resources, how they would gather data and control its use. They suggested that communities should evaluate projects relative to their own goals, and use appropriate measures. In this way they would be relevant, practicable and sensitive to particular conditions and be acceptable to users.

At the outset of the project we had the impression that similar concerns and confusions existed in the UK. Balanced against this was a steadily growing recognition in the field of the need to measure the effects of alliances in a meaningful way by the application of agreed sets of indicators. We also acknowledged that the expertize in alliance working resided in alliance workers, and that any measurement tool would need to be acceptable to both users and experts, and that results would be both project specific and generalizable. We planned the research to be participatory, recognizing there would need to be co-operation between the "researchers" and the "subjects" to solve the problem of how to evaluate alliances, and that our role would primarily be that of facilitator of the research process (Hall, 1975; Reason, 1981). Our relationship with the field was as a colleague and co-producer of learning, considered to be more likely to produce a high level of uptake of results (Elden, 1981). It was hoped that the project would lead to a better understanding of how to evaluate alliance work and have an impact on practice. Diffusion-Innovation theory, widely used in health promotion, shows that dissemination of innovations can be improved through the involvement and participation of the intended audience (Green and Lewis, 1986). Thus the research methods employed followed both the principles of participatory research and good practice in health promotion.

A steering group was established with membership from the UKHFA Network, the Office for Public Management, the DoH, and public health physicians as well as the funding body and researchers. The research was conducted in two phases each of one year's duration. The aim of the Phase One was to develop a set of measures to evaluate healthy alliances. It involved over 200 people and was conducted in three stages. First a telephone survey was undertaken to gain an overview of the extent and focus of alliance work in the UK, and to identify examples of good practice in evaluation. As it was primarily to select participants for the next stage the survey was not comprehensive. The sample was drawn from existing networks of practitioners in health and local authorities, including the UK Health for All Network, the National Environmental Health Promotion Network, and Directors of Public Health. It was allowed to snowball to capture interested participants and a total of 129 full interviews were taken.

This stage also served to highlight the main issue of the research, and opportunities were taken to discuss the plans at meetings of these networks. Practitioners were particularly anxious about the use to which the research would be put, and the relative roles of the funding body and the researchers. For it to succeed it was essential to engage practitioners and every effort was made to defuse tensions at this point.

Six small workshops were held in three locations around the UK with 38 participants drawn from the survey on the basis of their experience or ideas about evaluation, grouped according to the health topic of their projects. Debate was encouraged to draw on the participants' knowledge and experience of the characteristics of effective healthy alliances and ways of measuring success. Discussions were recorded on flip charts and audiotape, and subsequently two sets of indicators were developed describing the processes and outputs of alliance work, using the participants' words and meanings. A draft document was then presented at a consensus forum for a wider group of 74 participants and stakeholders. Critical examination was encouraged leading to agreement on the content and shape of the materials. It was agreed that a framework for evaluation should be user friendly and encompass both process and output indicators. An important feature of the workshops in this phase was the clarification and consensus about terminology used and the meaning of underlying concepts. As practitioners ranged from health to non-health, and from expert to lay user, it was vital that different perceptions were aired and considered from sometimes opposing viewpoints, resulting in lively and productive argument.

A draft self assessment pack, "Towards Evaluating Healthy Alliances", was produced and tested in phase two in five pilot sites in England. These were selected from applications to provide a range of alliance types across the country. Written confirmation of agreement to participate was sought from each alliance. The intention was to learn about how to apply the pack in practice, and to assess how generalizable the indicators were across projects and alliances.

Testing started with a three month familiarization period during which workshops were held and an implementation plan for each site was developed. It was important that each site approached the evaluation in their own way, both to ensure ownership by the participants, and for us to learn about different evaluation processes. Over the five months of testing the sites had ongoing access to support from the research team. Sites chose which projects to use for testing, and which aspects of process or output indicators to study and in what depth. At the end a focus group was held with the key contacts from each site to identify main concerns which were compiled into a questionnaire sent to each person who had participated in the testing.

The draft pack had also been sent to all involved in the first phase, and to anyone who requested it during the year to stimulate evaluation activity widely in order to gain additional feedback from unsupported alliances. A postal survey of all recipients of the pack was undertaken. An additional workshop was held during the final review period with representatives of purchasers of health care to ensure that their views on evaluation were also captured.

The pack was reviewed in the light of all these comments to include more guidance on evaluation process to provide a clearer path for planning and evaluation, emphasizing the choices available to customize the framework for local use. The resulting pack "Towards Healthier Alliances - a tool for planning, evaluating and developing healthier alliances" was distributed to all individuals who had been involved at any stage of the research (Funnell et al. 1995).

The pack describes five process indicators; commitment, community participation, communication, joint working and accountability, broken into a major category description, main elements and detailed indicators in question format (see Table 33.1). The five major categories and their main elements are as follows:

Table 33.1
The process indicators

Category	Main elements
Commitment	Group purpose, resources
Community participation	Liaison, empowerment
Communication	Shared information, accessibility
Joint working	Strategies and action plans, flexibility
Accountability	Responsibility, evaluation

In a similar way, output indicators have been defined into six major categories falling into two main groups dependant on whether they impact the health of the population indirectly or directly. The six major categories are policy change, service provision and environment change, skills development, publicity, contact and knowledge, attitude and behaviour change.

These are also presented with detailed questions to be considered when planning or reviewing evaluation activity. Crucially these represent the outputs of alliance work which aim to lead towards changes in health outcomes where the impact of alliance activity may not be immediately measurable in health terms. Exercises to aid users in the planning of evaluation and the selection of appropriate indicators are provided, as are indicator assessment sheets to record the findings of evaluation. Particular emphasis is placed on the cycle of evaluation to guide users through what is for many a complex and unfamiliar process (see Figure 33.1).

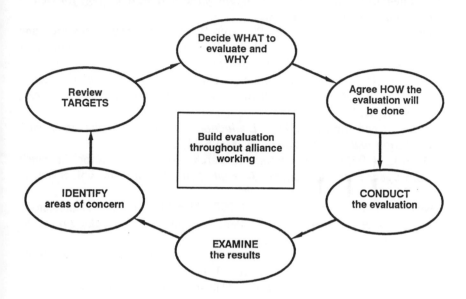

Figure 33.1   The evaluation cycle

The Mult-sectoral Collaboration for Health: Evaluative Project has thus enabled a wide ranging and yet focused debate on the evaluation of a complex and increasingly important area. The process of the research has allowed the many constituencies inherent in this type of work to become engaged in and to influence the production of a practical tool. It has brought the users along with the researchers and vice versa, and allowed us to analyze and formulate solutions to a difficult problem. In the course of the research it has been clear that not only has there been an increased understanding of evaluation but also a better awareness and acceptance of the varied concepts and values by which different practitioners operate. By openly acknowledging these differences and encouraging debate it has been possible to use conflict productively to develop a tool for general use. The key to its further acceptance lies in the commitment of individual alliances to continue the

391

debates at local level to develop better and more effective alliances for health.

References

Ashton, J. (1988), "Tying Down the Indicators and Targets for Health for All", *Community Health Studies*, vol. xii, no. 4, pp. 376-85.

Department of Health (1992), *The Health of the Nation: a Strategy for Health in England*, Cm. 1986, HMSO.

Elden, M. (1981), "Sharing the Research Work: Participative Research and its Role Demands" in Reason, P. and Rowan, J. (eds.), *Human Inquiry. A Sourcebook of New Paradigm Research*, Wiley, Chichester.

Funnell, R., Oldfield, K. and Speller, V. (1995), *Towards Healthier Alliances - a Tool for Planning, Evaluating and Developing Healthy Alliances*, HEA/WIPHM.

Green, L. and Lewis (1986), *Evaluation and Measurement in Health Education and Health Promotion*, Mayfield, California.

Hall, B.L. (1975), "Participatory Research: An Approach for Change", *Convergence, an International Journal of Adult Education*, vol. 8, no. 2, pp. 24-32.

Hayes, M. and Manson Willms, S. (1990), "Healthy Community Indicators; the Perils of the Search and the Paucity of the Find", *Health Promotion International*, vol. 5, no. 2, pp. 161-6.

Kar, S.B. (1988), "Indicators of Individual and Community Action for Health Promotion", *Health Promotion*, vol. 3, no. 1, pp. 59-66.

McQueen, D. and Noack, H. (1988), "Health Promotion Indicators; Current Status, Issues and Problems", *Health Promotion*, vol. 3, no. 1, pp. 117-25.

Noack, H. and McQueen, D. (1988), "Towards Health Pomotion Indicators", *Health Promotion*, vol. 3, no. 1, pp. 73-8.

Reason, P. (1981), "An Exploration in the Dialectics of Two-Person Relationships" in Reason, P. and Rowan, J. (eds.), *Human Inquiry*, Wiley, Chichester.

WHO (1981), *Global Strategy for Health for All by the Year 2000*, WHO, Geneva.

WHO (1988b), *Five-Year Planning Framework, WHO Regional Office for Europe, Healthy Cities Papers, no. 2*, Copenhagen.

WHO (1988a), *A Guide to Assessing Healthy Cities. WHO Regional Office for Europe, Healthy Cities Papers, No 3*, Copenhagen.

WHO (1992), *The Multi-City Action Plan on Baltic Cities and Indicators*, WHO Regional Office for Europe, Copenhagen.

Ziglio, E. (1991), "Indicators of Health Promotion Policy: Directions for Research", *WHO Regional Publications*, European Series no. 37, WHO, Copenhagen, pp. 55-83.

Section 6   Arts in health promotion

Some readers may be uncomfortable about finding that, with the exception of passing reference to a few examples such as the Drumchapel evaluation (see Chapter 16), the reports on art and drama have been placed in a separate section of this book. It may, perhaps, be seen as a manifestation of a false distinction between the "art" (as a way of viewing society and human experience) which we have already encountered in earlier discussion of research methods, and "the Arts" (represented here by community art work and drama) which are artistic forms. Our purpose in doing this however, has been to draw attention to the existence of art, and the Arts, in the midst of a volume on public health research and practice.

We have argued that the traditional polarization between scientific research traditions needs to be melted down and refashioned into a continuum of techniques which complement each other. So too must we extend our perception of what qualitative research and participative practice have shown to be valuable about understanding and building on human experience, to a fuller acceptance of the capacity of art to both describe and move. Art, not simply as decoration or individual therapy, but as a tool for understanding and bringing about change in the wider context of community health, should be valued and promoted to the full.

Included here are two very different expressions of art which nevertheless have much in common with each other, and crucially, much in common with the research and policy experience described so far. In the first example, Rebecca Kilbey describes the work of the First Bite Theatre Company, including the use of theatre in health promotion work in schools, dealing with relationships, drugs, smoking and alcohol. It is interesting that the evolution of participation in their activities echoes some of the more general experience of how participation has developed in community health research and policy work. Another important theme is the way in which artistic expression, principally through drama in this instance, can be employed as one method

393

for researching knowledge and understanding. It can contribute to the portfolio of methods that are available. In terms of effectiveness this work is focused on the process rather than longer term outcomes, but we can see again the benefit of persisting with involvement and participation - in this case of the pupils and teachers. Furthermore, the point is made that approaches to health promotion through drama should not be seen or used in isolation, and the implications of this for assessing outcomes in considered further in section eight.

The second paper is by Mike White, who examines the concept of "Art as Health" through the work of Celebratory Arts, an organization using art work, community celebration and other techniques to explore and promote health. Here, art is contributing to the expression of the often complex determinants of health, providing "mediating images" that allow people to be touched in a more gentle and meaningful way than has characterized more traditional approaches to health education. Much of this work is also participative, in which the involvement of communities and individuals leads to creativity and momentum in partnership with, for example, primary care. These are concepts that have become familiar in the chapters on research and strategy, and here art offers yet another dimension which can contribute to the common goal of health promotion.

34 Out of this world: Drama in the research and promotion of health

Rebecca Kilbey

The First Bite Theatre in Education Company was formed in 1988 by five graduates from Middlesex University. Initially the company aimed to create health education theatre productions which engaged, informed and educated young people between the ages of five and thirteen years. The company's first production looked at dental health and was devised by the company in partnership with Kings College School of Dentistry. "The Nashers" toured for 18 months and led to a follow up production, "Choppa's Army", which was commissioned by Liverpool Health Authority's Department of Community Dental Health and seen by over 17,500 eight to eleven year olds in Liverpool between May and June 1990.

These two productions, whilst very successful with the majority of audiences, were created for young people by First Bite in partnership with health professionals. Evaluation questionnaires showed that the productions were missing approximately 20 per cent of the audiences who generally did not relate to the content, approach and style of the performances. This evaluation process, coupled with the fact that the company had decided to move away from dental health to general health and welfare, led to the setting up of First Bite's first in school residency at Breckfield JML School in Anfield, Liverpool. The three week residency was backed by Liverpool Education Department and aimed to use drama to explore "health" in its widest sense across the curriculum. The key aspect of this project was that First Bite now worked with two top junior classes for three weeks to identify what "health" meant to them, to identify areas of misinformation, explore key issues in more detail and devise coping strategies for difficult and potentially hazardous situations.

The results of the research project were used as a basis for First Bite's production "Tickers" which looked at peer pressure, confidence, self esteem, healthy living, smoking and the heart. Evaluations from this production (and demand for the company's work in general) demonstrated the success of this working process which is now carried out as part of every First Bite health education project.

The sucess of this new approach was built on in the development of our subsequent production about relationships, which was called "Out of this World".

Researching and developing "Out of This World"

First Bite spent three weeks working with 13 year olds from three different secondary schools in Liverpool. The three schools were selected by the Education Department from different areas of the city to ensure the research project accurately reflected the views and concerns of young people across the city. Each of the three schools allowed First Bite to work off timetable with a class for the whole week. A key member of staff from each school was also attached to the group for the week.

At the beginning of each week, after a warm up and "get to know you" session, we brainstormed the word "relationships" in small groups. Each group was then asked to select the three most important words from their brainstorm and to create and present still images of the words. This introductory session enabled workshop leaders to identify key areas of interest to the group and structure the rest of the week accordingly. The group from the Catholic High School, for example, was most interested at looking at teenage relationships (pregnancy, birth control, peer pressure etc.). The other two schools concentrated on the issues of substance abuse and peer pressure. All three schools identified the concept of choice and decision making as a potential problem area for young people. Throughout the week, drama exercises, creative writing, discussion and debate were utilized to explore what the young people already knew, identify areas of misinformation and devise coping strategies for potentially difficult or threatening situations. At the end of the three week project the three groups came together to share their work with each other and with an invited audience of health professionals, educationalists, parents and other young people.

These three weeks of creative research with the children resulted in a wealth of material, including character and scene studies, lyrics, potential plots and a list of over 500 words from the "relationships" brainstorms. All of the material was analyzed by the research and development team (senior staff from First Bite and Chris Ball from Liverpool Educational Advisory Agency), which eventually selected the following key themes for inclusion in the one hour long performance: teenage pregnancy/relationships; friendship; fmily relationships; peer pressure; substance abuse; alcohol; image; confidence; self esteem; trust and responsibility.

From the start of the project, First Bite was anxious that the final production should be used in school as a teaching tool and not simply seen by staff and a one off piece of entertainment. Chris Ball (drama advisor for Liverpool Education Department), who scripted the performance for the company, came up with the idea of using the central character of "Trauma", an alien scientist from another planet, as a controlling device for isolating key themes and "decision points" and then exploring them in more detail through action replays, slow motion etc. The final product, "Out of This World", told the story of John, a 14 year old, who's life was being examined by Trauma as part of her thesis. Over the course of the play John gets deeper and deeper into trouble, and more out of control, as a result of making a series of bad judgements and hasty decisions.

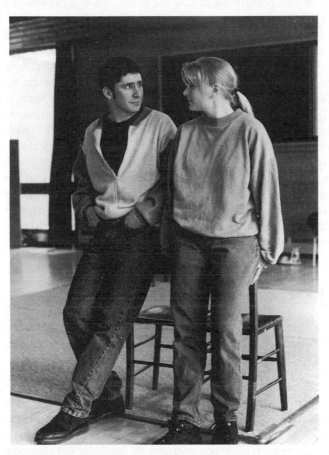

John and Jackie's first date, a scene from "Out of this World" before John takes a series of bad decisions that end his relationship and land him in trouble with the police

At the end of the play, because of the bond she has formed with John, Trauma decides to rewind the action with a view to giving him a second chance. Teachers are then encouraged to use the notes which accompany "Out of This World" to replay the action in class and discuss what John could have done differently, what choices were available to him, who could have helped him, and how he could have dealt with his problems.

Drama as a health promotion exercise

When First Bite began touring health education projects in 1989, the majority of schools booking performances saw the event as a one off health promotion exercise. Often, once the performance had started, teachers would leave the hall altogether, and those that did stay either watched in five minute relays or caught up with their marking at the back. After a year of working in this way the company redesigned its contract with schools to include a clause requiring all teachers to watch the production with their pupils with a view to following up the themes in class time. Initially this clause was unpopular! Traditionally, theatre visits seemed to be regarded as free time which staff were understandably reluctant to relinquish. Now, five years on, our evaluations show that staff look forward to watching the performance with their pupils. More often than not, particularly in secondary schools, the production and optional follow up workshops are written into the school's annual personal and social development programme. The First Bite production is experienced by both pupils and teachers and is used to spark off debate, discussion and follow up work on the themes presented, and on other issues which may have been identified during the group discussions.

Assessing the contribution of drama to health promotion

Some examples of comments from schools illustrate the ways in which the performances have been appreciated:

> I am writing on behalf of the pupils and staff of Linlithgow Academy to congratulate your company on their performance and workshops. The pupils said the play was "brilliant" magic! In the workshops pupils participated well and enjoyed exploring the issues raised in the play. The staff involved also felt it was a very worthwhile experience. Staff expressed their commitment to continue development of these issues and welcomed the enthusiastic approach of the Theatre Company (Linlithgow Academy, West Lothian).

398

I write to express my warm thanks and appreciation to your company for the wonderful production, "Out of This World"' recently performed at our school. All of the 250 Year nine and ten students (ages 14-15 years) who saw the performance were enthraled throughout. This is certainly due to the extremely high quality of both the script and the cast. The Relationships Programme was the perfect vehicle to further the work our staff have been discussing with the students during their personal and social education lessons (Newton-le-Willows High School, Merseyside).

First Bite has not attempted to evaluate the effectiveness of its health education programmes on each individual member of the audience. The programmes are designed as part of an overall strategy for the health education of young people and many other individuals and organizations (personal and social development staff, parents, health promotion departments, community police units, local education departments, etc.) are included in the process. What is clear from First Bite's evaluation of key staff in each school is that tremendous importance is placed on the personal and social development of young people and that both staff and pupils benefit when programmes are enriched by input from outside organizations providing tried and tested, relevant, appropriate health education material.

35 Art as health

Mike White

> Factors which make for health are concerned with a sense of personal
> and social identity, human worth, communication, participation in the
> making of political decisions, celebration and responsibility ... the
> language of science alone is insufficient to describe health; the
> languages of story, myth and poetry also disclose its truth (Wilson,
> 1975).

Over the last seven years, working with artists from Celebratory Arts for
Primary Healthcare, I have helped set up a number of pilot projects for arts
in primary health care, in the West Midlands and recently in Gateshead where
I work as Arts Officer. Much of the work has been in or for General
Practitioner (GP) surgeries, and has been developed with regard to health
education, public health, and useful complementary practice that encourages
creative participation. From this I have become drawn to an idea of "Art as
Health". I can see a new aspect to local arts and community development that
has a lot to offer and a lot worth evaluating. The work I have been involved
with has been mainly funded outside the arts funding system: for example in
Gateshead, The King's Fund provided a major grant award for a two year arts
development project, called "Prime Time", to explore links between creativity
and health in older people. Part of this programme involved artists from
Celebratory Arts working with older people and schools.

Some key points arising from their project work to date, I suggest are:

1. The role of arts in health in the community is different from the role
    of arts in health in hospitals (commissioned art works and creative
    therapy).

2. Surgeries and the localities they serve should be places where we learn
    to be healthy.

3.   The arts (and friendly artists) can shape contexts in the community to provide mediating images for health education so that people are "touched" rather than indoctrinated.

4.   The re-integration of art into health checks the dehumanization of medical science and is essential for both mental and physical health promotion.

This is a creative opportunity too for public health to assert its important role in medicine. There is a relationship between creativity, and well being, and to encourage people's latent creativity, arts in primary health care should be domestic, communal and celebratory.

The development of arts in health care has to date been mainly confined to the arts in hospitals movement. The development in tandem of arts in primary care is equally necessary and challenging. For hospital admissions form only a fraction of those in need of medical treatment or health consultation. The "front line" in preventative medicine is primary care.

Medicine is an art as well as a science. It can take advantage of the ability of art to crystallize metaphor and assist explanation. Artists need not be aliens to doctors and health workers but fellow practitioners. The primary health care environment could benefit from dedicated arts that can mediate between the sum of medical knowledge and the complexity of everyday life and individual patient experience. In these terms, a health service without artists is perhaps like a cathedral without stained glass. Applying functional arts, crafts, music and story telling to surgery spaces is more than a pleasant diversion for patients. Indeed, what is needed is not a superficial face lift but a re-orientation of thinking for a better alignment of medical utility and social values. How can this be achieved?

Arts in primary care

Work in the field of arts in primary health care includes: use of arts in health promotion; improving the quality of the health environments; use of arts activities to connect health services with communities they serve; arts in health service training and arts as a tool in health needs assessment

This is a new field for arts work, and examples of good practice need to be carefully nurtured and developed in a range of primary care settings and social contexts. Arts in primary care is fun and accessible, may relieve stress and improve the health care environment.

Arts in primary care work is essentially participatory, so we are keen to assess its impact through group activities promoting the health of the community. We are therefore looking through and beyond the therapeutic benefits to the individual, or performance indicators in a clinical environment. We are taking an outward looking approach to community development rooted in local health services, providing friendly arts support for people to value their health and to be informed participants in primary care services.

Befriend don't frighten

The involvement of artists and communities in the production of quality health promotion material may have tangible benefits for local health services and regional/national health campaigns.

Health information, like all information, is being treated as an increasingly commodity and sold to the consumer through the persuasive tyranny of advertising. Health campaigns, such as that for AIDS, assume the authority of diagnosis and appeal to the indeterminate viewer in terms of threat and sentence.

Why does a strong health message have to be unfriendly? The series of health posters which artists Alison Jones and John Angus of Celebratory Arts created for Brierley Hill and later Gateshead speak personally and mythically to the viewer. The immediate conversion to more healthy living which their message encourages is likely to be more effective than the future nemesis proposed by cause and effect health propaganda. Furthermore, using artists in this way as a catalyst between the health information worker and the patient can point up that a right to health care goes hand in hand with a right to expression.

The Gateshead project

On a damp March evening in Gateshead a few hundred school children, each accompanied by a parent or granny, carried their newly made sculptural lanterns through a bleak housing estate with the local street band playing a Latin Geordie arrangement of "Teddy Bears Picnic". Local residents switched off the peak time TV "soaps", roused their babies, and came out to share their astonishment with neighbours. The procession wound up at a primary school where a giant "Heart of Community" lantern was illuminated with pyrotechnics against the night sky, looking like a large belated Valentine. Health promotion nurses distributed heart shaped wholemeal rolls made by a local baker in an outdoor kiln and the town brass band played a specially composed tango. As one teacher's husband recovering from a recent coronary put it, "seeing that big heart light up made my own heart feel better." It was an event to remind even the most hard bitten arts worker that this is a great business we are in. Or as dramatist Bertholt Brecht put it, "the most difficult art of all is the great art of living together."

I am reminded by contrast of the former Secretary of State for National Heritage Peter Brooke's comment that the functions of his department are concerned with "what people do when they are not working." This somewhat flippant remark belies a pay for view approach to culture as a permissible form of idleness. In Gateshead there are many people who are "not working" all the time, so the choices they can make in a leisure economy are limited. The local authority's arts subsidy is directed towards creating access to the arts in opportune contexts.

In recent years we have best achieved participation in three activity areas: through education initiatives within an art in public places programme that has gained national awards; in long term community residencies for artists of all disciplines and through the concept of art as health.

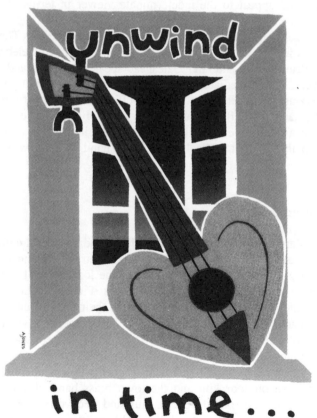

One of the posters produced by Celebratory Arts (Alison Jones)

In the last two years our biggest direct programme funder has been a health foundation, The King's Fund. Their major grant award to explore links through the arts between creativity and well being in old age has resulted in the Prime Time project, possibly the most ambitious arts programme for older people in the country.

Prime Time has drawn in additional funding from the Health Authority who have seen its significance for the Community Care plan, and attracted business sponsorship worth over £40,000. An Urban Programme project being developed in parallel to Prime Time by Equal Arts with Social Services has made dance and ceramics a norm of activity in residential care homes. In Prime Time over 300 pensioners have created extraordinary art works ranging from ornamental benches to embroidered changing screens for GP surgeries, to animated films and an interactive soap opera for day centre clients. The lantern procession originated from a group of older people with heart conditions working with school children on a "healthy heart" campaign, led by artists from Celebratory Arts for Primary Healthcare. Art works with health messages created with older people have adorned billboards on Tyneside's Metro transport system, with sponsorship from Merck Sharpe and Dohme.

Arts activity makes for good health?

As the "Carnegie Third Age" report revealed last year we are rapidly moving to a society in which 40 per cent of the population will be of pensionable age. Our Prime Time project attempts to promote access and participation by responding to this changing demography at a local level. The person centred evaluation of Prime Time has been useful in seeing the impact of the arts in terms of mental and physiological change in individual participants. It has begun to touch upon a major and relatively unexplored issue (outside of therapy) as to whether arts can keep you healthy. Increasingly I see health as a shaping metaphor for the development of arts in the community, and that the arts can have a benign influence on the pathology of the environment. If arts led health promotion could tap one per cent of the NHS drugs bill (currently over £3 billion a year) projects like Prime Time could be established in every health authority. The role of the arts in health development is potentially as valid an argument as that made for their role in economic development, and just as qualitative in effect.

With the lanterns event we were looking to achieve a combination of visual poetry and practical welfare. The Heart of Community image was chosen because Gateshead has the worst morbidity record for coronary disease in England.

Arts were used to create lateral connections around this issue rather than just colourful hectoring. The Health Promotion Mobile's staff are staying on at the estate for six months, using the lantern event as a talking point. Already children and adults are together growing organic vegetables in the school grounds. Next year we will have another lantern parade to celebrate and measure the change in health awareness.

Note

Mike White is Assistant Director - Arts for Gateshead Libraries and Arts Department. The views expressed here are personal and not necessarily those of Gateshead Council.

Reference

Wilson, M. (1975), *Health is for People*, Darton, Longman and Todd, pp. 59-60.

Section 7   Funding research for health promotion

Much health promotion activity is innovative, cuts across traditional disciplines, and includes participation of the "community" or "service users", and as has been explored in the foregoing chapters will inevitably challenge the current research orthodoxy.   The evaluation of such activities in turn requires a range of research, much of which needs to be innovative, multidisciplinary and participative.   Since these approaches and methods cut across generally accepted views of and structures for research, it can prove difficult to secure funding for such projects.   This is one reason why there is a paucity of research into the processes and outcomes of the majority of urban community health initiatives.

This paper has drawn on experience of research and community development in the UK and Australia, but many of the observations will be familiar to those promoting urban health elsewhere, and some common themes are drawn out.   Successful strategies for overcoming barriers to obtaining funding for research are shared in the hope that others may derive benefit. Obviously, such approaches will need to be tailored to local circumstances.

Principal sources of funding for health research

Research into health and factors affecting health in the community is typically funded from either biomedical sources, or from social science funding agencies. Far more total resource is involved in the biomedical sector, as this encompasses most public sector health related research funds, the majority of health related charities (whose activities are usually based around a disease category such as asthma, heart disease, arthritis, etc.) and the enormous budgets for research and development in the pharmaceutical and medical technology industries. Social science research funding comes from the much smaller base of central government funding, and from a relatively small number of philanthropic institutions. Consequently, the majority of research which comes under the broad umbrella of health research is disease oriented, hospital or specialist service based, and methodologically is usually of a quantitative, "hypothesis testing", nature. Relatively little research is qualitative, looking for the "how and why", rather than the "how many". Very little research is directed at questions which are important for Health for All, such as: how can we reduce inequalities? How can we encourage greater participation? How can we overcome the barriers to interagency working?

Within health services, there may be a specific budget destined for research or evaluation, for instance, in Australia it is common for ten per cent of new project funding to be devoted to evaluation. In the UK, a research and development (R and D) strategy for the National Health Service (NHS) has been developed over the last five years, and there has been a shift from biomedical and/or basic research, to addressing areas relevant to the provision and evaluation of health services. The overall health service budget devoted to R&D remains small when compared to the total expenditure on health related research within the UK, but at least there is now an acknowledgement of the importance of research that is more relevant to health policy by the government.

Areas missed by "usual" health research funding

As a consequence of the predominance of the biomedical model of health in most funded research, the broader approach of interacting social and environmental factors tend to be under researched. Among the areas and types of project for which it has been difficult to secure funding are:

1.   Research on community development projects: the local nature of these projects places them outside the interest of research councils and charities concerned more with what they see as generalizable scientific research. Among more locally oriented funders, health authorities may be helpful but do tend to think of this work as more within the remit of local government, and not a priority for health. Local authorities, however, are less used to commissioning and using research than health authorities, as decisions about the development of these initiatives are usually more overtly political. What tends to happen is that the research falls between and across the various funding opportunities, and in the current structure is essentially homeless.

2.   Research on health promotion (salutogenesis) as opposed to disease management - this type of research would for instance include the

identification of factors that keep individuals healthy, and that make communities safe.

3. Research on multi-sectoral/interagency working - even within a single sector, it has been the "norm" for research to be conducted in one setting, and not to integrate, for example, hospital and community health provision.

4. Research on environmental issues and health - due to the complex interactions of factors in the environment (for example, that the poorest housing is also usually where industrial pollution is heaviest, and where the highest concentration of cigarette smokers live, unemployment is worst, etc.) research becomes complex and therefore requires a multi-disciplinary team approach. Such an approach is still relatively uncommon in the academic research world.

In addition to the subject area posing difficulties for the research establishment, the research methods of choice for many projects are unfamiliar to the membership of grant making bodies and ethical committees from which approval is sought. Participative action research, for example, in which the subjects become involved in the research design and execution, compounds this issue further, as it is impossible to say before the research in undertaken exactly how it will progress. One researcher recounted that the secretary of an ethics committee looked with dismay at his proposal to use qualitative methods, stating that the committee only felt comfortable dealing with clinical trials. Other researchers reported that committees wanted to see "the final questionnaire" before approval was given for health service users to be contacted.

Incompatable timescales and competing resource needs

Cultures and timescales often clash - particularly if researchers have been employed for a specific and short period of time, as is almost universally the case, and are working to a tight deadline. Community members will be far less interested in short term outputs such as a research report, and much more interested in the continuing developments in their area. The agenda of a local community group will not always coincide with the agendas of local or national governments, nor does it necessarily match the agenda of the academics who are trying to produce publications which will be credible among their peers.

The cost of carrying out research is often under estimated, particularly by those working with communities who are in economically deprived areas.

Adequate research takes time, and that includes time for background reading and preparation. Researcher time will not be expensive when compared to the costs of, for instance, management consultancy, but to a community project existing on a shoestring, it will be a substantial investment. To evaluate a project in an academically rigorous way would often cost more than the project itself.

Strategies which may encourage the funding of appropriate research

Education

The key to securing more funding which uses a broader range of methods and investigates areas of social policy concern must be education. This education will need to be targeted at individuals who have traditionally been thought of as very highly educated, but whose education has in reality been intense but rather narrow. It is hardly surprising that reductionist scientific research gains the great majority of the funding when it is the proponents of this approach who generally sit on the funding bodies. To reach those positions, the scientists will have undertaken higher degrees which encouraged specialization and achievement of the individual researcher. Members of grant awarding committees should be developed into their role, with much wider experience of and respect for different research methods and settings. This is particularly relevant for those making decisions about funding research in the field of (urban) community health, and research which is designed to achieve more effective translation into policy. It needs to be recalled that the notion of relinquishing absolute control and working with the agendas of others - in at least part of their research portfolios - can be difficult and threatening for the researcher concerned.

There are many reasons why this is difficult, some of which reflect traditional working practices and career development imperatives, but there is also the very real concern that loss of individual control means uncertainty about the quality of research. It is important in this debate however, not to confuse the approach to the type of research and its context with the attitude of the researcher towards the quality and validity of what they propose to do. As is evident in this volume, many researchers in the field do care about the validity of what they are doing. Furthermore, the reality of conducting research which promotes more informed policy development pushes research into unfamiliar territory, and the old rules and yardsticks don't easily apply. Funding bodies need to acknowledge that researchers in this field want to ensure that their research is of good quality, and are striving to develop the theoretical framework and practical methods for achieving this. Funders can contribute by improving their own understanding of the issues, and thereby promote the whole research development process.

Joint working

The means of instilling a greater flexibility in the minds of the research establishment are many. Members of funding bodies should consider working alongside members of communities who are actively trying to find ways to bring about improvements in health and social conditions, so that they can engage in the dialogue that is so much needed in order to achieve an exchange of ideas. One method suggested for "broadening horizons" is to encourage all senior researchers to engage in at least one truly collaborative project before serving on any major grant awarding body dealing with this and related fields of research in particular, but probably also to the benefit of all health research.

"Lay" members

The citizens, on whose bahalf senior scientists are appointed to be the guardians of public and other research money, should ensure that they have their say in how it is spent. This is not about technical details, but about the priorities for and approaches to research. The customary single lay member of a board may not always be sufficient and can become little more than a token presence.

Some encouraging moves are being seen, for instance, one of the recently established Research and Development committees in two districts of the UK has ensured that about a third of the membership is made up of non-health professionals, but including representatives from social services and the voluntary sector. Their lack of expertize can be overcome by using technical experts to assess the scientific merits of an application, but involving the non-technical members of the panel much more in the assessment of the relevance of the project and methods.

Targeting grant awarding bodies

Those interested in changing attitudes in the research establishment may wish to target their lobbying towards the major bodies administering public research funds, and the main charities. The social sciences need to engage more with the medical establishment, and press for greater representation of sociologists and qualitative researchers on the major biomedical grant giving bodies.

Developing the research skills of project workers

It is probably fair to say that most workers who are engaged in community development and healthy city type initiatives are not researchers. And yet they are often expected to evaluate the projects they are working on. One suggestion, which might help overcome this problem, was to provide some training in basic evaluation at the start of new initiatives, with visits by an experienced researcher for support. This training is not envisaged as anything too elaborate, but may include simple techniques such as maintaining a diary for the project in which key events are recorded in a systematic way. Logging clients, or requests for help, or whatever measure of process would be appropriate for the project in question helps gives some information, and could provide a sampling frame for a more indepth and technically rigorous study should funding become available later in the project. Encouraging project workers to enrol for short courses and higher degrees will also help them develop their research skills.

Promoting examples of good practice

Examples of where a multi-sectoral approach has led to much better resolution of an issue should be made more widely available. Those involved in education could use these as examples in their teaching, and researchers preparing bids could cite studies using a similar approach in their bids. When researchers have been involved in successful multi-sectoral projects, they should disseminate the results not only in the medical and sociological literature, but also to local health authorities and grant awarding bodies.

Taking the evolution of audit as an example

In the UK, what started in the National Health Service (NHS) as medical audit (involving doctors only) soon broadened to become clinical audit (involving other providers of clinical care such as nurses and the professions allied to medicine), as it was widely acknowledged that the medical component of a patient's care was only one aspect. Currently the NHS is encouraging "interface audits", which include not only a range of disciplines within one setting (for instance a hospital) but across settings (for instance hospital and primary care and social services). Those preparing bids for funding of community health initiatives may wish to refer to these developments to strengthen their case for "interface" work involving participation and multi-sectoral collaboration.

Conclusion

In summary, the situation for funding of research for health promotion is in many ways a product of the innovative, challenging and collaborative principles that underlie health promotion itself. Researchers and teachers can contribute to raising the awareness of funders to the importance and value of this developing field of research. The pace of change will however be very slow if at the same time those who allocate research funds do not make an effort to work with those engaged in the practice of health promotion, and show greater openness to the variety of research methods that are required. In doing so, they will be able to make a valuable contribution to the development and quality of the research that needs the financial support they control.

Acknowledgements

With thanks to all the workshop participants, especially Fran Baum and Janet Henderson.

Section 8   Discussion

A common concept of health

An important element underpinning all the papers in this volume and the conference it represents is that they all share a common understanding of the concept of health.   That understanding is firmly based in a socio-environmental model of health, a view that draws heavily on the Ottawa Charter and Health for All ideology.   This view is not a universal one.   It is not generally shared for example, by the medical establishment which tends to view health as the absence of disease, and health promotion as the prevention of disease through screening and risk factor modification through medical treatment or targeted education.   While good quality health care and screening programmes have an important part to play, sometimes offering the only recognized strategy for prevention in the current state of knowledge (for example, the use mammography and appropriate treatment in breast cancer), there is a pressing need to shift the generally held view of health promotion into this much wider arena.

This socio-environmental approach is also not a dominant view among some sections of the health promotion field, or among those on the right of politics who prefer to see health as the responsibility of individuals and its promotion rooted in changing behavioural risk factors primarily though health education, and through limited advocacy for healthy public policies such as workplace smoking bans.   The socio-environmental approach, whilst acknowledging the contribution these other factors to health, is concerned with a much wider focus which takes in issues such as poverty, lack of opportunity for education and employment, environmental pollution, and psycho-social problems such as social isolation.   Health promotion seeks to create better living conditions and reduce the constraints on choice which hinder the adoption of healthier lifestyles.   It is for these reasons that the strategies for health promotion described here focus on personal empowerment, community development, healthy alliances and political action. It is not that these are the only strategies we require. Rather, they are seen as the fundamental and necessary strategies for achieving improvements in population health, and perhaps of greatest importance, in the inequalities that remain such a prominent feature of contemporary society.

What has been achieved?

The application of the Health for All strategy in recent years has yielded rich and diverse experience, and this is an appropriate time to take stock of what is being achieved. Much has already been done in the field of research that examines the structures and processes of this work, and in developing the techniques for this assessment. Many of the authors have argued that understanding the processes is important and valuable, not least because these are an integral part of what is being sought. In that sense, the processes are not simply a means to some distinct and far more significant ends, but are part of the constellation of outcomes which are desired.

We now need to build on this experience, in particular what it has taught us about the need to recognise a "plurality" of outcomes and the value of participation in research and action. This leads on to an issue which we have touched on already in section four and must be examined further, that is the concept of the effects of these programmes on health. This may be expressed by the question "Does the application of Health for All principles improve the health of communities, and is it cost effective?" There are a number of reasons why we need to address this question, including the following:

1. Sooner or later there is going to be a political and financial reckoning on the part of hard pressed funding agencies, and there will need to be some demonstration, or at least examination of, costs and benefits.

2. The strong commitment to this work could in time lead to a degree of complacency, and it is important to maintain a sense of open mindedness and willingness to modify practice in the light of more fundamental assessment.

3. The work on participative evaluation has demonstrated the value of building up knowledge and expertise among the participants, and seems to strengthen the ability of those concerned to directly influence the course of policy. There is no reason why this would not apply to research conceived in the same way which focused on costs and health benefits, thereby advancing the capacity of the participants address these issues and the relevance of policies to deal with them.

416

What are we trying to achieve with evaluation?

A seemingly major difficulty for those adopting the broader based approach to health described above is the problem of proving that the activities which are advocated for improving health actually do so, and more importantly what worked and why? Alongside this is the question of what effects can be attributed to which policy actions. The answers to these questions will be neither simple nor precise.

Thus, it is very difficult to unravel the complexity of the factors involved, to assign a relative value to each of the elements that contribute to change and acknowledge what may be a synergistic effect. In addition, few real outcomes, either short term or long, term have been systematically documented. The reasons for this are many (Springett et al. 1995). Even when evaluation does take place it is often after the event and is not clearly related to the aims and objectives of the individual projects concerned or the broader issues of long term change. Moreover, with the inevitable resource constraints, there is a tension between the need for action and need for evaluation reinforced by the failure to adequately resource evaluation. Thus, sophisticated evaluative research is rare and much evaluation is anecdotal.

Study design

Traditional approaches to study design for examining the outcome of a given intervention, in purest form the randomised controlled trial, are really not helpful in the situation we are facing. The nature of the interventions that we are considering means that these are neither discrete nor amenable to containment, and this simply adds to the problems already experienced by controlled community intervention studies investigating much more clearly defined actions (see for example Egger, 1983). There are many reasons why a simplistic approach to study design for outcome evaluation will not be helpful, including the following:

Identifying and defining health and other "outcome" indicators

We should begin by recognising that one problem for the development of satisfactory outcome indicators is the unrealistically short time scales prevalent in much evaluative work to date, which are reinforced by (if not actually the result of) managerial agendas driven by immediate considerations of efficiency and effectiveness, and the often short term funding of the projects themselves. This can often result in indicators that are largely quantitative and superficial, with little meaning in terms of community development or priorities on the ground. Such indicators often fail to capture the psycho-social aspects of health and the benefits to individuals that accrue during the community development process.

More generally, indicators of health and health determinants need to allow for a realistic time interval between the initiation of the community development process and assessment of outcome. For most traditional health indicators, this will be many years, although it could be argued that some measures of child health, or for example accidents which do not have the long "incubation period" of chronic adult illness, would be expected to respond more quickly. It is important too that indicators representing key health determinants, and measures of factors which can be shown promote health be included. If disease risk factors, such as smoking are used, it is very important that the context and meaning of such behaviours for the people concerned are also studied. For example, the unqualified finding that over a five year period smoking rates in young mothers were unchanged in a given community would not be helpful if the truth was that, although motivation to quit had increased, this had been counterbalanced by increasing socio-economic pressures and more targeted advertising during the period under study.

Complexity and unknowns in assessing costs

Measuring cost is complex and will almost certainly be incomplete. Whilst certain inputs such as project staff time and their resources can be costed, there are many other components such as the economic consequences of intersectoral working, the empowerment of members of the community who may go on to further training and employment, which would be very difficult to assess.

One attempt to respond to the pressure on health promotion agencies to demonstrate short term outcomes and proximal outcomes attractive to the government funders, has been demonstrated by the Federal Heart Health project in British Columbia, Canada (Frankish. J, personal communication). This community based health promotion project has included in the evaluation an assessment of economic gain, with the calculation of the return for each dollar spent in terms of office space, time and free publicity achieved from the estimated market value of the volunteers. This raises many questions about the roles of "volunteers", but does illustrate the directions in which these kinds of calculations can go.

Multisectoral action implies complex interacting inputs

Multisectoral working is by definition expected in applying the Health for All approach, and this results in complex, interacting inputs from many different angles which impinge on the community under study. So, even if a relatively distinct agency or "project" is promoting the initiative, a much wider range of people and organizations will be expected to play a part and it is unrealistic to isolate the individual and combined effects of their contributions.

External influences

Outside of the local arena of action for a given community, political, financial and social initiatives will have an influence. It therefore becomes convoluted to the point of absurdity to attempt to establish in a systematic way all the effects of specified local and city inputs as well as the external influences. That does not mean that describing what has gone on locally and more widely is unhelpful: on the contrary, it is very important to document this. The difference comes in the approach to interpretation of effects, and we are arguing here that a reductionist analysis - attempting to understand the effects of all the components - is doomed to failure.

To reiterate, one key reason for this is that very few of the "component actions" should be implemented in isolation, but rather as part of an integrated approach. As a result, the component actions would not be discrete entities and any attempt to define and evaluate them as such within a Health for All programme would make the study irrelevant. It is important to appreciate that this argument applies to the evaluation of the overall programme, and not to studying the health effects of more specific actions such as traffic calming, reducing exhaust emissions or improved house insulation. We still need to know how these affect health, and this issue is highlighted further in the following discussion.

A model for the evaluation of longer term outcomes

If the goal of a systematic, quantitative and controlled evaluation of the costs and health benefits of the Health for All approach is illusory, then is there any point pursuing the idea of evaluating outcomes and the economic efficiency of all this work? We would argue that it is both important and possible. The key is to use a variety of methods, and to be prepared to rely much more on a consensus of experience about how change has come about, how wasteful or efficient the processes have been, and so on. This component of the evaluation however, needs to be backed up by specific research including:

1.   Monitoring of the health, environmental and social indicators that have been identified as important to the agencies and communities concerned.

2.   Continued efforts to understand the health effects of the many
       components of an socio-environmental approach to health, such as
       environmental pollution, housing, work and unemployment, various
       aspects of transport, and many more.

Once we understand more about the changes that are going on, we can draw
on the results of these more specific research activities to draw inferences
about the value of what is being done in terms of policy. Furthermore, the
principle of participation in this evaluative endeavour should be maintained.
The effects of participation on the thinking and actions of the people involved
could be very substantial, and the debate generated about measuring "health
outcomes" and understanding "cause and effect" should to some extent at least
ensure these concepts become part of everyday pratice.

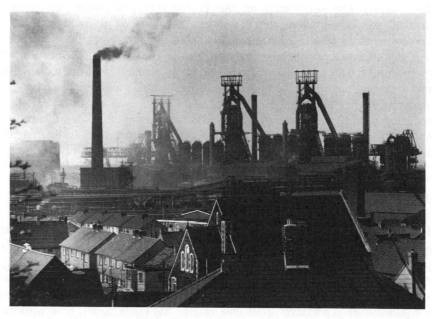

*Further research is needed into the effects on health of many aspects of the
social and physical environment*

An important role for the research community

The research community can play an important part in developing approaches to evaluation that look at long term outcomes but do so in a manner that engages all the stakeholders in the process. There is a need to maintain a balance between the perceptions and needs of policy makers and those who hold the resources on the one hand, and those who are involved in health promotion and research with communties on the other. The research community thereby has the opportunity to facilitate a closer relationship between these hitherto largely divided camps. Adopting a participatory approach to evaluation and research will make a significant contribution to creating opportunities for dialogue, and the resulting learning could enable a move towards a consensus about desirable and useful outcomes and their measurement. This should also go some of the way towards removing the distinction identified in section 4 between the type of evaluation that focuses on whether the goals of participants have been met, and that which addresses the needs perceived by funders and policy makers for measured change in prescribed indicators for a given financial investment.

This process will take time however, since consensus building is likely to be threatening to those who hold the power and currently determine the content and timescale of health research, as well as to communities and their support workers who still sense the pressure to get on with the action. The degree to which this can be achieved, and the ways in which the process can be encouraged, are considered below.

Defining a research agenda for healthy cities

A good deal has been written about the important role research has in the Health for All strategy and Healthy Cities (Davies and Kelly, 1993; WHO, 1985; WHO, 1988; WHO, 1991). Our purpose here is to build on this and present an agenda based on where we seem to be at present. This an overview rather than a detailed prescription, since in any given situation the refining of the agenda should in any case be the product of the needs and perceptions of the "stakeholders". It is hoped that this could be seen as a stimulus to that process, the main components of which should be:

1.   Consolidation of the techniques for needs assessment, employing a variety of methods, refining epidemiology further, placing greater emphasis than hitherto on qualitative research and the arts as a means of expressing ideas and experience, and using techniques such as geographical information systems which can integrate and display data from varied sources.

2.   There is a need for a more creative approach to choosing and measuring indicators of health and health promotion, and wherever

relevant the communities and individuals concerned should be involved in the whole process.

3. Consolidation of the techniques for process evaluation, compiling the findings, including the outcomes of participative evaluation for those involved.

4. Development of models and methods for assessing longer term and health outcomes, and economic aspects, which can help in the development of strategies for effective action, particularly with reference to reducing inequalities in health.

5. Compiling what is known, and filling in the gaps, about the social and environmental influences on health, with particular emphasis on those influences outside of the health service sector (for example, housing, transport, air pollution, etc.).

Although there is a need to continue working to shift attitudes about what constitutes appropriate research for health promotion, and to ensure this is refelected in education and training, there is nevertheless a good deal of commitment and expertise already. What is lacking are a framework and mechanisms for:

1. Determining the most relevant research agenda (at national, district, city, and community level), through structures and processes which involve the people whom it concerns.

2. Co-ordination of research activity to avoid unecessary duplication, and to make the best use of expertise.

3. More balanced funding, with a clearer link between funds that are available and the agreed agenda.

4. More systematic compilation, and effective dissemination, of the experience gained in the methods and findings of research and policy, making this experience available beyond the worlds of the pure academic and academic practitioner.

At the city level, the City Health Plan initiative of Phase II of the WHO Healthy Cities project does provide the framework for at least some aspects of all these points (Bruce et al. 1994), although individual city level initiatives may have little influence on national policy and funding opportunities, at least in the short term. As more and more cities become involved however, and

422

with better dissemination of the experience and findings of research, their influence should grow. The dimension of international collaboration and communication will also help.

Achieving effective community participation

Particpation of the community, however the term "community" is defined or understood, has been a central and fundamental issue throughout this book. It is possible to draw out from this experience some of the key issues that appear to help in achieving more effective participation.

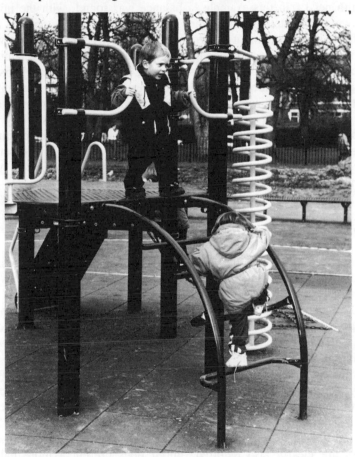

We need to be more creative about the indicators we choose. Parents and children, as just one example, think that safe play areas are very important, and they can contribute to assessing need and planning change

Getting the balance right

In Chapter 12, Joop ten Dam has clearly articulated a matter identified by other authors in this book and which must be of concern to many people, particularly those whose responsibilty is to take a strategic view of need within a city or district. He highlighted the dilemma of how to proceed with a community with manifest need, but little effective organisation. Waiting for an appropriate community initiative may be too slow, while if the statutory sector takes the initiative there is a danger of imposing the wrong policies. The capacity of different communities to begin the process will vary within a city, and may not necessarily be related to the extent of social, economic and health need. In this example, a balance was found, with the initiative being taken by the statutory sector and participative research acting as a vital means for building community expression and capacity. This offers a way of addressing the problem, and although this principle may be quite familiar to those involved in community development, it does serve to emphasise that differing levels of input are required to encourage and support participation and that this is a dynamic process which cannot simply be set up and then left alone. Achieving an appropriately distributed response across a city which will typically have areas of greater need and varying levels of community organisation and readyness to participate, requires a strategic and sensitive approach and the necessary resources to establish and maintain the support that is needed.

The capabilities of communities are important too

Much has been said about the "needs" of communities. The processes of measuring these and developing policy responses, where this has been participative, have drawn attention to the capability of communities. This may take the form of personal empowerment which was beyond the expectations of those who thought they knew the individual, or activities and services set up by groups of people including for instance health forums, credit unions and counselling services. These have the potential to serve communities in an appropriate way, but should also emphasise to those in the statutory sector that what may appear to start out as committing resources for needy communities to express demands for further expenditure can actually lead to development of capacity within that community. That is not to say that statutory agencies are then "let off the hook", since their expertise and resources are clearly also required, but it does present a more balanced prospect for constructive partnership.

424

Research for change

It has been frequently observed that many of the findings of research and evaluation have not found their way into policies programmes or practice (Green, 1992). As a result there have been a number of calls for increased cooperation between researchers and practitioners to support health promotion in practice (Kok and Green, 1990). The aim of this conference was to move some way towards such cooperation. The papers presented here offer only a small sample of the type of research and action taking place within the urban community health setting. In many respects they are somewhat biased, representing as they do a mainly European and Western perspective and more particularly a British one. In Britain, ironically, the wider policy context has run counter to the forces which encourage urban community health; local authorities have relatively little local power over the health enhancing social factors and research is largely ignored, as David Hunter argued, when it runs counter to conviction politics. But even if the political context of action varies this does not negate the more universal themes that emerge, at least in western societies.

The complexity of the changes currently taking place in society and the rapidity of that change is beginning to have an impact on the way we do research. The traditional scientific method has come under increasing criticism for failing to take account of the complexity of the social world. Although still not completely accepted, new approaches to research which incorporate action research and qualitative as well as quantitative methodology and which give value to the lay perspective are increasingly being used. The role of the researcher is changing to one of facilitation and technical support rather than detached expert, but this change is still marginal. Health promotion practitioners do have interests and preferences that differ from those of researchers. They also, like researchers, often have their own hidden agendas. Nevertheless, the seeds for cooperation can be planted. One way researchers can help practitioners is to join forces with them to record and write up their experience. Another way is for researchers to reach out to the practitioners and produce journals that cross the divide, as this volume attempts to do and as do new journals such as the Journal of Contemporary Health. For their part, practitioners need to open a dialogue with researchers and respect their needs and problems too - and there is evidence that they are increasingly ready to do so.

Changing perspectives

In the final session of the conference participants were asked to write down how their perspectives had changed as the result of the conference (research) and what action they either in their personal or working lives they would take as a consequence (change). It was clear from the responses that the art and drama elements had a major impact on many of the participants and encouraged them to adopt some of the ideas in their own work. This is not surprising. There is a tendency for most research and action to engage only the left half of the brain. Yet as human beings we respond to other forms of activity and become whole beings by integrating all aspects of ourselves: mind, body and spirit. Art and drama touch our souls, which science and rational thought since Descartes, has denigrated as an unworthy component in our search for knowledge about the world. This spiritual dimension is only now beginning to be recognised as a key element in understanding and promoting health (Seaward, 1995).

Many participants at the conference also reported on how they had come to recognise the quite different role research can play in change from that which they had been led to expect. They could now see how the actions of researchers and the process of research itself can have an impact rather than the product of research merely being a tool to inform policy implementation. The conference also gave hope and support to those struggling with participatory action research methods. One participant wrote:

> It (the conference) has stimulated many practitioners to reopen the dialogue with researchers and researchers to do likewise with policy makers.

Taking the community's example into organizations

The focus on community in bringing about change for health means that there has been much focus on community development in this volume. Indeed internationally, Healthy Cities has been as much about healthy communities as about cities. Although there has been some recognition of the need for organizational change and development, if community development is to bring about long term change, little parallel development has been undertaken within organizations. While working collaboratively comes naturally to some, many individuals working in organizations do not know how to work together and need support and training to help deal with the threats to power and control that new ways of working imply. Giving up power is an issue of self empowerment too and requires a different attitude towards change from that hitherto held by bureaucratic organizations. The rapid changes taking place in municipal government represent an opportunity for organizational change in the right direction but also a complex managerial challenge. This suggests that a new role is required for local government with more emphasis on technical support and facilitating others through support mechanisms such as networks and other organizational forms shaped by the participants needs (Lewin, 1993).

Can the barriers to change be overcome?

The blocks to such change are numerous. Many politicians, senior managers and professionals are, for example, reluctant to relinquish or share power, central governments seem largely unable to work intersectorally and the political ethos seen in many countries, especially during the 1980s, by its nature emphasized individual competetition rather than co-operation. So, could the ideas and action reported in this volume yet be doomed in the same way as the UK community development movement of the 1960s? (Farrant, 1991). Will it remain worthy, interesting but marginal: a kind of "challenging projectism" that dances provocatively around the bastions of financial, political and academic power, and never succeeds in being anything more than that? This could be described as a situation where "the organizationally powerless meet the socially powerless" (Labonte, 1992). Or is there a more positive trend in which the ever more visible evidence of people with these new attitudes and ways of working reaches a critical mass, in the long run able to change the everyday practice of the majority?

The power of stories

An important contribution can come from the stories people tell and the way they interpret their experiences through the meanings they put on events. Cognitive science has demonstrated for example that the way members of organizations understand and interpret events influences both their individual response and organizational functioning (Bartunek and Moch, 1987). As the number of stories increase so learning takes place and the meaning placed on events begins to change.

An example of this is the way the ideology of participation in health planning and health promotion has changed over time. Early expressions of ideology were directed mostly at cooperation in implementation of plans already formulated. This moved towards looking at participation in terms of health service use and then to involving people in decentralized planning and evaluation. In its most effective form, however true participation involves much more complete and substantial involvement in the learning process by all parties from diagnosis, through setting priorities to change and evaluation. This is what true empowerment is, involving critical self awareness, self determination and development. But such activity will ultimately be of limited value if it does not proceed hand in hand with the development of

427

appropriate policies regarding the broader social and environmental context in which such empowerment takes place. This is why an integrated approach to both research and action is so important.

Conclusions

The field of health promotion is inherently multi-disciplinary. This can potentially create a vulnerability in its theoretical base, the diversity of which has been reflected in the papers in this volume. The desire to make research more relevant, accountable and useful inhibits the critical perspective which such theory can generate. Potentially too, the absence of a philosophical and theoretical dialogue can prevent long term knowledge development. That knowledge development will be greatly enhanced as both practictioners and academics come together as part of wider learning community and as they acknowledge and value each others perspectives. In this way the delicate balance between the needs of theory and those of practice can be enhanced and brought together.

This volume represents a chance to reflect on progress in the application of the ideas embodied in the Health for All strategy. It certainly is not comprehensive, but we hope largely representative of what has been achieved in those societies, mainly European, that are included. There is no question that this progress has gone far beyond the well argued theory, and the often heard, worthy but otherwise insubstantial rhetoric. In many different settings, and in a variety of countries, this new approach is poised to engage, or has actually engaged, in modifying mainstream practice. The extent to which it succeeds will depend on many factors, some of which we may have very little control over, but will nevertheless require an appreciation of the complex and challenging nature of what is involved as well as the breadth of change. The experience reported here demonstrates that, so far as desirable changes in both the practice and union of research and policy are concerned, some substantial foundations have been laid.

References

Bartunek, J.M. and Moch, M.K. (1987), "First Order, Second Order and Third Order Change and Organisation Development Interventions: A Cognitive Approach", *The Journal of Applied Behavioral Science*, vol. 23, no. 4, pp. 483-500.

Egger, G., Fitzgerald, W., Frape, G., Monaem, A., Rubinstein, P., Tyler, C. and Mackay, B. (1983), "Results of a Large Scale Media Antismoking Campaign in Australia: North Coast "Quit for life" Programme", *British*

Medical Journal, vol. 287, pp. 1125-8.

Farrant, W. (1991), "Addressing the Contradictions: Health Promotion and Community Health Action in the United Kingdom", *International Journal of Health Services*, vol. 21, no. 3, pp. 423-39.

Green, L. (1992), "The Health Promotion Research Agenda Revisited", *American Journal of Health Promotion*, vol. 6, no. 6, pp. 411-3.

Kok, G. and Green, L. (1990), "Research to Support Health Promotion in Practice: A Plea for Increased Co-operation", *Health Promotion International*, vol. 5, no. 4, pp. 303-8.

Labonte, R. (1992), "Health Promotion and Empowerment: Practical Frameworks", *Issues in Health Promotion Series 3*, Centre for Health Promotion, University of Toronto,

Levin, M. (1993), "Creating Networks for Rural Economic Development in Norway", *Human Relations*, vol. 46, no. 2, pp. 193-218.

Seaward, B.L. (1995), "Reflections on Human Spirituality for the Worksite", *American Journal of Health Promotion*, vol. 9, no. 3, pp. 165-8.

Springett, J., Costongs, C. and Dugdill, L. (1995), "Towards a Framework for Evaluation in Health Promotion: The Importance of Process", *Journal of Contemporary Health*, vol. 2, pp. 54-63.